THE
OLDEST
CURE
IN THE
WORLD

ALSO BY STEVE HENDRICKS

A Kidnapping in Milan: The CIA on Trial

The Unquiet Grave: The FBI and the Struggle for the Soul of Indian Country

THE
OLDEST
CURE
IN THE
WORLD

Adventures in the Art
and Science of FASTING

STEVE HENDRICKS

ABRAMS PRESS, NEW YORK

Published in 2022 by Abrams Press, an imprint of ABRAMS. All rights reserved. No portion of this book may be reproduced, stored in a retrieval system, or transmitted in any form or by any means, mechanical, electronic, photocopying, recording, or otherwise, without written permission from the publisher.

Library of Congress Control Number: 2022933711

ISBN: 978-1-4197-4847-9
eISBN: 978-1-64700-002-8

Printed and bound in the United States
10 9 8 7 6 5 4 3 2 1

The medical information contained in this book is not intended as a substitute for the advice of skilled medical practitioners. The publisher and author accept no responsibility for any liability, loss or risk, personal or otherwise, which is incurred as a consequence, directly or indirectly from the use and application of any of the contents of this publication.

Abrams books are available at special discounts when purchased in quantity for premiums and promotions as well as fundraising or educational use. Special editions can also be created to specification. For details, contact specialsales@abramsbooks.com or the address below.

Abrams Press® is a registered trademark of Harry N. Abrams, Inc.

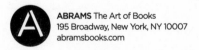

ABRAMS The Art of Books
195 Broadway, New York, NY 10007
abramsbooks.com

For Jennifer, naturally

CONTENTS

In the sciences, that which has been handed down or taught at the universities is also looked upon as property. And if anyone advances anything new which contradicts, perhaps threatens to overturn, the creed which we have for years repeated, and have handed down to others, all passions are raised against him, and every effort is made to crush him. People resist with all their might; they act as if they neither heard nor could comprehend; they speak of the new view with contempt, as if it were not worth the trouble of even so much as an investigation or a regard, and thus a new truth may wait a long time before it can make its way.

—Johann Wolfgang von Goethe

CRIMINAL QUACKERY

Ten years before she found the lump in her groin, cancer took Ivonne Vielman's father. It started in his lungs, although he had never smoked, and chewed through his body with such swiftness that by the time it was diagnosed there was nothing to be done. He died at fifty-seven. In the decade since, Vielman—a mother, wife, and corporate secretary, aged forty-two and living on the exurban fringe of San Francisco—had harbored a barely suppressed dread that cancer would someday come for her too. The knot in her groin felt like her fear made manifest. Big as a golf ball and nearly as hard as one, it must have been fast growing because she hadn't noticed it the last time she massaged the area, which she had done regularly after a bladder surgery left the spot tender. Since her father's death, the mere mention of cancer had disquieted her, and she tried to push the word from her mind in the days she waited to see her doctor, but it got a toehold in her thoughts and wouldn't be budged.

The doctor, a by-the-numbers sort whom we might call Hughes, felt the node and asked whether anyone in Vielman's family had had a lump before. Vielman barely got the story about her father out before Hughes picked up a phone and told someone on the other end that she had a patient who needed emergency CT scans—today.

The next day Vielman went back to Hughes's office for the results, her husband along for support. The doctor said the scans showed tumors on both sides of her groin and in her right armpit, and they hadn't been there when she was scanned prior to the bladder surgery two years earlier.

There was little doubt they were cancerous, and she referred Vielman to an oncologist. *Oncologist* was another word whose mention unnerved Vielman, four syllables that struck her momentarily dumb. But she composed herself, turned to her husband, and said with as level a voice as she could manage, "We are going to take care of this. I'll be fine."

Then she burst into tears.

The oncologist, whom I'll call Greenfield, biopsied one of Vielman's tumors and told her there was no doubt it was follicular lymphoma, a cancer that attacks the white blood cells of the lymphatic system, the network of vessels and organs whose dual duty is to fight disease and rid the body of waste. Vielman's tumors were in her lymph nodes, and the diagnosis contained good news and bad news. The bad news was that because the lymphoma was in both the upper and lower parts of Vielman's torso and on both the left and right sides, it had to be considered advanced, stage III out of IV. Worse, there was no cure. The good news was follicular lymphoma grew very slowly. Four out of five people at Vielman's stage were still alive at least a decade after diagnosis, and a sizable number lived two decades or more. Greenfield said she could reasonably hope for another twenty years. It was a death sentence but one that carried a long stay of execution.

Greenfield didn't recommend treatment, not yet anyway. For the moment, chemotherapy and radiation were poor options because they could only slow the cancer, and since it was slow growing already, the toxic side effects of the treatment would far outweigh the modest potential for benefit. Once matters grew dire, such therapies might make sense, but for now he suggested they simply monitor the cancer with checkups every three months. There was, he said, nothing more to do.

*   *   *

Vielman was of another mind. A few years before her diagnosis, her fear of dying young like her father had driven her to look for ways to live more healthily, and her search led her to an odd little clinic in Santa Rosa, just ninety minutes up the road from her home. In lectures she watched online, doctors from the clinic argued that many of the chronic diseases that had become epidemic in the developed world—type 2 diabetes, cardiovascular disease, hypertension, obesity—were caused by eating the standard American diet and could frequently be reversed simply by eating a healthier diet of minimally processed plants. For those wishing to speed up the healing process, another treatment usually helped: prolonged fasting. The doctors had some science to back their claims. In one study they published in a peer-reviewed journal, 154 of 174 patients with high blood pressure who fasted for a week and a half on nothing but water normalized their blood pressure. Doctors elsewhere were talking about managing hypertension, cardiovascular disease, and diabetes—incurable, lifelong conditions, to hear most doctors tell it—but the doctors at the TrueNorth Health Center were talking about getting rid of those disorders for good.

In 2010, four years before her cancer diagnosis, Vielman had driven to TrueNorth and consulted with Dr. Michael Klaper, one of the fathers of the modern vegan-health movement. She didn't think she needed to fast, but Klaper's suggestion to eat more plants made sense to her, and she went home and began eliminating meat, dairy, and eggs from her family's diet. She didn't go as far as Klaper and colleagues advocated—the TrueNorth diet was also free of salt, oil, sugar, and processed foods—but even with a lesser veganism, for the first time in a long time Vielman stopped gaining weight and then started losing a few of the 180 pounds she had packed onto her five feet, five inches. She felt more energetic and thought she was on the right track until cancer came calling. When she walked out of Dr. Greenfield's oncology clinic in 2014, she had no doubt what she was going to do: she was going back to TrueNorth to fast.

On a gloriously sunny Monday in November she presented herself, suitcase in hand, at the doorstep of the clinic, a former apartment block on a nondescript thoroughfare in a not especially distinguished precinct of Santa Rosa. She planned a fast of fourteen days, which seemed dauntingly long but in fact proved rather easy, even buoying. Toward the end of her second week, she got to chatting with another patient who said her own fast of several weeks had healed a traumatic head injury. The clinic was swirling with stories like hers, fantastic-seeming tales of rheumatoid arthritis and lupus and colitis either going into remission or being greatly lessened with fasting. A theme of the stories was that the people who healed most thoroughly usually fasted the longest. The woman with the head injury, for instance, said she hadn't begun to get well until the third week of her fast. Vielman thought of her two sons at home who, she would later write, "needed me to stick around longer than the expiration date traditional medicine had given me: 20 more years. I would be 62 by then, and I certainly did not want to die the day after I retired."

She asked Dr. Klaper if she could fast three weeks instead of the planned two, and after checking her vitals and lab work, he said he saw no reason she shouldn't. A day or two later, as she was palpating her largest tumor, she thought it seemed softer and smaller. Then again, she was losing roughly a pound a day, and what seemed a shrunken tumor might just be the dwindling of fat around it. But as the days passed, the lump continued to shrink, and the diminution seemed out of proportion to her weight loss. She asked Klaper to check, and when he did, a wide smile broke across his face. He checked her other tumors, found them in retreat as well, and patient and doctor exchanged a great bear hug. For the rest of Vielman's stay the tumors continued to wither, and by the time she broke her fast after twenty-one days, they were gone.

"When Ivonne came to us," Klaper would later say, "those tumors were the size of hen's eggs. And in the end they just melted away."

Vielman broke her fast twenty-two pounds to the good, weighing 152. Her body-mass index (a ratio of weight to height expressed in kilograms over meters squared) was a smidge above 25, the traditional dividing line between normal weight and overweight. She went home and reformed her diet further, now staying away from added salt, oil, sugar, and highly processed foods like white flour and white rice. Within a year, she had knocked off another twenty pounds.

Some weeks after her fast, she returned to Dr. Greenfield, the oncologist. He palpated her groin and armpits, evinced little surprise, and said follicular lymphoma sometimes did that: it fluctuated a lot, now flaring, now subsiding, even to the point of seeming disappearance. Spontaneous remissions, as the withdrawals were called, occurred in ten to twenty percent of patients, but the disease always came back. One hint Vielman's would was that her white blood cell count remained quite low—one of lymphoma's calling cards.

Dr. Alan Goldhamer, the founder and director of the TrueNorth Health Center, had a contrary view. In his three decades treating some very sick people, he believed he had seen many "incurable" conditions go away not through chance but through the restorative biochemistry of water-only fasting. He thought Vielman's case a particularly important instance, not just because her turnaround was so dramatic but because patients only rarely came to him with "before" scans like hers confirming her lymphoma diagnosis. Those scans could help document her remission, provided she could also get "after" scans showing the tumors were really gone, not just lurking sub-palpably. If the after scans indeed showed that, Goldhamer thought he could publish a report of her case in a high-impact medical journal.

But Dr. Greenfield, who would have to order the scans, didn't want to. He hadn't been enthusiastic about Vielman's fast in the first place, although he hadn't opposed it. This was Northern California, after all, and certain allowances had to be made for the alternative treatments his patients sometimes pursued. (His tolerant ambivalence was enlightened compared to the reaction of Vielman's family physician, Dr. Hughes, who had told Vielman before her fast that any studies claiming fasting was effective had to be phony and she was delivering herself into the hands of criminal quacks. Hughes wasn't the least interested later in discussing the possibility that the fast had chased her patient's lymphoma into remission.) When Vielman asked Greenfield for scans, he said it made little sense to subject her to more radiation just to confirm the disease was in temporary abeyance. But the doctors at TrueNorth had coached her in persistence, and Greenfield eventually relented and ordered the images, which showed no lurking tumors. Vielman's lymph nodes had shrunk back to their normal size, her cancer to all appearances gone. In the coming months her white blood cell count normalized, and at her next checkup with Dr. Greenfield three months later, the tumors still could not be palpated. Nor was there a sign of them at the next three-month checkup, nor at the next.

Goldhamer and Klaper wrote a paper about Vielman's case and submitted it to *BMJ Case Reports*, an arm of the *British Medical Journal*, one of the world's oldest and most widely read medical reviews. In late 2015, the paper was accepted. Before it was published, Goldhamer wrote Greenfield to ask if he would like to sign on.

"I said to him," recalled Goldhamer, who has a puckish streak, "'Thank you for the confidence you've shown in referring your patient to us for therapeutic, water-only fasting. As you know, and I'm sure as you expected, she's gone into remission, . . . and because we have a paper that's been accepted for publication in the *British Medical Journal*, we'd like to invite you to join us as coauthor.' I haven't gotten a reply yet, but it's only been six years."

The offer of coauthorship was not extended to Hughes, who wouldn't even release Vielman's medical records to the criminal quacks at TrueNorth.

At the end of 2016, two years after her tumors disappeared, Vielman had another round of scans, which again came back clean. A year later she went back to TrueNorth and fasted nineteen days as a sort of housecleaning measure. Scans following that fast came back clean as well. In lymphoma, most spontaneous remissions will un-remit well before three years have run, so Goldhamer sent a follow-up to *BMJ Case Reports* demonstrating Vielman was still cancer-free. One of the journal's two external reviewers recommended the editor publish the paper, but the other did not. The gainsayer said Vielman's cancer had to have disappeared through spontaneous remission, not fasting, but offered no reason why; apparently fasting was just too crazy to contemplate. The editor, who held the tie-breaking vote, published the article anyway. Nearly eight years have passed since Vielman's tumors disappeared, and they have not come back.

*   *   *

Ivonne Vielman's story is not unique, as I hope this book will make clear. In fact, the only unusual thing about it is that it received a measure of attention in "serious" circles. The history of therapeutic fasting is largely one of neglect, skepticism, and ridicule punctuated by brief intervals of understanding and acceptance, which makes the moment we're living in—a time when fasting is suddenly much in the news, to good notice—at once anomalous and splendid. Not all that long ago, you couldn't get anyone to take fasting seriously. In 2011, I pitched an article on the history and science of fasting to several of the nation's leading highbrow magazines. One editor I corresponded with, who was sympathetic, said his colleagues thought the pitch well written and well researched, but it just didn't *seem* right. Like the reviewer of Goldhamer's article, the editors could point to no weaknesses in the science I presented. They just felt it couldn't be. It was, I gathered, simply too counterintuitive to think not eating could make you healthier. Other editors told me in nearly so many words that fasting was on the wrong side of respectability, something akin to crystals and chakras and not far removed from

Eye of newt and toe of frog,
Wool of bat and tongue of dog.

In the end, the piece found a home at *Harper's*, where it played a small part in the modern revival of fasting.

What a revival it has been. If there is a periodical or podcast, a website or blog, a TV or radio show that covers health or medicine that hasn't discussed fasting, I don't know of it. Enthusiasm for fasting is outpacing skepticism (which, however, persists, especially among doctors), and now all sorts of astonishing claims are made on fasting's behalf, some of them true. It is true, for example, that fasting seems able to send follicular lymphoma into remission. It is also true that fasting can lessen or entirely do away with asthma, psoriasis, eczema, lupus, ulcerative colitis, Crohn's disease, irritable bowel syndrome, rheumatoid arthritis, migraine, type 2 diabetes, Hashimoto's thyroiditis, some forms of schizophrenia, and many other bothersome disorders. Just about everyone with high blood pressure who undertakes a prolonged fast can, under the supervision of a doctor experienced in fasting, taper off their hypertension pills. In fact, the greatest drop in blood pressure ever recorded in a peer-reviewed publication came not from medications, exercise, or changes in diet but from fasting at TrueNorth in the study mentioned above. On average, patients with severe hypertension enjoyed a staggering drop of 60 mm Hg—*sixty*—in systolic pressure, the top number in a blood pressure reading. And in one of the most exciting developments of the last decade, fasting has even been shown to make chemotherapy more effective at killing certain cancers while protecting patients from chemo's worst side effects.

But for all that, there's much that fasting cannot do, no matter how many incautious boosters say otherwise. Fasting cannot by itself kill most cancers. Indeed, fasting alone can probably cure only a very small handful of cancers. Nor does it seem likely that fasting can reverse advanced cases of multiple sclerosis, Alzheimer's, or Parkinson's, although it may help us avoid those diseases in the first place, might check their advance in the early stages, and might provide relief of a few symptoms even in advanced cases. Nor, for all the hype of clickbait headlines, will fasting make us young again, even if it will slow some of the worst effects of aging.

Fasting, in short, is astoundingly and variously useful, deserving of the enthusiasm it is finally getting but deserving as well of being treated with sensibility and discernment. What follows is, I hope, a fuller chronicle of fasting than has been told before, one that neither hides its enthusiasm nor relinquishes its judgment. In addition to telling stories like Ivonne Vielman's, which illustrate why the new science of fasting is so thrilling, I give several chapters to the history of fasting, which is as old as the written word. I've done so partly because I wanted to answer a question that has long interested me: why, given fasting's use throughout history, has it taken until now for therapeutic fasting to come into its own? Put another way: what forces prevented this most simple of remedies from being more widely adopted? The answers span nearly three thousand curious, confused, and contentious years in which intelligence and ignorance have squared off time and again with stakes of life and death. It's a tale in which both despair and hope abound, but as you'll have gathered from Vielman's case, hope may at last be ascendant. After a hundred false starts and blind alleys, scientists are finally unlocking the health-giving secrets of fasting, and we are fortunate indeed to live in a time when anyone can benefit from this knowledge.

CHAPTER 1

TANNER'S FOLLY

Two weeks after a Fourth of July at the end of Reconstruction, a doctor in Minneapolis resolved to cure himself of the several illnesses from which he was suffering or die trying. By one account, he was indifferent to the outcome. The doctor, Henry S. Tanner, had lately succumbed to what he called a gastric fever, which may have been a stomach flu, as well as cardiac rheumatism, which was inflammation of the heart, and nervous exhaustion, which was something not far short of a nervous breakdown. He had other troubles of longer standing. His wife had left him some years earlier in favor of Duluth, which may have spoken to the quality of his husbandage, and his final effort to reacquire her had failed just that week. He had been a lecturer on temperance but not a rousing one, had owned a Turkish bathhouse but not a successful one, and was, per a friend, "not over particular as regards the orderly arrangement of his wearing apparel or of household or office furniture." In the past when he had succumbed to minor illnesses, he found relief in abstaining from food for a few days, and he now thought a fast of ten or twelve days might rid him of his complaints. If it failed, it would surely rid him of his life, for the consensus among men of science was that a human could survive no more than eight to ten days without food. Christ may have fasted forty, but his was thought a special case.

So it was that on July 17, 1877, Tanner drank a pint of milk and repaired to a lounge in the Minneapolitan home of his friend and fellow physician, one A. Moyer. He passed some days, hungrily. Dr. Moyer urged him to eat, but Tanner held his resolve and only water crossed his lips. Presently things happened that most doctors would have considered odd—indeed, most anyone would have considered odd. Tanner's hunger vanished, and he stopped thinking of food. Day by day his ailments began to ease. By the tenth day, which should, by the wisdom of the moment, have been his last, all of his complaints had fallen away. His countenance was brighter, his eyes clearer, and far from nearing death, he felt a renewed strength. It had been his custom to walk one to three miles twice daily, and after the tenth day he resumed these constitutionals. If his step was shaky at first, it quickly grew steady. Soon he judged his recovery complete and bade Dr. Moyer, who had kept a nervous vigil, bring him food.

But while the food was being prepared, Tanner turned to a thought that had lately danced around the edge of his consciousness: if a man might not merely survive but indeed thrive after ten foodless days, what would be the limit of his unfed endurance? Twenty days? Thirty? More? And what would the answer say about mankind? Did it imply, for instance, that we were meant to live on less food than we commonly took or that we should take food less often? If so, what were the consequences of our overeating? It was the sort of teasing enigma that will gnaw at a person of a certain turn of mind until he must have an answer, and by the time Moyer brought his meal, Tanner had come to another resolution. He would forgo gratification of the stomach for gratification of the mind. He told Moyer to remove the viands and stood firm in the face of his friend's protestations.

Ten fasted days became fifteen, then twenty, then twenty-five. Tanner noted no great changes in his person save loss of weight, a bit under a pound a day. He acknowledged a slight slowness in cogitation, chiefly on complicated subjects, but otherwise his mental powers were undiminished, and he enjoyed long talks with Moyer about his fast and the science of acquiring good health. On reaching four foodless weeks, he celebrated by walking six miles of riverbank to Minnehaha Falls and a more circuitous seven miles back. Several days later he circumambulated Lakes Calhoun and Cedar, but after drinking from those bodies, he contracted gastritis and spent the next two days retching. As he grew visibly more frail, Moyer once more urged him to end his fast, and he at last relented. On the forty-first day, he took a few sips of milk. Henry Tanner had bested Christ.

*   *   *

Tanner had no inclination to advertise his feat, which is odd in light of later events, but Moyer thought his friend's attainment should be trumpeted and with his permission sent a dispatch to the *Chicago Medical Times*, which published it. Disbelief ran high, and certain residents of the Twin Cities impugned the integrity of both doctors for embarrassing the metropolis. Even so, a few correspondents wrote the local press to say they too had made prolonged fasts for health, which suggested therapeutic fasting was not an entirely unknown art.

The disbelief so irritated Tanner that he announced he would prove his bona fides by fasting another forty days, this time under a public watch, provided the skeptics put up a purse of $5,000. Upon completing the fast, he would give $4,000 to Mrs. General Van Cleve's house of reclamation for the unfortunate of her sex, while the remainder would stick to him for his trouble. At the time, $1,000 was better than the average yearly wage. There were no takers.

Tanner's fast might have been lost to history, and the course of modern fasting set on an entirely different and perhaps quieter path, but for another challenge, at first unrelated to Tanner, that was issued the following year by an acclaimed Manhattan doctor and former surgeon general of the United States. Dr. William Hammond had been vexed by the publicity attending one Mollie Fancher, a Brooklynite who claimed to have lived for years almost without food. A decade and a half earlier, Miss Fancher had become bedridden in a streetcar accident, which, however, was said to have endowed her with miraculous powers. She allegedly passed months subsisting on air alone, and on the rare instances when she took more customary nourishment, she ate only enough to feed a finch. She was also believed to have the power of clairvoyance, to read books without opening them, and in one instance to construe the contents of a ripped-up mining report sealed inside an envelope.

Dr. Hammond wrote Miss Fancher a check for $1,000, placed it in an envelope, and announced the draft was hers if she could divine the number of the check, its date, and the name of the issuing bank. Furthermore, if she would fast for a month under the observation of doctors, taking neither food nor water, he would add another $1,000 to her fortune. Miss Fancher spurned the check-reading challenge on grounds that her divinatorial powers could not be rented, and she declined the fasting challenge on grounds that decency did not allow her to be examined by (male) physicians. Learning of Miss Fancher's demurral, Tanner wrote Hammond and offered to take up the fasting part of the challenge, albeit modified to allow him to drink water. When Hammond failed to respond, Tanner entrained to New York to engage him from closer quarters. For weeks the two doctors communicated with growing rancor through reporters and letters to editors, who, knowing good copy when they saw it, gave prominent coverage to this wrangle between a pillar of cultivated New York society and a short, stout eccentric from the provinces who claimed a marvelous fasting power.

Ostensibly the two doctors quarreled over details like Tanner's wish to fast on water, but the real source of their bunfight, the one that drew the public eye, was that Tanner was an eclectic doctor, something like a naturopath today, while Hammond was a conventional MD. In that period, unlike now, both were allowed the title "medical doctor," but the divide between conventional and unconventional doctors was cavernous and seldom crossed with friendly intent. The "regulars," as the conventional physicians styled themselves, believed they stood for science and institutionalized learning, while the irregulars charged the medical emperor had no clothes. The "science" of the regulars, they said, was a sophisticated screen for bilking clients and was no more curative, and often quite a bit less, than the folk cures and other remedies favored by irregulars. The irregulars were largely right—medicine was still emerging from a most appalling primitivism, and its science was often more akin to pseudoscience—but the press usually sided with the establishmentarians. One journalist wrote of Tanner and his kind, "They would like to demonstrate that the world is square and flat, that the moon is made of green cheese, or any other absurdity that might seem to invalidate regular science, and so to make room for their own irregular pretensions." Some newspapers went so far as to add mock quotes to Tanner's honorific—"Dr." Tanner—even though in that era the curricula of irregular medical schools were often more rigorous than those of their regular counterparts.

The dispute came to a head when Hammond insisted the observers who would watch Tanner during his fast be mustered solely from the ranks of conventional doctors, preferably from the membership of the New York Neurological Society, of which Hammond was a leading light. Tanner said Hammond's societarians were more than welcome to run the watch, but he refused to exclude physicians of other schools, whose presence, however, Hammond would not abide. When the two failed to come to terms, Tanner proceeded at his own cost, securing a public lecture hall in Manhattan at the United States Medical College and a cadre of the college's professors and students to monitor him round the clock. He raised Hammond's dare from a month of fasting to the biblical forty days—no doubt calculating to stimulate the public imagination—and he would permit himself water. Because the medical college was eclectic, establishmentarian doctors eschewed the affair. Then as now, establishments liked nothing so little as progress not established by themselves.

And so on a summer's morning in 1880 the unlikely Tanner—squattish, thinning of hair, outstanding of mutton chop—his person having been examined for hidden food and his vitals recorded for statistical baseline, took the stage at Clarendon Hall on East 13th Street. His furnishings consisted of a cot, a cane-backed rocker, and a gas-fired chandelier set within a railed-off enclosure. The spareness of the set and the glow of the chandelier were meant to dispel suspicions he had secreted food about him. At the stroke of noon, he took a seat in the rocker and proceeded to do—nothing. This he supplemented, as the hours passed, with a little reading, a little drinking of water, and a little chatting with his public, the size of which would be familiar to a short-story writer on book tour today.

After two days, he felt so fine that he declared he would continue his fast in the Hammondian manner, without water. By the third day he had lost 10 of his 157½ pounds. New York's newspapers ran well-nourished reports on his progress morning and evening, papers all over the country republished the dispatches, and Tanner's appeal grew so steadily that by the fifth day the doors at Clarendon Hall were thronged. Among his visitors on the sixth day were more than a hundred physicians of every school—"allopathic, homœopathic, electric, eclectic, hydropathic and physiomedico electricians." A doctor named McDonald who oversaw the lunatic asylum on Blackwell's Island (Roosevelt Island today) pronounced Tanner's condition extraordinary. Dr. Hammond was not among the callers, but when his opinion was solicited by the press, he declared himself incredulous and the faster "a fraud." His condition was "too good . . . to have been absolutely without food," and in any event his experiment was "of no scientific value."

Fascination with Tanner grew all the same, particularly as he inched toward the fatal window, the limit of man's unfed endurance, which would open on the eighth day. The *New York Herald* supplemented the collegiate watchers with its own platoon of fourteen reporters detailed in pairs, seven shifts a day. They tasted Tanner's every jug of water, inspected his many missives for contraband, even checked under his fingernails for sustenance furtively passed in a handshake. A few days later, as Tanner was becoming the most talked-about man in the country, members of Hammond's own Neurological Society set up a watch, and they would soon declare the little faster from the Middle West a man of probity, his fast genuine.

Without water, however, he began to deteriorate. A dry fast would have been a tall order in any season, but the July heat simply desiccated him. He passed long hours torpid and irritable and called frequently for wet cloths on his forehead and wet sponges for his hands. These reviving him, he would be "lively as a cricket" for a few hours, only to sink again. He survived the critical eighth and ninth days, but on the dread tenth he was described, with a bit of tabloid license, as near delirium. Certainly he looked a candidate for expiration, wan and weakening, his cheeks and eyes sunken, his frame sixteen pounds lighter than when he began. "At this time his sufferings had become so terrible to witness," a dispatch in the *Times* read, "that his physicians were sometimes moved almost to tears."

But the eleventh day dawned with Tanner still extant, and he was prevailed upon to take a little water. Feeling renewed, he declared he was strong enough to continue with no more liquid henceforth, but his sufferings grew so pronounced that on the sixteenth day he took water again and said it had been foolishness to fast without it. He recovered his vigor almost immediately and over the next two days gained four and a half pounds, a sign of how desperate his dehydration had been.

Viewers by the thousand were now paying two bits a head to wonder at the awful spectacle of "The Stomachless Man," as the press fashioned him. Young ladies played the piano for his amusement or serenaded him with duets, children recited merry rhymes, and professional actors elevated the divertissements with off-Broadway performances. Other entertainments were less welcome. "A strong minded female" wanted to read a tract titled "Have You a Soul to Save?" but stronger minds induced her to leave off, and a young man who sang off key "was informed that if he continued a general alarm would be sent out and the engine company next door requested to turn the hose on him."

Tanner's mailbag contained up to four hundred letters a day, among which were several gentle proposals from members of the fair sex. A Miss Lillian Irvin of Philadelphia invoked leap-year privilege as she offered her hand and was candid her motive was kitchen heat: "What woman, this weather, would refuse to idolize a man who comes home from business and who does not think of eating." Other correspondents enclosed contraband—a slice of roast beef, a bottle of gin, another of claret—which Tanner's watchers removed. Rare lilies, a nightshirt, a hammock bed, and Indian clubs (the trendy exercise gear of the day) were allowed to pass.

As the stream of visiting doctors grew to a mighty freshet, Dr. Robert Gunn, president of the US Medical College, adjudged its constituents "rude almost without exception. One man insisted upon feeling Dr. Tanner's arms and legs; another wanted to feel his pulse; a third demanded a view of his tongue; a fourth declared food must be given to him surreptitiously, else he would be dead; a fifth wanted to search his pockets; the sixth asserted [on] his professional reputation that there was fraud about the whole business[;] the seventh had some patent surgical, or other appliance, which he wished to test upon the patient; and yet another wanted to analyse even the water he used, before the faster drank it."

Tanner's effort brought out other fasters, a few in the flesh, most by post, which again suggested fasting was more widespread among the public than the regulars cared to admit. A Dr. Smock of Staten Island said he had once fasted fifteen days, and a Dr. W. B. Lee of Marion, Illinois, claimed to have fasted twenty-four. (The reasons for their self-denial, presumably therapeutic, were not recorded.) Imitators also arose. A medical student in Fort Wayne, Indiana, announced he would fast thirty days but failed, and a James H. Rindley of Princeton, Illinois, aimed for twenty days with no food but all the beer he could drink, also without success. A certain Signor Goldschmidt, "known in Naples as a singing master, as a marvellous swimmer, and as a vegetarian of some years' standing," said he would outdo Tanner's forty days with a fast of fifty, but I could find nothing of his triumph. Tanner's most serious mimic was a fellow named Charles Livingston ("The Other Fasting Idiot," the *Washington Post* dubbed him), who went so far as to rent a hall in Brooklyn and arrange a relay of watchers for what he said would be a Tanner-beating fast of forty-two days. He quit nine days into the effort after his wife, despairing of his abstinence, claimed to have swallowed poison only to miraculously recover when he agreed to refeed. The copycats prompted *Scribner's Monthly* to call on a thousand fools to fast forty days. "Think what a saving of the materials of life would be effected! And then think how surely the whole batch would die, and relieve the world of their useless presence."

A few fasters had already done just that, for reports of macabre fasts also emerged. The *Argus* of Albany, New York, recalled the long-ago starvation of twenty-seven-year-old Reuben Kelsey, who in July of 1829 said he wasn't hungry and that he reckoned the Almighty would furnish him with an appetite when it was His will he should eat again. Kelsey grew so vigorous during his fast he decided food wasn't required for life, but eventually he turned blue, then blackish, and finally looked "so ghastly that children were frightened at the sight of him." He died after fifty-three days.

Tanner's own demise was regularly forecast. On the fourteenth day, per one correspondent, "all physicians who have been consulted predict his SURRENDER OR HIS DEATH before the seventeenth day." But come the seventeenth, one of the habitual forecasters, a Dr. Miller, said, "I am about giving up my theories." By the start of the twentieth, everyone agreed Tanner cut a better figure than he had on the tenth: "a smiling,

good-humored old gentleman, with a keen, bright eye and strong, reso-
lute voice, sitting up on the end of a cot, and exchanging jokes with the
corps of watchers."

His survival put two questions on the tongue in every town in America
and many abroad, the same two that had moved him to undertake his first
great fast three years before: How long could he endure? And what did his
survival mean for human biology?

*　　*　　*

Tanner was born in 1831 in Tunbridge Wells, Kent, thirty miles south
of London, and at the age of seventeen emigrated with his family to
Painesville, Ohio, thirty miles up Lake Erie from Cleveland. There he
plied his father's trade of carriage-making before running a small fruit store
and finally enrolling in the Eclectic Medical Institute of Cincinnati. In his
youth, Tanner had been exposed to fasting as a remedy for acute illness,
and in his medical practice he sometimes encouraged patients to go a few
days without food, with what success we cannot say. But his failure with his
wife on that score was total. On occasion when he fasted, per one report,
"he generously invited Mrs. Tanner to bear him company. But she firmly
refused." In Tanner's words, "She would eat fat pork and cabbage three
times a day. She had a habit of gorging herself, and was always sick and bil-
ious. I would mildly remonstrate with her and hint that she could expect
nothing else, and that, in fact, it served her right for eating so much." These
mild remonstrances went over about as well as you might expect and led
ultimately to Mrs. Tanner's departure for Duluth without including Mr.
Tanner among the movables. He eventually followed, but his only reward
was divorce.

Tanner may have been a misery as a mate, but many of his ideas about
the science of fasting and health were uncannily sound. "The whole thing
is in the recuperative power in man," he said, and he explained that most
disease arose from two sources that were within the body's power to reme-
diate. "The first source," as one observer summarized, "is the excess of food
taken over the body's needs. The second source is the debris of the worn-out

tissues of the body itself.... Dr. Tanner's plan is to allow nature to clear away the debris by relieving the body of the constantly replenished excess of food over requirement.... In this way, Dr. Tanner claims, is brought about the purification, or, as he sometimes terms it, a new birth."

Neither doctors nor patients shared his assumptions (which would prove correct) that fasting could clear away the debris of worn-out tissues and give birth to new ones. The doctors' blindness hardly surprised Tanner, for, as he said, "The thing that makes doctors in good demand and well paid is the belief in the curative powers of medicine"—and few doctors cared to lessen the call for their services by letting the body heal itself. But their patients' rejection of his creed wholly mystified him because in that era they were more apt to be harmed than healed by the doctor's kitbag. "It is very strange to me," he mused, "that people can't understand this and cease to be such faithful devotees of burnt toads and dried flies."

Yet it was Tanner, not his brothers in physic or their patients, who was roundly lampooned as unscientific. The distinguished Charles-Édouard Brown-Séquard, known today for the paralysis that bears his name (and soon to be infamous for a cockamamie claim to have rejuvenated his sexual prowess with injections of animal testes), groused that because Tanner didn't measure the air he inhaled and exhaled, the sweat he gave off, and everything else he excreted, "the scientific results of the experiment are absolutely *nil*." In fact, Tanner's urine was collected, studied, and found unexceptional, and he produced no feces. But even if every possible measurement had been made, the science of the day was so crude that most of the readings would have told little of fasting's promise, which was an idea far grander than anything hidden in his excreta. The body, Tanner was declaring, could heal itself. What was true of a nick of the skin was true of a rheumatoid heart or the common cold: give the body a chance to rest, and it would restore and renew its ailing parts. Doctors, blinded by their fixation on measurements, couldn't see the forest Tanner had led them to and could but stumble over the twigs.

We can get an idea of just how rudimentary the science of the age was from the fact that scientific minds couldn't agree on the substance on which Tanner's body was surviving. Though his fat melted away before their eyes, only a minority of experts thought it fueled his organs. Many thought the air alone nourished him. One lecturess accused Tanner of choosing New York for his fast because the rich metropolitan atmosphere, unlike that of Minnesota, was filled with life-giving particles exhaled by its two million inhabitants. Other learned minds maintained, as Dr. Hammond had from the start, that water nourished him. The spring in Central Park from which Tanner drew his water was said to be rich in life-giving *animalcula*— microscopic animals—although when it was examined under a microscope, it proved freer of microbial life than the water from the Croton Aqueduct that sustained most New Yorkers. (The spring, which arises west of the Great Lawn, is to this day known as Tanner's Spring.)

Tanner himself sometimes said he was sustained by an almost mystical, hibernation-like process, the same that allowed Indian fakirs to be entombed underground and unearthed alive months later. But in more sober moments he held, as one journalist synopsized, "that whoever had a surplus of adipose tissue had a reserve stock of food to draw upon, as much as if he had laid in a stock of provisions in the cellar." Here, again, Tanner was on the money.

* * *

As Tanner's "Terrible Task of Endurance" approached a month, his fame grew even more immense, and his exploits were sketched in the columns of multiple London papers, the *Times of India*, and the *West African Reporter*. *Scribner's* wrote without embellishment that "there is hardly a spot in the civilized world that is not acquainted with his name," and the Baltimore *Sun* asserted, "Even the Presidential candidates pale before this abstentious monstrosity," although in truth James Garfield and Winfield Hancock would have paled before a three-legged hamster. A New York playhouse offered Tanner $700 a week to complete his fast in their theater, and a museum in Maine offered to stuff and exhibit him should he expire during his trial. These offers and more Tanner declined, although he eventually agreed to a post-fast lecture tour for an emolument in the thousands of dollars.

Amid the circus, there were medical lessons to be learned, brief flickerings that might have sparked scientific thought for any with eyes to see. One came from an Irishman in Cincinnati named O'Halloran, who fasted to cure an illness of an unstated nature. He succeeded in going only five days without food, but "for the next 11 days Mr. O'Halloran ate very sparingly, and found that his condition improved out of all proportion to the amount of food he took." He had, it seemed, discovered what is today known as a fasting-mimicking diet, a regimen of very few calories that yields some of the curative benefits of fasting.

An even more dramatic case was that of Agnes Dehart of Mariners Harbor, Staten Island. Miss Dehart, aged twenty-one, had "for several years been distressed by ulcers of the stomach, and . . . applied in vain to the most skillful physicians for relief." When one of those physicians told her a fast of thirty days might give her stomach the break it needed to heal itself, she stopped eating on the same day Tanner did. She also stopped drinking and solved the problem of dehydration through the peculiar means of bovine lavage: "two pounds of beef tea, which was administered in the form of an enema every six hours." She passed a difficult first week hungry, nauseated, and vomiting but finally settled into a cheerful fast. Unlike Tanner, who went for chaperoned walks and rides, Miss Dehart spent most of her time abed. She slimmed from 123 to 96 pounds and broke her fast on four raw oysters. Her ulcers disappeared entirely.

These were promising suggestions that Tanner's theory of regenerative fasting might be worth looking into, but there's no hint in the public record that anyone did so. The press, for its part, all but ignored O'Halloran and reported Dehart as simply another endurance wonder. As so often in science, the clues lay invisible in plain sight.

*   *   *

On the twenty-fifth day of Tanner's fast, a Dr. Alley in Atlanta told a reporter that if Tanner continued much longer, "he will begin to eat himself or those around him."

"In the event that he becomes a cannibal," the reporter asked, "what part of himself would he first attack?"

"I think he would masticate his fingers and toes."

He did not, but the following day he complained of nausea for the first time since returning to drinking water. The next day he was better, but on subsequent days he was again nauseated and became weak and irritable, and for the remainder of his fast he suffered on and off from fever, headache, cramp, and several varieties of gastrointestinal distress. Now and then he vomited bile and mucus. "His worst battles," per one witness, "were fought the last four or five days, when slightest exertion caused the eructation of wind from the gastric region." His burps were tremendous.

On the thirty-fifth day, Tanner was much heartened by a telegram from Paris from one of the era's most illustrious and regular of physicians, Marion Sims. Sims was the father of modern gynecology, equally ingenious and notorious (latterly anyway) as a monster who perfected his surgical techniques on enslaved women whom he didn't bother to anesthetize. Sims told Tanner, "Your experiment watched here with great interest by scientists; ridiculed by fools. . . . Courage, brave fellow; hold on." Praise from such an eminence ruffled to no end the proud plume of Dr. Hammond, who said the transmission must be an imposture and that if his esteemed friend could indeed "cable such trash," he would endeavor to forget him. But the cable was genuine, and eventually even Hammond came around, acknowledging a few days before the end that the fast had been fairly conducted and had caused him to revise his views of starvation. Tanner, he said, had "great pluck and endurance, commanding admiration." The flagging Tanner gloated over Hammond's admission a whole day.

On the final morning, Tanner was revived in spirit and color, but when he tried to rise from his bed at ten o'clock, he was too weak and had to be carried to a large armchair. The collegians weighed him at 121½ pounds, 36 fewer than when he began. His other vitals were interesting only for being uninteresting; his pulse was calm, his respiration normal. As the minutes edged toward his midday breakfast, he seemed to gain in vigor, no doubt stimulated by the thousand people gathered inside to witness it. Outside, the street was mobbed from curb to curb with a thousand more.

For days Tanner had been showered with advice about how to break his fast. Queen Victoria's physician urged him by cable to start with no more than five or six drops of milk. A doctor in New York said such a meal was far too hearty and counseled no more than a single lick of a postage stamp, while another warned such a feast would overtax his system and prescribed a good long sniff of well-done toast. After speaking with several authorities of a somewhat more serious nature, one reporter concluded, "It is not thought likely he will be able to eat an ordinary meal before the lapse of a week or ten days." A few experts said he would never eat an ordinary meal again, that his digestion had been irretrievably ruined, and from his first bite his days would be numbered few.

"Judge of their surprise, then, when . . . he practically resumed his relations with the dietary table where he left off 40 days ago." As the factory steam whistles blew noon and the steeples chimed their assent, Tanner, ignoring all advice, stood before an open window and brought a peeled peach to his mouth in front of the multitude in the street below. Their roar as he took an enormous bite could be heard blocks away. So lustily did he attack the peach that Dr. Gunn, the college president, reproached him, but Tanner waved him off and continued his assault until nothing was left but the pit. He then proceeded to the lecture hall to such deafening cheers and general pandemonium that only with great effort did the constables keep the barriers between the faster and his admirers from being reduced to splinters.

Stepping nimbly onto some low tables that had been set up as a dais— gone was his earlier feebleness—Tanner surveyed the scores of gifts laid out in a kind of edible homage. They encompassed "every variety of fruits and delicacies," from half a dozen of the season's largest watermelons and several bottles of Russian kumis (a libation of fermented mare's milk) to fresh-baked loaves of breads and prize chickens. The wag who sent a box of shingle nails was probably intimating that Tanner, like the ostrich of proverb, could digest even nails. If so, he or she was prophetic.

Tanner called over the roaring crowd for a glass of milk and drank the goblet passed to him in nearly one gulp.

"I tell you that tastes good," he cried, and the crowd cheered and stamped "until Clarendon Hall trembled."

After a second goblet, he commanded, "Now bring on the Georgia watermelon." As one of his watchers heaved forward a colossus of forty pounds, a horrified Dr. Gunn protested that Tanner was waltzing with the Reaper.

"Look here," Tanner retorted, "I have been through this mill before. Just stand aside and let me have my own way."

His demolition of a formidable slice of the melon brought another boisterous ovation, and amid that clamor he proceeded on the arm of Dr. Gunn to a waiting carriage, their progress slowed by incessant pawing and a raucous shaking of hands. When the cab finally pulled away from the horde, children chased it for blocks.

Tanner convalesced in the home of Dr. Gunn, and in the succeeding hours he added to his stomach a modest half-pound of broiled beefsteak, a like amount of sirloin, four apples, and for lubrication Hungarian wine and Bass Ale. By the following evening, not having slackened his pace, he had reclaimed eight and a half of his lost pounds. After three days he would regain nineteen and a half, and after eight days he would recoup all of the lost thirty-six. The question of which was the greater marvel—surviving his starvation or surviving his wanton refeeding—remains, in light of what we now know about fasting and refeeding, open to debate. At the time, however, his ability to recover bulk was a credit in fasting's ledger, proof that a voluntary famine need not sap a starver. The *Kansas City Review of Science* did his anatomy no less than justice when it said, "We are inclined to regard the Doctor's individual stomach as the most remarkable organ on record." Incredibly, at no time during his refeeding did he feel nausea or indigestion. His only complaint, throughout the first night, was that "he felt like a bee-hive all over, and there was not a grain of tissue in him that was not at work." To every outward appearance, neither forty days without food nor promiscuous refeeding had done Henry Tanner a jot of harm.

* * *

The significance of Tanner's fast was as hotly disputed in its aftermath as it had been during its progress. The *Times* labeled his achievement "Tanner's folly," which shows the predictive power of the establishment press hadn't improved in the thirteen years since it had declared Seward's folly. "It may be of use to the shipwrecked, or to persons who are lost," the *Chicago Evening Journal* opined of the fast, but not to anyone else. Overseas critics were even harsher. An editorialist for the *Times of India* struck the self-satisfied chord of indignant superiority in which British colonials excelled: "An excitement to Americans is something like what the horse is to the Arab, or the dog to the Esquimaux: they can scarcely do without it." But such grotesquerie did not "find favour with the more phlegmatic, and in some things more practical, Britons," who evidently preferred their starvation inflicted phlegmatically and practically on an entire subcontinent they were looting.

One hindrance to Tanner's didactic mission was that he was a pitchman without product. Three years earlier in Dr. Moyer's Minneapolis chambers, his fast may well have healed his digestive tract, his heart, and his nerves, but in New York he hadn't so much as a hangnail to cure. A healthy man whose health survives forty foodless days may be a wonder, but he is no cripple who has arisen and walked again, and only a few men of letters subscribed to Tanner's belief that fasting could be therapeutic. One of these, an editorialist for *Scientific American*, wrote, "Dr. Tanner may not have proved that everybody can fast forty days, but if he has only proved that man can fast longer than has generally been supposed, that we are all eating too much, and that for a family remedy, fasting affords a better, safer, and more economical cure than the taking of all sorts of patent medicine, to which many people are so much addicted, he has done really good work."

Dr. Gunn took the argument further by questioning the then-prevailing medical dogma that said the ill should be pushed to eat. "We have been disposed to urge the taking of food to 'sustain life,' even when the patient protested against it. . . . Now, it becomes a question whether food thus taken when the system did not demand it had any effect in sustaining life; and whether nature is not the best guide as to the necessity for food being taken into the stomach.... If we have an inflamed arm or eye we give it rest, and it is rapidly restored. The same treatment adopted for diseases of the digestive organs must necessarily be followed by equally good results."

It was the rare conventional doctor or scientist who conceded the merit of such ideas. Among them was a writer for the *St. Louis Courier of Medicine and Collateral Sciences*, who went so far as to say that starvation might be used to treat some illnesses and who postulated a curative mechanism that could hardly be stated better today. Fasting, he said, forces "the body to use up its own reserved stores and then feed upon itself, searching out every available molecule," after which the stripped-down body was "reclothed with a fresh and consequently unimpaired tissue material—a sort of new birth."

Those who wanted evidence of this new birth would have found the start of it in Tanner's blood. Dr. Peter Henri Van der Weyde, a chemist and contributor to *Scientific American*, drew Tanner's blood in Clarendon Hall just before he took his first bite of peach and was shocked by what he saw under his microscope. Tanner's red blood cells had shriveled in size by about a third and had assumed a desperately irregular shape. Healthy red blood cells are smooth disks with a gentle depression in the center—they look remarkably like undeployed condoms—but Tanner's were as scalloped and knobbed as a fruiting prickly pear. "This ragged appearance was so common in all of them," Van der Weyde wrote, "that there was scarcely a smooth corpuscle among them, except the white ones, which had very nearly the normal size and were smooth."

In a typical person, Van der Weyde found one corrupted red blood cell among every twenty or thirty, but in Tanner nine out of ten were in such bad shape they appeared on the verge of breaking up. Almost all of them were covered by what looked like fungoid spores, a type of growth Van der Weyde had seen before in victims of typhus and consumption. He hypothesized that as the red blood cells decayed, a fungus preyed on them in the same way mold preyed on a decaying sandwich.

Van der Weyde was in for a pleasanter surprise when he looked at Tanner's blood the day after he broke his fast. Many of the irregular, fungoid cells had disappeared and been replaced by "fresh and small corpuscles, looking very smooth and perfect, and bearing the stamp of youthfulness." Either the unhealthy cells had shed their spores and healed themselves, or, as Van der Weyde thought more likely, they had been destroyed and replaced by new cells. The next day, new red blood cells made up about half of Tanner's total count. A day later, almost all of them looked new.

This was a most astounding finding. Ordinarily, a red blood cell lives four months before being dismantled and replaced, but Tanner had apparently swapped out nearly his entire complement in just a few days after his fast. An inquisitive mind might have wondered about the therapeutic implications of the discovery. Would certain illnesses benefit from replacing every erythrocyte in the body? Had other cells been broken down and replaced too? If so, with what effect? Was Tanner, in short, right that fasting tore down the body only to rebuild it better than before?

Van der Weyde cautiously hailed Tanner's "contribution to science" and begged it "should be acknowledged," but it was not to be. Doctors and scientists ignored the view from his microscope, laypeople weren't primed to understand the meaning hidden there, and the journalists who might have enlightened them were already chasing the next story that would enrich their employers. The brief uptick in interest in therapeutic fasting ticked right back down again after some months.

All the same, a seed had been planted. It would take a generation for its shoots to become visible, and generations more before they bore lasting fruit, but Henry Tanner had just sired modern therapeutic fasting. Its speedy disappearance from the public eye would not have surprised a historian of fasting, had one existed. Across three millennia, small hints that fasting might be curative had emerged with some regularity and just as regularly faded away. But the idea never stayed dead. Fasting was too simple, too readily available to anyone to be ignored indefinitely. It is to this rich and instructive story that our chronicle now turns.

CHAPTER 2

"I FORGET I HAVE FOUR LIMBS"

Crack open nearly any book about fasting, and before you've even had the chance to dribble a few crumbs in the crease, you'll learn the practice has a long and proud pedigree. Pythagoras, Hippocrates, Plato, and Plutarch, to name just a few, are said to have fasted for health and spirit and to have urged pupils and patients to do the same. Such lineage is recounted to reassure the apprehensive novice, and when I first began dabbling in fasting fifteen years ago, that suited me just fine. It may be hard to recall now that fasting is fashionable, but in the first decade of this century anyone who forswore a meal, let alone five or six, soon found himself the recipient of dark counsel. People with pill organizers the size of pizza boxes, the type who wouldn't walk around the block without packing a Double Whopper, would tilt a head gravely and say if your abstinence didn't fell you by sundown, you'd surely keel over in a year from scurvy or a decade from Parkinson's.

To know the sages of antiquity fasted was welcome ballast against the doomsayers and also ennobled the effort. By fasting, you weren't just aligning yourself with grunting primitives of the Paleolithic who skipped meals when winter ran long and food ran short. No, you were following in the steps of fellows who knew a thing or two about a hypotenuse, thinkers of rare perception who somehow grasped that going without food could cure what ailed and maybe even guard against future illness. If, over the millennia, humanity had foolishly cast aside their simple remedy, your fasts made you one of its savvy rediscoverers. This delicious self-righteousness was almost universal in the literature of fasting, and I wallowed in every word of it.

So naturally when I finally examined the claims about ancient fasting, most of them proved so much offal and dross. Even writers smart enough to have known better got suckered. One brilliant and frankly dashing reporter named Hendricks must have given the fact checkers at *Harper's* some terribly authoritative-sounding sources for the frauds he perpetrated—that Pythagoras made his students fast forty days, that Plutarch said, "Instead of medicine, fast a day"—because they appeared in a story he wrote for that august journal in 2012. But as I was to discover, while the actual history was less fortifying to the fasting ego, it had the compensation of being much more human, which is as it should be for a practice older than the oldest human civilization.

*   *   *

Two things are certain about early humans and fasting: they did it, and we have almost no direct evidence they did. We know they did only because they must have and because our biology implies it. Before the development of agriculture around 10,000 BC, few places on Earth guaranteed nutritional abundance year after year, generation after generation, which meant that over the millions of years of hominid existence—including the three hundred thousand years of *Homo sapiens*—drought, flood, and infestation ensured that times of plenty alternated with times of want. Nearly every hominid who survived into adulthood must have gone hungry for days, maybe weeks, and even in our agricultural era only in the last century or so has most of humanity known nutritional abundance year in and year out.

Archaeological artifacts tell us nothing of fasting because they attest only to what people did, not what they didn't do. The knife among mastodon bones, the trace of bark between a pair of hominid teeth tell us what and how people ate but nothing of when they didn't. Scientists have hunted for markers of fasting in the isotopes of human bones but in the main have turned up little. At best, bones might reveal their owners starved to death or survived times when food was short or nutrition poor, but how short or poor and for how long we can only guess. A possible exception was discovered in 2020, when researchers studying the hominid remains at the Sima de los Huesos, the Pit of Bones, in Spain's Atapuerca Mountains, reported odd stop–start patterns in the development of many of the bones. The bones belonged to cave dwellers who lived 450,000 years ago and were part of a group from which both we and Neanderthals arose. The scientists believe the bone patterns show the Atapuercans survived the winters of their harshly glacial age by hibernating, much as bears do. The adults weren't overly harmed by this curious behavior, but the adolescents got diseases of nutritional deficiency like rickets. They did, however, survive. The extent of the hibernation is hotly debated—in fact, it's not even clear it can be called hibernation—but what does seem likely is that our near relatives endured substantial periods with little or no food by living off their fat stores, just as fasting humans do today.

But even if scientists had never found a bone that gave the slightest hint about prehistoric human fasting, we would know it occurred from the fact that virtually all species have the ability to do it, and for the same reason: when food ran out, those that couldn't withstand the deprivation died off before they could pass on their genes, while those that could fast survived until more food turned up, and transmitted their genetic code to the next generation, which transmitted it to the next. You, I, and everyone you know hails from a very long line of these evolutionary winners—one of the longest winning streaks on the planet—which explains why the mechanisms of fasting in humans are so similar to those in yeast, with whom we last shared an ancestor a billion years ago.

Scientists have a good idea how this must have played out in the everyday lives of our hominid progenitors. When nutrition ran short, some of them, thanks to an unlucky mutation or two in their genes, would have become desperately weak and slow of mind while others, profiting from a billion years of fasting-friendly evolution, would have been a little less enfeebled, their brains less poky, their muscles less spent. These perkier primates would have been better able to find the next berry bush and had a better shot at living long enough to beget descendants. Meanwhile with each hard season a few more of their sluggish cousins would have died off. This culling, again and again over the fifty thousand thousand years of primate existence, ensured that humans were a species who not only could fast but whose mental and physical faculties were actually a little sharpened by the absence of food, their eyesight and sense of smell honed, their reflexes a little snappier, their minds alert, all in service of spotting a sprig of carrot poking through the grass that they otherwise would have missed.

Fasting gave our forebears other advantages less immediately helpful but no less important for long-term survival, and none was more crucial than the body's ability to repair itself when fasting. We'll explore the astonishing biology of this healing mechanism in depth later, but for now it's enough to know that a very long time ago in our evolutionary odyssey, long before primates existed, one of our ancestors, undoubtedly a creature of a single cell, took the opportunity when deprived of food to do some internal tidying up, perhaps fixing a damaged protein or a breached membrane or a piece of wayward DNA. Most organisms make these kinds of repairs all the time but usually only at a modest rate because they're busy with the many other tasks of life, above all digesting nutrients and putting them to work. But when this unknown predecessor of ours was denied food, it got a reprieve from that work, and the repair it undertook made it more resilient and longer lived.

The organism, of course, didn't "figure out" how to repair itself. It just caught a lucky break from a chance mutation in one of its genes that resulted in an improved corpus. More than a billion years of such mutations have followed, and the repairs that cells can make when they fast have become bewilderingly complicated. Skip dinner tonight, and by the time you rise tomorrow, your body will have spent a few hours making the most intricate fixes to cellular components that were damaged during the day, and it will have recycled other parts too far gone to be fixed. Defects that might have turned into cancer or a stroke will have now, thanks to a little deprivation, been refashioned to yield a healthier cell. These processes occur in us every day even when our only fast is from the midnight snack to breakfast at dawn, but they're accelerated enormously when we extend the nightly fast, and fasting for multiple days supercharges them.

At some point prehistoric humans, with their impressive brains, would have noticed one or two improvements that ensued from fasting. When a fever got better after the food ran out, somewhere an early savant must have thought to take away food when the fever struck again. This, at least, is what Europeans occasionally found when they first made contact with aboriginal peoples. In the nineteenth century, for example, the Yámana of Patagonia were said to have four ways of treating illness: drinking cold water, applying heat, massaging, and fasting. An observant priest wrote, "They entertain high hopes for the curative effects of a complete fast of twenty-four hours when they suffer from indisposition, whatever its cause may be; everyone looks forward to that fast." Unfortunately, the practice of fasting therapeutically seems to have been extirpated from the region along with the Yámana. In North America, more than one colonizer wrote of indigenous tribes whose hunters fasted before setting off for the kill. The tribesmen said they fasted for purification or to appease a spirit, which they surely believed, but it was also true the fast persisted because it sharpened the senses and heightened awareness, thereby improving the hunt—gifts of the spirit made manifest. Of course, just because modern aboriginal peoples fasted for such reasons doesn't prove prehistoric humans did hundreds of thousands of years ago. A lot of evolutionary water has flowed over that land bridge. But the fasting of recent aborigines does show that unlettered peoples lacking in the scientific method were astute enough to identify how fasting improved body and mind. It's reasonable to suppose something similar probably occurred elsewhere across the ages.

Yet at the dawn of the historic era, rarely did anyone claim to fast for health, at least in the documents that have come down to us. When the first systems of writing emerged around three thousand years ago, fasting made early appearances, but always as a religious practice, not as a therapy (although not many of the ancients would have drawn the distinction between religion and health that we do today—to most of them, body and spirit were one). It's no surprise that fasting, so powerfully at odds with normal existence, took a religious color. Here was a condition, hunger, that you ordinarily strove to avoid but that could also, if sufficiently protracted, give you powers that must have seemed paranormal. Those who went without food for a very long time—weeks, say—or without food and water for even just a few days could become outright hallucinatory. To an archaic mind that conversed with gods in dreams and saw the supernatural daily in omens and portents, these hallucinations were portals to the spirit world, which is why in nearly every ancient religion, fasting played a part. Sometimes it was a minor part, more commonly it was profound, and here and there it was altogether terrifying.

*   *   *

Fasting first emerges in history during the thousand-year run of the Vedic religion in India that began around 1500 BC. Every month the Vedics observed a handful of *upavasathas*, holy days on which everyone stopped working and abstained from two of nature's most urgent and delightful preoccupations—eating and mating. Liberated from these cares, Vedics made offerings to the gods and kept a vigil at the sacred hearth as a show of gratitude to the deities who watched over them.

When Hinduism evolved from Vedism in the middle of the first millennium BC, it incorporated the upavasathas and added more fasting holy days—a lot more, for early Hindus were smitten with fasting. The Mahabharata, the lusty, blood-soaked Sanskrit epic that serves as one of Hinduism's bedrock texts, declares, "It was by fasts that the deities have succeeded in becoming denizens of Heaven. It is by fasts that the Rishis"—enlightened beings—"have attained to high success." Fasting was so commendable in the Mahabharata that just telling someone how to fast earned the teller a holy reward. "The man who teaches another the merits of fasts has never to suffer any kind of misery," one passage holds, while another says that merely letting someone else tell *you* about fasting could emancipate your soul: "The man who daily reads these ordinances [about fasting] or hears them read becomes freed from sins of every kind." You're welcome.

Ancient Hindus thought so highly of fasting because it eased an existential burden shouldered by every being. In Hindu cosmology, life was

dominated by suffering, the root of which was attachment, which led people to cling to things that would inevitably be snatched away—a harvest,
a child, the admiration of one's neighbors. To avoid suffering, a believer
needed to be attached to nothing, to have literally nothing to lose, which
required the eradication of desire. If you could pull that off, you could find
a state of consummate peace known as nirvana. Humans, however, were
weak and nearly always failed to reach nirvana, hence were doomed to die
unfulfilled and be reborn, whereupon they suffered and died again.

Most ancient Hindus did not expect, nor were expected, to eradicate
all desire from their lives. Their lot was not to reach nirvana in this incarnation but to do a little better and be born next time into a more worthy
caste. They worked their way to enlightenment on the installment plan.
In the here and now, the typical Hindu settled for eliminating small luxuries or needs—a task for which fasting was ready-made because any Hindu
could do it at any time. Each meal willingly denied was a mark on the right
side of the karmic ledger.

Nearly all ancient Hindus fasted. At least, that's the impression left
by Hindu calendars, some of which eventually contained a whopping 140
days of fasting a year. Many Hindus fasted yet more days as the need for
penance or purification arose. Originally both men and women fasted, but
the men who developed Hindu theology came to think women either better suited to it or more in need of it, and fasting evolved into the province
of women. Evidently the fragile male body required a more constant association with food. Fortunately for women, over the centuries fasting came
to mean not complete abstinence but only skipping a meal or avoiding a
single defiling food, like eggs or meat.

While fasting practices were probably flexible among laypeople, some
Hindu monks embraced it with a feverish asceticism. Many monks were
voluntary mendicants who wandered from town to town with almost no
possessions or obligations, not even ties to family. The idea was that if you
could give up food, sleep, shelter, clothing, and community, you would be
all the more immunized against desire, and even simple indulgences—a
bed, a bath, a dessert, a mother's embrace—would hold no temptation. It's

among these extreme ascetics that we read for the first time of prolonged fasting, a kind of athletic training for the soul.

With fasting so integral a part of early Hinduism, it was inevitable that the two great religions that grew out of it, Buddhism and Jainism, would have to wrestle with how to incorporate it. The first faster of Buddhism was its founder, the pampered young prince Siddhartha Gautama, who in or around the fifth century BC lit out from his family's palace in the Nepalese–Indian borderlands in search of enlightenment. Gautama, so the story goes, had so little idea where to look for insight that he threw himself into nearly every spiritual practice of the day: mendicancy, meditation, controlled breathing, yogic postures. For years he tried such feats as wearing rough hemp that savagely abraded his skin, going long spells clothed in not a stitch, sleeping out of doors in the fiercest weather when not sleeping indoors on a bed of spikes, drinking his own urine, even eating his own excrement. But these pursuits brought him no closer to enlightenment, and he turned at last to starvation. For long months he lived on a single kola fruit a day (the same from which Coca-Cola was first derived), while at other times his daily board was but a grain of rice. The scriptures say his limbs became like vines, his spine like corded beads, his ribs like the rafters of a tumbledown barn, his buttocks like a camel's hoof. So deeply did his eyes sink into their sockets that their feeble gleam was no more than that of a flicker on the water at the bottom of a well. Today when Westerners think of the Buddha, it is usually of the amiably doughy fellow of a million cross-legged figurines, but there's a lesser-known statuary of starving Buddhas that depicts him in all his emaciated glory, every rib and artery, every tendon and sinew urgently visible, his face the very embodiment of pained endurance. The best of them are like woodcuts cast in stone and to my taste are far more human and moving than any number of serene Gautamas.

Extreme fasting, however, brought Gautama no nearer nirvana, only nearer death. "Surely there must be a better way to achieve enlightenment!" he is said to have cried, and then suddenly a memory came to him. He saw himself a child sitting in the shade of a rose-apple tree on a radiant day, a moment when ecstasy had descended on him every bit as effortlessly and unbidden as the memory came to him now. The adult Gautama felt the supple tranquility of that long-ago moment, the almost supernatural coolness of the shade tree despite the heat of the day, and he realized such joy was not harmful, no matter what the desire-killing sages of the day taught. He understood this memory to be a foretaste of nirvana, which would not be found in trying to eradicate natural human pleasures, and he abandoned his fasting that instant.

I have sometimes wondered whether it was important to Gautama's hagiographers that although fasting was not sufficient for enlightenment, the insight they believed got him there nonetheless arose while he fasted—not while he meditated or mastered his breathing or did yoga or carried out any of his other asceticisms. Nor did his insight come to him *after* he broke his fast, as inspiration came to Proust with his madeleine. The revelation occurred during his abstinence. Did his followers sense, as fasters past and present have, that going without food can not only still the mind but generate thoughts more clear and generous than thoughts on a fed belly?

Whatever the case, after his realization Gautama sat under a fig tree with the resolution not to move until he found nirvana, which he is said to have achieved that very night. The path to it he called, with admirable directness, the Middle Way, which consisted of doing nothing too self-indulgent nor too self-mortifying—the Goldilocks principle of just-right moderation that remains one of Buddhism's hallmarks. The Buddha, as Gautama was called after his enlightenment (*Buddha* means "Awakened One"), gave his followers plenty of leeway to decide how much of any action to do, and this was especially true of fasting, which he left in a complicated state. Formally, he discouraged prolonged fasts, but he also said, or at least certain disciples said he did, "While the body is wasting, the mind gets more tranquil, meditation gets more steadfast, and understanding deeper." And the first thing he did on finding Nirvana was to fast for either four or seven weeks (depending on which text you credit), during which time he meditated almost continuously and proved his enlightenment to doubting gods by performing some rather showy, un-Buddha-like miracles, like conjuring a golden skybridge on which he walked in unfed contemplation for a week.

With such precedent, his followers could not ignore fasting, and after an apparently lively debate, they decided to treat it as a helpful but by no means essential adjunct to self-discipline and meditation. Some scholars think Buddhists chose this relaxed path in order to distance themselves from Jainism, which traveled a more austere road. In any case, Buddhist monks simply reduced their meals to either one or two a day, and lay Buddhists fasted rarely, if at all. It was as compassionate a take on fasting as existed in ancient religion.

* * *

Jainism, Hinduism's lesser-known issue, made fasting its very own iron maiden. To an ancient Jain, even the most zealous of Hindu ascetics must have seemed dilettantes. In Jainism the body was not a companionable host for the soul, nor even its troublesome but useful shell, but its literal prison. Jains believed all living organisms, plant and animal, were composed of particles of karma, which they conceived of as tiny atom-like bits that were the physical manifestation of good and bad deeds from past lives. Because the mass of human acts was far more bad than good, the soul was coated in a weighty damnation that kept it from floating up to its heavenly reward. If that wasn't alarming enough, mere existence presented Jains with a dreadful predicament: all organisms, even plants, had souls, and yet to live, one had to kill and eat them. Merely to walk on grass was to inflict violence. To an ancient Jain, life was one long horror of meting out suffering and slaughter punctuated by the recurring terror of having violence and pain inflicted on oneself. The best that most Jains could hope for in this existence was to minimize the new karma they accumulated and through good deeds to burn off as much old karma as they could.

Self-denial allowed them to do both. Jains went in for all of the asceticisms the Buddha tried, only they didn't abandon them as he did. They even added a few of their own. One discipline, known as *kesa-loca*, required the ascetic Jain to slowly, one might say masochistically, pull five handfuls of hair from the scalp, a practice still used today to initiate nuns and monks into certain Jain orders. Sometimes every last hair is pulled from the nov-ice's head. In the Jain sect of Svetambara, adherents wore cloths over their mouths and noses more or less their entire lives to keep from inhaling an insect. (Of all the world's peoples, the mask-wearing Svetambaras of today may have been the least inconvenienced by the great coronavirus pandemic of recent years.)

Jains were passionate fasters. In Jain lore, the saint Rishabhanatha went an entire year without food, although, if I may be permitted an imper-tinence, since he lived several million years, his feat, scaled to a human life, amounted to skipping midday snack. Jains of more normal constitution emulated Rishabhanatha's feat by fasting every other day for a year. Eating nothing from sunset until sunrise thirty-six hours later, they took one or two meals before sundown, when the cycle started again. *Varshitap*, as the practice is known, is still observed, and sometimes hundreds of Jains make a simultaneous show of it, the achievement capped by a feast for thou-sands, some would say ironically. For less karmically ambitious Jains, scrip-tures prescribed fasts of a day, a few days, a week, or a month, and as in Hinduism it was women on whom the duty eventually fell.

But the type of fasting with which Jains truly distinguished themselves was *Sallekhana*—starvation unto death. Suicidal fasting was and remains a horror to non-Jains, but in Jain philosophy it makes perfect sense. In fact, one might ask why, if life is nothing but the giving and receiving of pain, Jains don't just end it all by ceasing to live immediately. One answer is the practical obstacle Jim Jones ran up against: it is difficult to continue the faith when all the faithful have drunk the Flavor Aid. A more philosophi-cal answer is that the wish to end one's own suffering is itself a selfish desire, so to indulge it would saddle the suicide with the worst kind of karma and ensure a truly ghastly reincarnation. Sallekhana was apparently used spar-ingly, permitted only to those who had achieved enlightenment or gotten as close to it as they could in this life but were in some way kept from get-ting closer. Such people were supposed to have attained, or nearly attained, right knowledge, right belief, and right conduct and to have freed them-selves of every desire, to have fulfilled every obligation, and to have done all the good they could.

The virtues of Sallekhana were preached by the principal founder of the religion, a rough contemporary of the Buddha known variously as Mahavira or Vardhamana. Mahavira's life followed the same saintly Indian trope as the Buddha's: the royal who renounced worldliness for asceticism and found enlightenment while meditating under a tree. Mahavira didn't practice Sallekhana himself—his person was apparently more valuable in its incorporated form—but he urged the ritual on the worthiest of his disciples, many of whom obligingly starved themselves to death. How many less celebrated Jains did likewise over the centuries is impossible to say, but they were numerous enough that the practice became highly regulated to ensure purity of motive. Eventually the vow of Sallekhana was extended to the terminally ill on the notion they had burned off all the karma they could in this life and would gain nothing by needlessly suffering. Today somewhere between a few dozen and a few hundred Jains take the vow annually. Observers say that while their deaths are not entirely painless, they are more free of pain than not. It is a peaceful route that today's euthanasiasts, in the absence of a legal right to give pills, might consider. The American writer Sue Hubbell, no Jain, chose this way out in 2018 when dementia began to steal her faculties. She ate a last grapefruit and died thirty-four days later.

Both Hinduism and Buddhism felt the pull of Sallekhana, with tiny sects adopting their own versions. A few Buddhist temples today still display the startlingly lifelike remains of self-starved monks, robed, seated in lotus position, and fitted with sunglasses to cover their desiccated eye sockets. They're playfully eerie. But the practice never spread in Hinduism or Buddhism, whose moderation is a big part of why today there are more than a billion Hindus and half a billion Buddhists while the extreme self-denial of Jainism has attracted just six million followers.

Fasting, in sum, was an extraordinarily malleable tool that the three enduring Indian religions of antiquity put to work for their own particular ends: as a modestly rigorous purifier in Hinduism, a gentle aid for calming the mind and training the body in Buddhism, an astringent purgative in Jainism. What's missing in each is fasting for physical health. Ancient Indian texts contain few suggestions that fasting does a body good, and not until nearly modern times would fasting find a small space within Ayurveda, the Indian medical practice that dates back at least to the Mahabharata. Given the abundance of religious fasting on the subcontinent, this oversight is hard to explain, but it was not an omission limited to India. Other Eastern peoples thought even less of fasting, for either body or soul.

* * *

It's no coincidence that the major religions of today all originated in a single era, the period historians call the Axial Age, which ran from roughly 800 to 200 BC. The Axial Age was a time of great social, political, and intellectual upheaval across an enormous arc of the eastern hemisphere stretching from the Mediterranean to China. The unrest led to great suffering that was not addressed by the existing ways of thinking or the gods that embodied them, and the most important replies to this failure were the three Indian religions, Confucianism and Taoism in China, Zoroastrianism in Iran, Judaism in the Levant (with its later elaborations Christianity and Islam), and the great early philosophic schools, most notably in ancient Greece. Fasting, as I've said, had a role in nearly all of these.

In ancient China, its role was small, but Chinese sages nonetheless occasionally wrote of fasting with an elegance unsurpassed. The Taoist text *Zhuangzi*, first committed to print around the fourth century BC, contains a beautiful tale of a woodworker named Qing who carved a wooden bell-stand so exquisite, so perfect in every detail, that everyone who saw it said it looked as if it had been made by the gods. When Qing was asked how he, a mere man, had created an object so divinely beautiful, he replied, "When I am going to make a bell-stand, I never let it wear out my vital energy. I always fast in order to still my mind. When I have fasted three days, I no longer have any thought of congratulations or rewards, of titles or stipends. When I have fasted five days, I no longer have any thought of praise or blame, of skill or clumsiness. And when I have fasted seven days, I am so still that I forget I have four limbs and a form and body. By that time the ruler and his court no longer exist for me. My skill is concentrated, and all outside distractions fade away. After that I go into the mountain forest and examine the Heavenly nature of the trees. If I find one of superlative form and I can see a bell-stand there, I put my hand to the job of carving. If not, I let it go. This way I am simply matching up 'Heaven' with 'Heaven.'"

We cannot say at this remove whether fasting for Qing meant giving up all food or only a sizable share of it, but his motive in fasting makes quite the contrast to the fasting for purification of Hinduism or for penance of Jainism. The philosophy of Qing assumes perfection lies within us, we need only access it, and fasting can help us do so—a view the Buddha would have understood. But Qing's tale may be anomalous in Taoism, for we have few surviving ancient Taoist scriptures that propose fasting as a skill to cultivate for so practical an end. Early Taoists seem to have used fasting chiefly to purify the spirit and perhaps thereby to endow the body with vaguely useful powers, but even this kind of fasting wasn't universally celebrated. In fact, many Taoist texts trivialize fasts of the body as inferior to fasts of the mind, by which are meant meditative emptyings of the psyche. This attitude shifted somewhat in later Taoism, when a text called *Zhonghuang jing*, perhaps written in the early centuries AD, laid out a rigorous form of bodily fasting to nourish one's *qi*, the universal life force. But this kind of ascetic fasting didn't become central to Taoism either.

Confucianism gave fasting even shorter shrift. Confucius himself appears to have fasted only as a very occasional discipline, like when offering a sacrifice to the gods. He didn't push fasting on his followers, who in the main don't seem to have done it much. Nor did ancient Chinese medicine give fasting any more consideration than Ayurveda did in India, and today the practice has only a minor role in traditional Chinese medicine.

On the other side of India, in Persia, the man known as Zoroaster or Zarathustra went Confucius one better by rejecting fasting entirely. Like the Buddha, Zoroaster at first flirted with fasting and other asceticisms but later decided a full life of the body—one might say a *deliciously* full life of the body—rather than just a pleasant Buddhist restraint, was needed to fortify the soul against evil. Zoroaster was rare among the great thinkers of the Axial Age in taking wives and siring children—three of the one, six of the other—and the sumptuous living he preached included eating well. In his view (or perhaps his followers'), fasting left the body too weak to cultivate fields, to produce vigorous heirs, or to demonstrate a sturdy piety, and was therefore a sin. The same went for other asceticisms. It is a curiosity of history that this mild, slightly hedonistic faith lost out to more severe religions, especially Islam. Today Zoroaster's flock numbers fewer than two hundred thousand, just one ten-thousandth the fold that Muhammad has posthumously gathered round him. A dissertation is waiting to be written on what this says about humanity's yearning for discipline over indulgence.

This tug between the poles of austerity and license, a conflict that gave little attention to fasting for health, would prove to be the great theme of the history of fasting. In the West, as we'll see next, its reverberations would be felt right up to Henry Tanner's day.

CHAPTER 3
CHRIST'S ATHLETES

When, near the start of the first millennium, the Roman emperor Augustus wished to boast of his stamina in fasting, he wrote to his adopted son, "Not even a Jew, my dear Tiberius, fasts so scrupulously on his sabbaths as I have today; for it was not until after the first hour of the night that I ate two mouthfuls of bread in the bath." One might gather from this that Jews were the most devoted of fasters, yet a couple of centuries after Augustus, a certain Rabbi Sheshet in Jewish Babylonia (in what is now Iraq) sneered at scholars who let fasting interfere with their study of the Torah. "Let the meal of a student who fasts be given to the dogs," he groused. As it happens, both glimpses of Jewish fasting are accurate. The chosen people's attitude toward fasting was, like so much else in their religion, complicated.

The Hebrew Bible, assembled between the eighth and second centuries BC, mentions nearly four dozen fasts, and the motives for them, especially in the early going, were as varied as you like. King David fasted in mourning after his ally Abner found the wrong end of a blade. Saul ordered his army to fast before giving the Philistines a good thrashing. Joel called his people to fast and cry unto the Lord for mercy after locusts devoured the crops in the fields and the fruits in the trees. And the barren Hannah fasted after her husband's other wife, fertile as a desert cottontail, taunted her with her fecundity. Hannah laughed last, with the birth of a child. If there was a unifying theme, it was that fasting was less an act of devotion or routine than an ad hoc response to crisis.

But after the fall of the First Temple in 586 BC, fasting became more ritualized, and Jews fasted more often to let God know how sorry they were for infracting one or another of his many divine ordinances. This was fasting as prophylactic penitence, a way of saying, "As you can see, Lord, we're doing pretty well at hurting ourselves—no need for a plague upon our houses." These penitential fasts became institutionalized in the annual Day of Atonement, Yom Kippur, when from sundown to sundown Jews went without food, drink, and (in the manner of the ancient Vedics on their fast days) coupling.

Fasts of this period tended toward the showy, with much wailing and smearing of ashes and rending of garments because Yahweh was both an inattentive deity who needed an extravagance to catch his eye and an insecure one who when sinned against needed to be appeased with self-abasement even more than atonement. As in Hinduism and Jainism, fasting in Judaism exhibited an expansionist creep, and with each century the Jewish calendar sprouted more fasting days. By the start of the Christian era many Jews were also fasting every Monday and Thursday, possibly because on those days Moses was said to have ascended and descended Mount Sinai. Some Jews observed the biweekly fasts as strictly as the fast of Yom Kippur, with neither food nor drink from sundown to sundown. Others simply ate fewer or lighter meals. There must have been quite a few of the stricter fasters because several references to them, like that of Augustus, survive.

As a rule, Jews didn't remark whether their health improved while fasting. More often they kvetched about the inverse, as when Saul's son, in 1 Samuel, all but called his father a fool for forcing his army to fast before battle or when Judas's scrappy guerrilla forces, in the apocryphal 1 Maccabees, fretted that their pre-battle fast had weakened them before Seron's legions. God lifted both of those hungry militias to victory, but neither text makes fasting before warfare seem shrewd with anything less than a celestial being backing you up.

Perhaps because of these concerns for health, Jews only rarely took fasting to the extremes of early Hinduism. The few great fasts of the Jewish Bible, like the forty-day deprivations of Elijah and Moses, had divine support and were clearly intended, and certainly taken, as acts to be venerated rather than emulated. The exceptions to this moderation are invariably delightful. In the *Testaments of the Twelve Patriarchs,* compiled around the second century AD, Reuben fasts seven long years to atone for a lusty tumble with his father's concubine, Joseph fasts seven years to atone for the mere thought of a tumble with Potiphar's wife, and Simeon fasts two years to conquer envy. The disparate penalties say something about the hierarchy of sin in old Israel. In the main, though, early Jewish thinkers cautioned against taking fasting to such lunatic extremes—and sometimes against fasting at all, as Rabbi Sheshet preferred. That sort of nuttiness, they increasingly said, should be left to the Christians.

* * *

Christians didn't start out nutty about fasting. In fact, the first Christians fasted less ardently than their Jewish cousins, in keeping with Jesus's decidedly subdued view of the practice. Like other Jews, Jesus must have fasted regularly, but the only glimpse the New Testament gives of it was his forty foodless days in the wilderness during the temptation. As a literary device, the fast marked him both as heir to those forty-day fasters of old, Moses and Elijah, and as a superior specimen because he not only fasted without his heavenly father's assistance but did so while swatting away Satan's seductions.

We might expect early Christians to have imitated Jesus's fast in some lesser way, but just as Jews regarded the fasts of Moses and Elijah as more symbolic than imitational, the earliest Christians didn't think Jesus's heroic standards applied to them. (Lent came centuries later.) Jesus himself never touted his fast, and in the Sermon on the Mount he rejected the garish fasting of the day. Only hypocrites, he said, "disfigure their faces that they may appear to men to be fasting," whereas the pious fasted quietly, seen only by a watchful father above who appreciated their understated humility.

None of that is to say Jesus opposed fasting. His words make clear he accepted it as a given; he just wasn't a booster. When the followers of John the Baptist grumbled that Jesus didn't force his disciples to fast, he retorted,

"Can you make the friends of the bridegroom fast while the bridegroom is with them? But the days will come when the bridegroom will be taken away from them; then they will fast in those days."

From those two sentences a great deal of trouble would arise over the next fifteen hundred years.

*　*　*

The trouble wouldn't have had legs to stand on without the Greeks, who have a lot to answer for. This isn't at first apparent because the Archaic Greeks fasted infrequently. Priests sometimes fasted in preparation for carrying out rites, and laypeople might fast when consulting an oracle or being initiated into the cult of a deity, but most people probably fasted on only two occasions. One was mourning. Mourning fasts were recorded as far back as the *Iliad*, which was committed to writing around the eighth century BC. After Achilles's understudy Patroclus is killed, Achilles fasts three days not only to punish himself but to show his fellow Greeks the depth of his pain and to demonstrate to his dead friend how much he loves him. After Achilles avenges Patroclus by impaling Hector, it falls on Hector's father Priam to fast, which he does for twelve days, a length meant to impress but not overawe us. Apparently the Archaic Greeks were accustomed to long displays of grief.

The other widespread occasion for fasting was an autumn fertility festival called the Thesmophoria, which simultaneously celebrated the harvest and commemorated the goddess Demeter's painful loss each year of her daughter Persephone to Hades, lord of the underworld. Demeter's own mourning fast, of course, we know as fall and winter. During the Thesmophoria, women who were married and free of scandal sat on cushions of willow (the symbol of fertility and also, oddly enough, chastity) and fasted the day long. Greek men, evidently as brittle as Indian men, had no equivalent fast.

A robust fiction now entering its third millennium holds that fasting for health entered Western thought under the able stewardship of the Greek philosopher Pythagoras, who lived in the sixth century BC.

According to the legend, young Pythagoras traveled to Egypt for his studies and was made to fast forty days before matriculating. He complied, perhaps grumpily given the lack of fasting in his homeland, and was so transformed he later required fasts of all his students.

Sadly, not a word of it is true. The yarn was spun a few centuries after Pythagoras's death by followers of his mystical credo who wanted to bolster their man's reputation—the same lot who credited him with the mathematical theorem that bears his name but with which he had nothing to do. (The chap wasn't even a mathematician, just a numerologist.) According to another invention by his disciples, in his old age, weary of life, Pythagoras lay down and starved himself to death over forty days. One clue these stories are bogus is the forty days, a length to which hagiographers often turned to associate their champion with the greatness of Moses and Elijah, just as the hagiographers of Jesus did.

In fact, fasting for health first appears in the West in writings associated, appropriately enough, with Hippocrates, the father of Western medicine. Hippocrates is one of the most elusive characters of the ancient world. About all we can say of him for sure is he was born on the island of Kos around 460 BC, became a much-admired doctor and teacher, wrote either a little or a lot, and died about 375 BC. Sixty-odd texts known as the Hippocratic Corpus bear his name, but we don't know which of them he wrote, and it's possible he composed not a single one. Most scholars believe the bulk of the Corpus was written by his students and family, but whoever wrote it touched off the most stupendous revolution. Before the Corpus, disease was attributed to magical or supernatural sources—to an angry god, a mischievous spirit, a magic-wielding neighbor—but the authors of the Corpus said sickness was the result of natural phenomena that could be studied, sometimes understood, and often treated. This radical declaration set humanity on the 2,400-year voyage of medical discovery we're still on. Our debt is immense.

On the other hand, the Hippocratics got nearly everything wrong about how the body worked, which was unsurprising since dissection was taboo. Unable to root around among the organs, they invented theories that were spectacularly off target and that jockeyed and jostled uncomfortably against one another when they weren't in flat contradiction. After five disputatious centuries, one of those theories emerged supreme: humoralism, which held that health was achieved by balancing the body's vital humors or liquids, the most important of which were blood, phlegm, black bile, and yellow bile. When a humor was out of balance—too much phlegm brought on by a winter's storm, too much yellow bile after a raging argument—the Hippocratics turned to one of several therapies, the most common of which were dietary change, emetics (which caused vomiting), purgatives (which provoked diarrhea), and bloodletting. Rest, exercise, bathing, and other adjuncts rounded out the doctor's therapeutic stock.

There was comically little agreement on when to reach for one treatment over another. One author in the Corpus might treat a headache with an emetic and bedrest, while another prescribed bleeding and exercise, while a third wanted a purgative and a new diet. The dietary advice was particularly imaginative. Roosters, symbolically virile, were recommended to elevate the warm and dry humors, but so was the limp herb dill. A woman seeking to get pregnant—clearly a dry-humor case—needed moist fare, including, in one prescription, "boiled puppies and octopuses in sweet boiled wine."

It is the conceit of many who write about fasting today that ancient Greek doctors used fasting frequently and with a degree of skill, but in fact fasting wasn't much mentioned by the Hippocratics, and when it was, it was tethered to the same humoral twaddle as the rest of the Corpus and was discussed with irritating imprecision. One of the authors of the Hippocratic text *Aphorisms* declared, "Spasms are cured either by overeating or by fasting. The same is true of hiccups." More than one ancient reader, spasming or hiccupping, must have muttered, "Well, thanks, but *which* should I do—overeat or fast?" Another aphorism advised that when deciding whether to starve or stuff a patient, "the place and season, the age of the patient, and the nature of the disease must all be considered," but which places, seasons, ages, and natures were more conducive to fasting and which to stuffing were never specified. The *Aphorisms* were so rife with this kind of thing, it begs the question why its title was drafted into English to mean "a concise statement of scientific principle."

This isn't to say the Corpus was useless. One of the more thoughtful takes on fasting appears in *On Regimen in Acute Diseases*, whose author worried that when it came to fasting and feeding (and a great deal else), doctors didn't know what they were doing. To his mind, they often wrecked the health of gluttons by making them fast too abruptly, and they hurt moderate eaters by abruptly overfeeding them. "One must not without good reason order severe fasting," the author judiciously suggested, but on the other hand a doctor mustn't "give food when a disease is at its height and is accompanied by inflammation." The author worried the second part of this counsel—to continue fasting a patient through the worst throes of illness—was too counterintuitive for doctors to grasp. Instead, "they prescribe the change from fasting to gruel at exactly the stage when it is beneficial to reduce the diet even to a complete fast—that is, when the disease is approaching a paroxysm." Some doctors, it seems, were fasting patients until their illness reached a crisis, at which point they lost their nerve and refed them. Had they continued the fast, *Regimen*'s author was saying, they could have subdued the illness. His advice is strikingly similar to that of modern fasting doctors, who hold that for certain disorders (and under proper supervision) fasting *through* a crisis can often help the body heal itself.

Regimen's author, one of the most sagacious in all antiquity where fasting was concerned, was also on the right track when he cautioned, "Taking too much food after a long fast does much more harm to the belly than fasting from a hearty diet. The effect is similar to that of overexertion after a long rest." He also made what is probably history's first argument for intermittent, or periodic, fasting: "Just as the body should be given complete rest and idleness, and slackness should follow a long period of strenuous effort, so should the belly be given a rest from full feeding, as otherwise it will cause pain and distress throughout the body."

This was promising stuff, the foundation on which a medicine of fasting could have been built, but these passages were only a small part of *Regimen*, and there's no sign they were widely followed even among Hippocratics, let alone Greek doctors of other schools. Only occasionally over the next few centuries would a Hellenic doctor make a strong appeal for fasting. One of these was Erasistratus, sometimes hailed the father of physiology. In the third century BC, he tantalizingly wrote, "The patient suffering from epilepsy should maintain a regimen of constant physical labor and either fasting or minimal food." But two millennia would pass before his sound advice to fast epileptics was heeded.

Most Greek doctors probably stood with the writer of *Aphorisms* who held that "fasting, if taken to extremes, is treacherous," or with the Hippocratic author of *On Ancient Medicine*, a sky-is-falling type who warned that skipping even a single meal could cause "dire consequences, symptoms of prostrating weakness, trembling, faintness, hollowness of the eyes, the urine becoming paler and hotter, the mouth bitter, the bowels seeming to hang, followed by dizziness, depression, and listlessness ... accompanied by wild and troubled dreams." Heaven only knows what he thought of fasting a whole day.

Many of today's fasting revivalists ignore this rich struggle among early Greek doctors to make sense of fasting and instead summon a notional Hippocrates whom they quote as having written, "To eat when you are sick is to feed your sickness" and "Let food be thy medicine and medicine be thy food." No Hippocratic author ever penned those phrases, although a character in a German novel of 1740, written by a great-uncle of Goethe, claimed Hippocrates composed the first. On such scrawny nags does rumor ride.

*   *   *

Over the centuries, first in Greece, later in Rome, doctors erected atop the wispy foundations of humoralism an ever more complex and fanciful framework of diagnosis and treatment. By the early years of the Roman Empire, these medical fantasies provoked a backlash, one strand of which was a school known as Methodism, so called because it reduced the practice of medicine to a few simple methods. Methodist doctors glee-fully boasted that their techniques could be learned in just six months by virtually anyone—a sailor, a mason, a slave, even (here one imagines horrified shudders) a woman. Hippocratic doctors who had spent years in study were appalled in much the way orthodox doctors today are at chiropractors.

Most of the Methodists' methodology was grounded in ideas no more valid than those they rebelled against, but one of their most meritorious treatments was the *diatritus*, a fast of two to four days at the start of a fever or other acute illness, repeated if the illness persisted. Fasting must have been in the air because similar treatments appear elsewhere, for example in the encyclopedia of the brilliant Aulus Cornelius Celsus of the first century AD. Among much else that was light years ahead of his day, Celsus described a primitive plastic surgery using skin grafts and called for cleaning wounds with liquids that later proved antiseptic. (Then again, he also suggested rubbing the body with a bruised plantain to ward off elephantiasis, the mosquito-borne swelling disease.) "The beginnings of diseases call for fasting and thirst," Celsus wrote. "After that . . . moderation is required so that nothing but what is proper be taken, and not too much of that; for it is not fit after fasting to enter immediately upon a full diet." Excepting the bit about thirst, we now know the first sentence is true for some illnesses, and the second is virtually always true. Unfortunately, his encyclopedia tells us little of how he came to his conclusion, how many doctors agreed with him, and which illnesses his fasting prevailed against.

As Methodism spread throughout the empire, the diatritus went with it, but we know only the barest details because few Methodist precepts survive on the page and those that do are mostly in the works of their detractors. The most spiteful of these critics was the second-century polymath and physician Aelius Galenus, a towering figure in his own time who remains the most influential doctor ever to check a pulse.

*   *   *

Galen, as he is known to us, was one of history's outstanding characters, a man of erudition and insight who pioneered several aspects of physiology and was as keen an observer of the human body as anyone of his era. He wrote astutely of the difference between motor and sensory nerves, the link between mental disturbances and the physical state, and the surgical technique for removing a cataract. Breathtakingly prolific, he and the legion of scribes he employed to capture his genius left nearly two hundred surviving treatises totaling four million words. Hundreds more of his works perished. We have a greater intimacy with Galen's mind than that of almost any other person in antiquity.

But if we're being honest, that's a decidedly mixed blessing. Prolix beyond belief, maddeningly repetitious, Galen was also one of the world's preeminent egotists, a consummate braggart who hurled scorn at anyone who didn't share his ideas or his lofty opinion of himself. He would have made a fine surgeon general for Donald Trump.

Born in 129 in what is now western Turkey, he worked his way up from patching gladiators to serving as court physician to Emperor Marcus Aurelius, as he reminded his readers whenever the mood struck, which was often. His life's great work was synthesizing into a coherent whole the medical knowledge amassed in the half millennium since Hippocrates, and he largely succeeded at this enormous task. But in his almost worshipful reverence for Hippocrates, he made the fatal flaw of putting humoralism at the center of medicine, where it would regrettably remain for most of the next two millennia. The emetics, purgatives, bloodletting, and rude dietetics that doctors had inflicted on patients for centuries would, thanks to Galen, be inflicted on millions more. He spared no ink savaging rival theories, and Methodism, with its faddish, simplistic fasting prescribed without regard to bile or moisture or any of a hundred other considerations, caught the full force of his attacks. The Methodists, he said, were idiot cobblers who tried to make the same shoe fit every foot.

In one particularly withering account, Galen told of a sick young man who fasted fruitlessly under Methodist doctors until he, Galen, took over the case. The Methodists carped from the bedside that by feeding the patient, Galen was only dragging out his illness. When, as Galen wrote, "I could no longer bear the jabbering of doctors," he decided to prove the stupidity of the diatritus by returning his patient to his fast. The young man fell obligingly into a coma, and when the Methodists understood the depth of their failure, they "became paler and colder than the patient himself, and were considering a means of escape" until

Galen barred the door and harangued them for their asininity. He then gave a draft of barley broth to the comatose man, who again obliged by reviving instantly.

It was a potent tale, parts of which may even have been true, but what's impressive is that neither this attack nor Galen's other broadsides stopped people from using the diatritus, notwithstanding Galen was the most listened-to doctor of his day. The persistence of the fasting therapy for a couple hundred years beyond his death suggests it filled a deep need for a simple medicine and quite probably cured or eased many ailments. Eventually, though, Galenism's sovereignty among medical theories crowded out all comers, including the Methodist diatritus. In a time of intellectual darkness, with dissection banned by both Roman law and Church dicta, people clung to authority where they found it, and Galen's sweeping, forceful writings were as authoritative as they came. For the next fifty generations in Europe and much of the Near East, Galenism *was* medicine, and the consequences for fasting were disastrous. Although not entirely banished from the condensed Galenic canon that practitioners came to rely on, it was relegated to the bit part it had played in the Hippocratic Corpus—deployed only occasionally to calm an overactive humor or draw out a flagging one as the doctor's imagination dictated.

It's not hard to imagine a different trajectory for medicine. Had Galen not been so slavishly venerated, doctors might have adopted a Methodist-like response to acute illness in which patients fasted at least the first few days of their infirmity. No doubt some would have died from indiscriminate application, but in most cases fasting would have done no harm, and quite often it would have helped. In time doctors might have learned which disorders improved with fasting and which not, and in any event the therapy would have been far more humane than the lancets, leeches, nauseants, and diarrheics imposed on the multitudes.

But Galenism's staying power was so unfaltering that as late as 1890 Mark Twain could publish an essay, the delightful "A Majestic Literary Theory," about how little medicine had changed from antiquity to his youth. "Galen could have come into my sick-room at any time during my first seven years," he wrote, "and he could have . . . stood my doctor's watch without asking a question. He would have smelt around among the wilderness of cups and bottles and vials on the table and the shelves, and missed not a stench that used to glad him two thousand years before, nor discovered one that was of a later date." This was no exaggeration. As the historian David Wootton, of the University of York, has written, "For more than two thousand years medicine effectively stood still, despite all the progress in human biology, and a doctor in ancient Rome would have done you just about as much good as a doctor in early nineteenth-century London, Paris, or New York." By Wootton's reckoning, "For 2,400 years patients have believed that doctors were doing them good; for 2,300 years they were wrong."

But if fasting as medicine came to a standstill after Galen, fasting in general did not. The new sect called Christianity, whose influence was itself growing to Galenic proportions, was about to sound the depths of fasting as nobody in the West had before or would again. The Christian view of the practice developed from ideas that were one part Jewish, two parts Greek. The Jewish we have seen. One of the Greek parts was Hippocratic Galenism. The other originated with Plato, who in his own way sent us down a path every bit as far off course as Galen did.

*   *   *

It's a little ironic that Plato plays so vital a role in the history of fasting because there's no record he fasted at all. (The bogus quotation that modern fasting writers attribute to *him* is "I fast for greater physical and mental efficiency." The clues to its fraudulence are that mental efficiency hardly existed as a concept before the industrial era, and Plato never wrote in his own voice.) Born around 429 BC into a distinguished family of aristocrats—his father's people claimed descent from the god Poseidon—Plato founded the Academy that became the model for the modern university and wrote the sparkling dialogues that starred the tremendous intellect of a goading, playful Socrates. These were so deftly reasoned and so beautifully constructed that the British philosopher Alfred Whitehead famously wrote, "The safest general characterization of the European philosophical tradition is that it consists of a series of footnotes to Plato."

One heavily footnoted Platonic idea was dualism, the belief that human beings are made of two distinct parts: a body that ties us to the earth and a soul that links us to the divine. The body is by far the baser of the two, the ball and chain that keep the noble soul from soaring to heavenly perfection. If this sounds unremarkable, that's only because Western thought has so completely assimilated dualism that it's accepted today without reflection—alas. But it was a foreign concept in Plato's time, hardly present, for example, in ancient Jewish writings or the teachings of Jesus, who suggested the resurrection on Judgment Day would restore not just the worthy soul, leaving the tainted body behind, but rather the unified soul and body.

To Plato, the trouble with the body was that its appetites and passions were a nuisance to philosophy, whose purpose was to free soul and mind. Appetite for food was a particular problem. "The authors of our race were aware that we would be intemperate in eating and drinking," says the titular character of Plato's *Timaeus*, "and that gluttony would compel us to take a good deal more than was needed." Gluttony also had the power to "render the whole race an enemy to philosophy and music, deaf to the voice of our most divine part." Plato's solution was simple: eat sensibly, with restraint. He never called for anything so self-mortifying as a fast.

Unfortunately, a priggish Alexandrian named Philo picked up Plato's dualism and his concern about gluttony and gave them an unbecomingly zealous twist. Philo was a Hellenized Jew whose life bracketed Jesus's by a decade or two on either end. He must have achieved a modest political prominence because he once traveled to Rome in a delegation to Caligula, then at his most sadistic and sexually predacious. The prudish Philo must have been staggered. We know little more of Philo's life, but in his substantial writings he sought to integrate the Jewish precepts he took on deepest faith with the Greek philosophy he equally revered, above all the teachings of Plato.

Philo declared the body "a plotter against the soul," "a cadaver and always dead," and he believed "the chief cause of ignorance is the flesh and our affinity for it." To curb the flesh, one had to curb the intertwined passions of gluttony and lust. Tasty food created "unceasing irritations, itchings, and titillations" in the gut, which stimulated the nearby genitals. "This is apparently why Nature placed the organs of sexual lust where she did," for those organs "do not like hunger but are roused to their special activities when fulness of food leads the way."

Philo cast the blame for this awkward predicament not upon Nature or its creator but upon that stained part of creation known as woman, a succubus who brought ruin to God's otherwise obedient servant, man. To Philo, nonprocreative sex with this creature was a horror, and even procreative sex was but a repugnant necessity. Page after page, he sowed the seeds of a religious misogyny that would have gruesome repercussions.

His hero Plato may have had no use for fasting, but Philo had eight hundred years of it in his Jewish heritage, and he drafted the practice to quash both appetite and libido. A little surprisingly, though, it wasn't his first line of attack. Instead, he said with Plato that the passions were best controlled by eating sensibly and that fasting could be a useful complement. He nonetheless wrote admiringly of devoted fasters, including a small community of Jews called the Therapeutae, who were vegetarian, celibate, virtually without possessions, and terrifically observant in fasting. Some Therapeutae so engrossed themselves in religious study, they forgot to eat for three days running. "Others," Philo wrote, "so luxuriate in the banquet of truths that wisdom richly and lavishly supplies, they hold out for twice that time and only after six days do they bring themselves to taste such sustenance as is absolutely necessary." It is one of our first glimpses in the West of prolonged fasting for contemplation.

A paradox of Philo is that his thinking hardly influenced his fellow Jews, who took one look at what he was offering and left the goods untouched. Christians, on the other hand, went in for the package deal. They saw the sexual repression, the rank misogyny, and the fasting for self-control and decided this was exactly what Jesus had wanted all along. It

may have slipped Christ's mind to say so, but his inheritors wouldn't make
the same mistake.

*   *   *

The eventual Christian enthusiasm for fasting is a little odd because the
first Christians were no more interested in it than Jesus had been. Paul,
the epistolary co-founder of Christianity, said not a word of fasting,
and the general tenor of the New Testament is that Christians, their sins
having been washed away by Jesus, no longer required the Judaic fasts
of atonement. Christians "ate their food with gladness and simplicity of
heart, praising God," and Paul warned of "liars" who would arise and try to
command people "to abstain from foods which God created to be received
with thanksgiving."

And yet even from the outset there were signs of trouble. Influenced
by Philo, Paul was extravagantly repulsed by sensuality. He complained the
urges of his body were ever "warring against the law of my mind and holding me captive to the law of sin that dwells within me." He, too, called for a
rigorous self-discipline to guard against the titillation of sex. Later thinkers
would elaborate, again with Philo, that while sex was needed to propagate
the faith, it ought to be cheerless and generative, and the genitals should be
kept in check by suppressing the voracious gut. From there, it was no great
leap to turn to fasting for help.

Many Christians were already fasting or weren't far removed from it.
Most of them, after all, had lately been Jews, and they either stuck with
or revived the Jewish practice of twice-weekly fasting. The Christians'
fast days were Wednesday and Friday because, as one early text said, "the
hypocrites" (for which we can read Jews) fasted on Monday and Thursday.
Theologians skilled in rationalization would later give the days a mournful meaning: Christians fasted on Wednesday because that was the day
Judas betrayed Jesus and on Friday because that was when he was crucified.
Although many Christians fasted in a Pauline quest to quell gluttony and
lust, others saw in fasting either a Christlike sacrifice that could redeem the

lost, an expression of humility before God, or a demonstration of superiority to pagans.

Early Christians fiercely debated how severely to fast. At first, most theologians who railed against gluttony urged only mild fasting, as Philo had. Cutting the day's meals from three to two, or two to one would suffice, whereas a sterner asceticism would distract from God's works. The opposing view was loudly championed by Tertullian, a Latinized Berber of the second and third centuries who fulminated on all things Christian from what I like to envision as his dim grotto in Carthage. In his tract "On Fasting"—the first surviving Christian propaganda devoted exclusively to the practice—he chided his fellow Christians for lackadaisicalness. The prevailing custom for the stations, as the fasts on Wednesday and Friday had become known, was to eat lightly throughout the day before taking a substantial mid-afternoon meal, but Tertullian declared the stations must be observed in strict foodlessness till sunset. Such a sacrifice, he said, not only pleased God but atoned for man's original sin, which in Tertullian's creative mind was Adam's refusal to heed God's command to "fast" from the tree of knowledge. A severe fast righted that ancient wrong, and, what was more, "Abstention from food makes God tent-fellow with man—peer, in truth, with peer!"

Claiming equality with God won Tertullian no friends among the cautious bishops who controlled the early Church, and it wasn't his only heresy. He also called for an elite *militia Christi* to lead the masses, and their boot camp was to be the hunger and discipline of fasting. For those not devoted enough to join their ranks, fasting would still be a fine preparation for the martyrdom every believer should invite. The bishops must have been aghast. They thought the path to worldly power depended less on mobilizing a zealous vanguard to lead converts than simply winning the converts in the first place, and they were certain pagans wouldn't come to Christianity if the bar to entry required too high a leap. They rejected Tertullian for a heretic, but they couldn't check his influence. Although he wouldn't live to see it, the Church would become more his than theirs, and nowhere more so than where fasting was concerned.

*   *   *

The fourth century saw the birth of a new kind of biography that proved momentous for fasting. This was the immensely popular tale of the heroic Christian ascetic, one several degrees more masochistic than even Tertullian's idealized Christian. Among the most beloved of these yarns was Athanasius's *Life of Antony*, whose eponymous protagonist—known variously as Antony the Great, Antony of the Desert, and the Father of All Monks—was born in Lower Egypt around 251. In the manner of the Buddha, Antony forsook his wealthy upbringing and retreated to the wilderness, where for twenty solitudinous years he holed up in an abandoned desert fort to pray, fast, and grapple with the odd demon. When he finally emerged, his friends were "amazed to see that his body had kept its same condition" despite the decades of fasting and demonic battling. The Antony of Athanasius radiated such tranquility that the sick were healed by his mere presence, and his life thereafter was a perpetual martyrdom of hair shirt, unbathed squalor, and either fasting or eating a single daily meal of bread, salt, and water. The real Antony was a more muted bloke who warned that the Christian who fasted too vigorously risked straying "far from God," but reality was no match for the larger-than-life character who banished disease and hell's ogres through the power of asceticism.

Ordinary Christians didn't take their fasting to such extremes, but through the heroic biographies they developed a taste for asceticism, and a small number of fanatics were inspired to take to the desert themselves—Tertullian's militia Christi brought to life. Variously called "anchorites" (from the Greek *anakhorein*, meaning "withdrawal"), desert fathers and mothers, or "athletes for Christ," they soon gave rise to that most durable of ecclesiastical personae, the Christian monk. So numerous were their colonies in the wastes of Egypt, Palestine, and Syria that travelers spoke of cities in the wilderness. The citizens could be fiercely competitive in their asceticism, with one devotee trying to inflict more agony on his battered body than the next, and in their ever-escalating war against the self, their greatest weapon was the fast.

* * *

But let's leave their mortified frames in the desert for a moment and say a quick farewell to fasting among the children of Abraham. After the destruction of the Second Temple in AD 70, fasting for atonement increased among Jews. In the *Apocalypse of Elijah*, likely written shortly before Alexandria's Jewish community was destroyed in 117, the author says of fasting, "It releases sin. It heals diseases. It casts out demons. It is effective up to the throne of God for an ointment and for a release from sin by means of a pure prayer." His claim that fasting could heal disease was nearly unique in Judeo-Christian writings to this point, and we might safely guess it was influenced by fasting in Greco-Roman medicine. But the author's successors didn't pick up the thread, and therapeutic fasting never flourished in Judaism.

Nor did ascetic fasting, although now and then Jews flirted with it. In Babylonia, probably in the third century, after a certain Rabbi Hisda offended his teacher, both professor and pupil undertook forty fasts of atonement: the student for making his teacher suffer, the teacher for having taken undue umbrage. They were outdone a century or so later by another Babylonian, Rabbi Hiyya bar Ashi. For years, Hiyya lived separately from his wife in a show of chaste resolve, but one day she disguised herself as a harlot and seduced him. Even after learning her identity (post-coitally, for it seems the rebbe hardly knew his bride), he was so guilt-ridden he kept repeating, "But I meant to sin!" For penance he fasted until he died.

On the whole, though, ascetic fasting never captured the Jewish imagination, and most rabbis held with Rabbi Sheshet (he of "Let the meal of a student who fasts be given to the dogs") that fasting interfered with the study of scripture. Certainly Jews had less need than Christians to fast, for Philo's sexual repression was outside the main channel of Judaism, whose adherents never came to loathe the body the way Christians did. The more Christians fasted, the more Jews distinguished themselves by fasting less, and eventually the practice simply withered in Judaism to near irrelevance.

* * *

Across the Christian calendar, meanwhile, fasting enjoyed a positively Hindu expansion, starting with the paschal fast in the second century. A sort of poor man's homage to Jesus's foodless forty days, the fast lasted one to two days before Christianity's first and most important festival, Easter. A scriptural warrant for the abstention was found in Christ's pronouncement that the wedding guests would fast when the bridegroom was taken away—a passage that fasting zealots would point to again and again over the centuries to legitimize their peculiar enthusiasm. The paschal fast was a deeply mournful affair reflecting the enormity of both Jesus's sacrifice and the sinfulness of man that occasioned it. It spread quickly, both geographically and calendrically, and by the fourth century occupied the whole of Holy Week save for the joyous day of Easter itself. It was never a total fast. Mostly people just ate sparingly, but shops and offices were shuttered, public amusements prohibited, the poor provided for, and freedom sometimes granted to slaves and prisoners.

The paschal fast expanded again when Christianity metamorphosed into the state religion of the Roman Empire in the fourth century. To gain favor with the imperial government, Roman subjects converted in throngs, but many proved indifferent Christians, and when Church fathers decided to set some standards, they outdid themselves by turning the six-day paschal fast into a forty-day famine. They called it the Quadragesima, from the Latin word meaning "fortieth." English speakers would come to call it Lent for the season in which it fell: *lencten*, the Anglo-Saxon spring. During Lent, the faithful were to repent their sins and swear off some measure of food. Many Christians just omitted meat or other animal products and sometimes just for part of Lent, while the most observant fasted strictly during daylight hours for the whole forty days—a forerunner of Lent's Islamic successor Ramadan.* Not until the seventh century did Lent attain the shape by which we know it today, commencing on Ash Wednesday and requiring abstinence from only certain meats and alcohols.

---

* The history of fasting in Islam, although fascinating, developed well off the historical line of this book's main concern, a thread that runs from antiquity through western Europe and Henry Tanner and onward to the modern science of fasting.

In time, nearly every Christian feast would get its own antecedent fast, usually lasting only a day or two but sometimes much longer, as in the forty-day Fast of Advent or Nativity, the prelude to Christmas. Today Christians honor nearly all of the fasts by omission. In the case of Nativity, I have always suspected even the most devoted followers of Christ are privately of the same mind as my son Elliott, to whom the meaning of Advent is a thick calendar with small pieces of chocolate behind its many doors and a grand truffle on the glorious gift-strewn day itself.

* * *

Fasting caught Christians' fancy not just because of ascetic titans like Antony but because a steady stream of lesser desert fathers and mothers used it to prove the merit of a new idea: through fasting and other asceticisms, they could approach the *bios angelikos*, the life of the angels that good Christians would attain in the hereafter. In the bios angelikos, the body would be but slight, there would be no need to eat, and the reborn would exist solely to serve and worship God—the pious mind's idea of a rollicking good eternity. The anchorites' efforts to approximate the bios angelikos make uncommonly grim reading. Some spent their entire monastic lives in shirts of coarse goat's hair or iron plates that rubbed their skin to open sores and made muscles burn. Others went naked in the harshest weather. Still others immersed themselves in freezing water, rolled in thorns and nettles, genuflected so many thousands of times they could no longer walk right, or stood stock still hour upon hour in what the expert torturers of a later time would call stress positions. The minds behind this cruel science weren't seeking suffering for suffering's sake. They were pursuing self-discipline and distraction from the temptations of the flesh. They were athletes in training.

Their fasts could be competitive indeed. When Macarius of Alexandria, a fourth-century monk in Egypt's Nitrian Desert, learned that monks farther up the Nile ate only raw food during Lent, he took all his food raw for the next seven years. When he heard of an ascetic who lived on a pound of bread a day, he stuffed his own hard bread into a narrow-necked jug and restricted his diet to whatever meager scrap he could extract in one pull. When news of an even sharper asceticism came to him, he cut his weekly menu to a few cabbage leaves on Sunday. Another monk by the name of Heron, in an account equally hard to credit, was said to have regularly fasted for three months at a stretch on only the Eucharist and wild herbs. At the Egyptian monastery of Skete, a certain Abba Isaiah was supposed to have habitually taken the saucepan off the fire just as the lentils began to boil because the mere sight of them cooking was enough to sustain him. Throughout many of these accounts ran a desire to tame desire, especially of the carnal variety. A desert father of fourth-century Egypt known as John the Dwarf explained, "A king who wants to take possession of an enemy's city begins by cutting off the water and the food; so his enemies, dying of hunger, submit to him. It is the same with the passions of the flesh: if a man goes about fasting and hungry, the enemies of his soul grow weak."

But even among the anchorites, such severe ascetics were in the minority. Most abbots urged nothing more strenuous than light eating, which permitted their monks the energy to do the work a thriving monastery required. The extreme end of what was acceptable was probably marked by Shenoute of Atripe, the fifth-century head of Egypt's White Monastery, who never ate before sundown, never fully sated his hunger or slaked his thirst, but only occasionally went the whole of a week without food. Abbots warned their novitiates of the dangers of immoderate fasting with lurid tales of ruined health, like that of Battheus of Edessa, who fasted so long that maggots crawled from his teeth, or of Adolius of Tarsus, who grew so emaciated that visitors took him for a phantom.

But the most headstrong pupils would not be deterred, and none was stronger of head, nor more celebrated for it, than Simeon the Stylite. When he first arrived at a monastery in Syria in the early fifth century, young Simeon was an exemplary postulant, "serving all and loved by all." But one day he stole the rope from the communal well, wrapped it tightly round his torso as a kind of penance, and hid it under his hairshirt. A year later the rope had embedded into his skin and, by one account, "was covered by the rotted flesh of the righteous man. Because of his stench no one could stand near him, but no one knew his secret. His bed was covered with worms." He further irritated his monastic brothers by fasting more zealously than they: they ate every sundown, he every Sunday. When his stench at last became too much and the abbot ordered him stripped, the horrified brothers "found the rope wrapped around his body so that nothing of it could be seen but the ends. There was no guessing how many worms were on him." The monks had to soak Simeon for three days in oil and water to remove the garment stuck to his suppurating flesh, and it took two months to nurse him back to something resembling health. The abbot showed him the door.

Simeon fetched up in a small desert hut where, during one Lent, a friend walled him inside with only a few loaves of bread and a jug of water. At the end of the forty days, the friend unwalled the door and found loaves and jug untouched. Afterward Simeon marked Lent with various severe practices, like standing the entire forty days (a post supporting him while he slept) and likely taking no food at all. His feats brought him fame, and to escape the crowds who beat a path to his door he moved to a ruined stylite, or pillar, atop which he built a small platform. For the next few decades until his death in 459, he remained atop stylites, preaching to herds of pilgrims who sought him out anyway and corresponding with wisdom-seekers, among them the emperor and empress of Byzantium. Centuries after Simeon's death, imitators were still perching atop stylites across the Levant.

It is telling that Simeon was kicked out of the monastery by those who had to live with him and made a saint by those who did not. Severe fasting and other harsh self-denials have always been more appealing in one's idols than in one's familiars, let alone in oneself, which is why neither Simeon nor the other desert fathers and mothers stirred large numbers of people to practice extreme asceticism. They did, however, make lesser assaults on the body far more acceptable to laypeople, and once again fasting was the readiest weapon to hand.

* * *

The spread of this personal warfare brought a sinister dawn to the half of Christendom whose mistake it was to have been born ovarious. Misogyny, of course, had been long brewing in Christianity, ever since Paul demanded women submit to men. Subsequent theologians first insisted on and then fetishized female chastity as the symbol of that submission, and they quickly enlisted fasting as virginity's protector. Not only did fasting dry up the moist humors that begat female lust (Philo's influence again); it also wrecked the feminine beauty that stirred the loins of that easily tempted brute, man. The virgin's compensation for a life of fasting and celibacy was to become the bride of Christ, a phrase meant all too literally. In some of the creepiest writings of antiquity, Church prudes worked themselves into sticky, self-stimulated puddles with visions of Christ uniting in the hereafter with his fasting virgins. Evagrius Ponticus, a theologian of the fourth century, can still be heard panting through the pages on which he wrote, "The virginal eyes will see the Lord. The virgins' ears will listen to his words. The virgins' mouth will kiss their bridegroom, and the virgins' nose will rush towards the scent of his perfume. Virginal hands will stroke the Lord, and the chastity of their flesh will be pleasing to him." Evagrius's contemporary Jerome (of whom, more below) wrote in no less of a lather, "When sleep comes upon you, He will come behind the wall and He will put His hand through the opening and will touch your body. You will rise, trembling, and say, 'I languish with love.'"

The harsh calls to obliterate beauty through fasting were soon surpassed by calls to erase womanhood entirely—to wither breasts, pare buttocks and hips, and end menstruation by abstaining from food. Tales arose, many apocryphal, all instructive, to glorify the women who succeeded. One was of Pelagia, the most lustrous dancer and working girl of fourth- or fifth-century Antioch. Pelagia paraded herself through town richly made up and perfumed, draped in lavish silks and exquisite jewels, her alabaster skin sumptuous, her character shameless. "Her beauty stunned those who beheld her," her hagiographer wrote, and "incited everyone who set eyes on her to fall in love with her." But eventually Pelagia saw the perversity of her ways, repented, and became an anchorite. The diet she adopted was so meager and her fasting so strict that in a short time "her astounding beauty had all faded away, her laughing and bright face that I had known had become ugly, her pretty eyes had become hollow and cavernous. . . . Indeed the whole complexion of her body was coarse and dark like sackcloth." Other tales speak of breasts shriveled like dried leaves, cheeks deeply chasmed, and devotees who passed for men in monasteries until their deaths, unrecognized even by their own families.

These annihilations, the reader was to understand, were not piteous but laudable. Their most passionate advocate was Jerome of Stridon, whose career in vituperative misogyny is still waiting to be outdone. Born in Dalmatia in the mid-fourth century, Jerome started adulthood a hermit before abandoning the life anchoritic and bootstrapping his way up the Church hierarchy to become an adviser to Pope Damasus I. He is best known for translating the scripture into the Vulgate, the standard Latin Bible of Catholicism, but among his other obsessions were the problems of lust and the iniquity of woman. Jerome so despised the female form that he demanded girls and women forgo bathing lest they see themselves unclothed, and he said the ideal female was "one who mourned and fasted, who was squalid with dirt, almost blinded by weeping. . . . No other could give me pleasure but one whom I never saw eating food." The goal for womankind was to endure a lifelong gnaw of hunger from undereating, which Jerome held superior to even a long fast because the torment was perpetual, refreshed with every meal.

In Rome, he gathered round himself a circle of rich female followers, mostly widows, the inferiority of whose sex was made up for by the superiority of their social status. One dowager, Paula, had a daughter named Blesilla, a happy child unhappily widowed at the age of twenty, who fell ill with fever after she buried her husband. For a month she could eat almost nothing and nearly died. Jerome and Paula helpfully explained that God had sent misfortune to Blesilla "to teach her to renounce her overly great attention to that body which the worms must shortly devour," and they generously added that she should "mourn the loss of her virginity more than the death of her husband." They pressed her to continue the fast that her illness had imposed on her so as "not to stimulate desire." She agreed, and a delighted Jerome wrote, "Her steps tottered with weakness, her face was pale and quivering, her slender neck scarcely upheld her head." Blesilla became a nun and devoted herself to prayer, penitence, and harsh fasting—and was dead in four months.

Her death scandalized the elite of Rome, and in 385 a council of clergy banished Jerome from the city. The theologian Jovinian, a foe of harsh asceticism, spoke for many when he quoted Paul on the latter-day "liars" who would come forth to forbid the eating of certain foods. But Jerome's exclusion was temporary. The Church's appetite for austere fasting only grew with the years, and in the end it was Jovinian whom the Church condemned a heretic while bestowing sainthood on Jerome and Paula. Harsh fasts were elevated to the ideal. For men and boys it was an ideal only to be admired, but girls and women were browbeaten into thinking they should approximate a Pelagia-like obliteration and their failure to do so displeased God. The enormity of the anguish visited upon millions of girls and women across so many centuries makes for unbearable contemplation.

*   *   *

The news of the age, however, wasn't all dismal, for a few people turned to fasting to heal. Even in an era when intellectual pursuit was dominated by theological rather than scientific concerns, a handful of thinkers noticed fasting could be a boon not just to the spirit but also to the body. In the third century, the Christian philosopher Clement of Alexandria wrote that excessive diet "harms man by dulling the mind and making the body susceptible to disease. . . . Those who live on simpler foods are stronger and healthier and more alert." And in fourth-century Caesarea, on the northern coast of what is now Israel, Basil the Great wrote that doctors were prescribing fasts because they helped the sick throw off illness. A contemporary of Basil's whom we know only for who he is not—historians call him Pseudo-Athanasius—echoed the Jewish writer of the *Apocalypse of Elijah* when he wrote, "Observe what fasting does: it heals disease, dries up the bodily humors, casts out demons, chases away wicked thoughts, makes the mind clearer and the heart pure, sanctifies the body, and places the person before the throne of God." In the same period, Asterius of Amasea, writing from what is today central Turkey, offered an even longer list of the ways fasting "brings peace for body and soul alike," which included freeing the mind of vapors, making the step firm and the hands steady, clarifying speech, eliminating bodily waste, and improving veins, stomach, digestion, eyes, breathing, and sleep.

Clearly word was getting around that fasting was physically therapeutic, and in a few cases it was used not just as a remedy but as a preventive. Syncletica of Alexandria, one of the few desert mothers of whom we have a record (albeit one of dubious reliability), was said to have regularly and judiciously fasted in the fourth century to maintain her health. So successful did her habit prove that when she deviated from it, "her face was pale, and the weight of her body fell." She also gave wise counsel against extreme fasting, which she called prideful and insalubrious. Jerome must have thought her the Angel of Darkness.

The figure of antiquity most captivated by therapeutic fasting was John Chrysostom, the sainted archbishop of Constantinople in the fourth and fifth centuries. As a young man, Chrysostom damaged his constitution with harsh asceticism, but rather than reject fasting completely, he argued for a nuanced version. He observed that monks who ate just one meal a day were more quickly cured of illness than those who ate more often and that they awoke in the morning more refreshed because their sleep was less troubled by snoring and tossing. "For when the heart is not oppressed by excessive food, it soon recovers from sleep and is immediately awake." "Frugality, a plain table," Chrysostom held, "is the mother of health," and with uncanny perception he warned that the fruits of a full table were gout, palsy, headaches, dizziness, premature senility, dimmed vision, ruined digestion, a distended abdomen, lost appetite, overly frequent defecation, and a lifelong dependence on doctors and medicines. He got most of it right. Gentle fasting was one of his antidotes to gluttony, for "the person who fasts is light and winged." But Chrysostom's elegant and wise exhortations were too far ahead of their time to be heeded by more than a small fraction of Christians, most of whom understood fasting only in religious terms.

Other writers made much of fasting's calming effect on the mind. Basil, who longed for a community that nourished love of neighbor and who saw a path to get there through fasting, wrote, "If only everyone who needs a counselor would take her in"—that is, would fast—"there would be nothing preventing a deep peace from abiding in each house. Nations wouldn't attack each other, armies wouldn't engage in battle. Neither would weapons be forged if fasting ruled. There would be no point in holding court, prisons would be unpopulated, and evildoers would have no place to hide." His tender vision stood in sharp contrast to the dominant severity of the Church, which may be why it had few takers.

By late antiquity, fasting had spread so widely that Christian treatises on the practice seemed to sprout from every cove and cape of the Mediterranean. But the treatisers quickly ran out of things to say and began to repeat themselves, and since Christianity dominated Western thought, no one else in the West had much to say about fasting either. In the fifth century the theologian John Cassian, roaming wide in the Mediterranean littoral, synthesized the range of Christian thought on fasting, and it is a sign of how few subsequent theoretical developments there were that well into the modern era his work was still the go-to reference on the subject. (Cassian, incidentally, was fascinated by wet dreams and urged fasting to combat nocturnal disgorgement.) But although innovation in thinking about fasting stood still in the Middle Ages, Church fathers weren't anywhere near done fiddling with the form and scale of it. Nor were their subjects, some of whom devised clever ways to avoid it while others took it to even more rarified extremes. Thought may have stagnated at the end of antiquity, but the practice of fasting had only begun to burgeon.

CHAPTER 4

A LESSER ME

It is a thin imagination that would not be titillated by the tale of Henry Tanner's great fasts of 1877 and 1880, and at the time I became acquainted with them I was thin of neither mind nor body. Years earlier, for reasons subsequently puzzling to me, I had been a distance runner, but a pitiable knee injury ended all that, after which lard came upon me. Its accumulation was so gradual that I didn't perceive it until I saw a couple of family photographs. Who was that shapeless man holding hands with my wife? That doughy guy with his arm around my brother?

Vanity was not my only concern. Even at the time, fifteen years ago, the science couldn't have been clearer that fat was the forerunner of disease, decrepitude, and premature death. The odds of developing diabetes or high blood pressure, respiratory or kidney failure, thrombosis or embolism, gout or arthritis, migraine or sleep apnea, cardiac arrest or gallstones all increase with one's ballast, as does the chance of most cancers, including those of the brain and thyroid, bone marrow and esophagus, stomach and colon, liver and gallbladder, pancreas and breast, uterus and ovaries. One study found those who are overweight in middle age have about a one-third greater chance of becoming demented later in life. For the obese, it's 90 percent greater, and at just about any age there is a link between weighing too much and thinking less clearly.

Even the fat who are otherwise fit suffer. In an analysis of 3.5 million Britons, obese people with generally healthy biomarkers nonetheless had a 50 percent higher chance of developing heart disease compared to people of normal weight. And those who aren't even technically over-weight can still get grief from excess fat. Researchers had long believed a body-mass index between 18.5 and 24.9 was healthy, but we now know a BMI above even 21 or 22 is linked to greater risk of chronic disorders.* At a BMI of 24.5, risk of heart disease is double that at a BMI of 18.5, and at a BMI of 25 a woman's risk of type 2 diabetes is five times that at a BMI of 21.

The mechanisms by which surplus fat creates or abets disease are com-plex and still being worked out, but we know extra fat generates chronic inflammation, which is at the root of all kinds of maladies from irritable bowel syndrome to rheumatoid arthritis to cancer. Overweight people also tend to be awash in insulin, which, among other things, is a potent growth factor that accelerates the development of tumors. Excess pounds also make hearts work harder to pump blood, which strains arteries and causes blood pressure to rise, which brings another cascade of downstream harms. The list of fat's insults is long.

A poor draw in the genetic raffle makes some of us more susceptible to these ills, and at the time of my larding, my inheritance, to judge of my kin, was hypertension, heart attack, stroke, diabetes, chronic kidney disease, dementia, schizophrenia, and a colorful assortment of cancers. As the toll mounted with the years, it seemed less a coincidence that in silhouette we bore uncomfortable resemblance to the Liberty Bell, that our family reunions suggested the long-ago congress of a walrus and an avocado. Although I concurred with the fat-acceptance movement that no one should be made to feel miserable for the shape of their body and that overweight people can and should be as happy as anyone, psychological health is not physical health. I was of the same mind as the Zen master Shunryu Suzuki when he told one of his pupils, "You are perfect just the way you are. And . . . there is still room for improvement!"

By my late thirties, I had enlarged only to borderline fatness. My weight *in extremis* was somewhere in the loftier 160s, which, by the

---

* For someone five foot nine, which is both my altitude and that of the average American man, a BMI of 21 means a weight of 142 pounds. For a person five foot four, the height of the average American woman, a BMI of 21 means 122 pounds.

swollen American standard, hardly qualified as pudgy for a man of five feet and nine inches. But year by year I felt sluggier and schlumpier. My toes had begun to point out when I walked, and if you were unkind or honest you might have said I had the start of a waddle. I certainly had the start of a dunlop, so called because it done lopped over the belt and because Dunlop is the name of a tire, spare or otherwise. One might even say of my perimeter that my *peri* was becoming frighteningly close to a *meter*. Had my weight seemed likely to settle where it was, my concern might not have been great, but my gains gave no sign of slowing. As in a bad novel, I could see where the plot was headed.

I resolved to fast.

My ambitions were at first un-Tannerly. I fasted a day, and all went well. It wasn't hard. In fact, the sensation of hunger was pleasing in just the way a little discomfort is when running. Two weeks later I repeated the performance, with a similarly gratifying result. A few weeks after that, I fasted again, then again. Soon I felt myself master of the one-day fast.

Fasters commonly report it's easier to eat moderately after fasting because they have a better sense of how much food they need. They stuff themselves less. It was the same for me. My stomach felt smaller for a day or so after each fast, as if there was simply less room for food, and a similar, if metaphorical, contraction seemed to take place in my mind, which after a day off meals was less fixated on eating and more easily sated. Fasters speak of their fasts "resetting" their relationship with food, and that was just how I experienced it. I upped the stakes to a fast of two days, then three, and eventually, in what was a marvel to me, a week. I lost several pounds, and ambition crept upon me. I thought of a fast of weeks. The plural excited me.

I would aim for 140 pounds, my collegiate weight, although to reach it I figured I would have to fast to 135. Fasting is mildly dehydrating, and the faster, on returning to food, rapidly re-accrues a liquid pound or two. He also loses during his fast the pound or so of solid waste that is a semi-constant in the gut and a couple of pounds of gut bacteria that die off when starved. Both of these return in the days after a fast. The long-haul male faster, so I had read, typically loses about a pound a day (women, more adept at fat storage, lose a little less), so I figured I could reach 135 in a bit over three weeks.

I made my preparations. The short fast requires little or no ground-work, but longer deprivations, I had also read, are best undertaken after several days on a fibrous, low-fat diet, with fewer calories the last day or two. Vegetables, fruits, and whole grains are counseled, meat and dairy discouraged, the idea being to smoothly move what is in one's interior to one's exterior. To do otherwise is to invite meals to linger in the bow-els long after the fast starts, which can be painful at best, damaging at worst. Ordinarily these dietary rules would have been no hardship, as I was mostly vegetarian anyway, but during the preparatory period I hap-pened to be passing through Kansas City, home to barbecue joints of hal-lowed name to which I made occasional hajj. I have since given up eating animals and the fruits we unkindly take from them, but at the time I was filled with something approaching self-awe as I drove past the Brooklyn Avenue exit on I-70 without flickering my blinker. I stuck to the pre-fast plan and on a Sunday night had a last supper of whole-wheat riga-toni and marinara, bland but purgative. I weighed myself. The scale read 160 pounds—a round 160, you might say. I went to bed with visions of a lesser me dancing in my head.

* * *

I passed Monday morning, the first of my fast, with no evidence of appe-tite. By afternoon, however, my stomach—I use the term in its general, nonclinical sense—was encircled by emptiness. Soon I felt it contracting, and now and then it murmured aggrievedly. For redress, I felt none of the sleepiness I usually feel after lunch. Indeed, I was sharply alert, possibly because my body, not needing energy to digest food, was sending the sur-plus to my brain. My stomach grew increasingly resentful as the afternoon advanced, but I felt no hunger. This must sound odd to anyone who has skipped a meal or two in sorrow, but I had learned from my short fasts that the sensation most of us call hunger is less the body saying it needs food than that it *expects* it. The typical body—certainly the well-grazed

American body—still has plenty of energy to run on when hunger first calls. In fact, it usually hasn't stopped digesting the food from the last meal. The trick is to ignore the call to eat, and fortunately I had learned a few tricks of the antihunger trade.

One of my earliest teachers was Gandhi, veteran of seventeen hunger strikes and deviser of a set of precepts about fasting. The majority of the precepts—take regular enemas, sleep out of doors—I honored in the breach. Two, however, I held close. One was to drink as much cool water as possible, a rule later fasters improved by recommending the faster drink whenever a thought of food arises. The other worthy precept was simply to banish thoughts of food the instant they sprang up. At first I thought this advice insipid. It seemed to me a faster—at least a non-Mahatma faster—could no more will away a mental masala than an alcoholic could a mental whiskey sour. But latter-day fasters had again helpfully elaborated, in this case by likening thoughts of food to internet pop-up ads, which disappear with a simple click on the red X. A faster, my teachers said, had only to click the X and the thoughts would go away. It worked just so for me, to my appreciative surprise. The few times it didn't, I resorted to evasive maneuvers. Reading *David Copperfield*, I skimmed whenever Dickens waxed lascivious over a leg of mutton or a tankard of ale or even suet pudding. This last has never tempted me—its cognomen "spotted dick" doesn't help— but I didn't want to take the chance.

That first evening I sat to dinner with my wife and son, Jennifer and Elliott, who had before them a béchamel lasagna (Jennifer) and a macaroni and cheese (Elliott). My entrée was water. Jennifer put knife and fork to the lasagna and made slow, deep cuts through the heavy cream, through the top layer of noodle, the spinach, more cream, more noodle. Elliott slurped his macaroni. I hadn't seen food all day, and it looked scrumptious, but I felt neither temptation nor privation. I confess, however, to a few prophylactic swigs of water and wasn't saddened when the plates were cleared. At bedtime, I noticed my skin had grown more taut, my belly more shrunken—fair restitution, I supposed, and slept contentedly.

* * *

Next morning, thirty-six hours into my fast, I awoke feeling not quite right but in a way that is hard to capture in words. I was a little weak, or maybe a little light, and I had the sensation that my being was centered in my head or was trying to be, but my head was too full of other things to hold all of me. I did not, however, have a headache. The discomfort was remote, and the alertness I enjoyed the day before had abandoned me utterly. In its place was a heavy, insistent somnolence. I napped in the morning and again at teatime but did not awake from either slumber refreshed. I stumbled through the day lethargic.

Endurance fasters say the hardest part of their labor is from roughly the second through fourth days. Just before this window, the body wrings the last nutrients from the food in the gut and exhausts its reserves of glycogen, the compound that is broken into the sugar glucose, which in turn fuels the brain, among other organs. The brain is ravenous. Though just two percent of the body's mass, it uses twenty percent of its resting energy, and the body's other main sources of energy—amino acids, which are broken down from proteins, and fatty acids and glycerol, which are broken down from fats—ordinarily do not power the brain. This is a bother because most of us would just as soon burn our great flubbery pounds of fat after we run through our pound or two of stored glycogen. Instead, our brains demand more sugar, for which they are on a nearly constant prowl. It is an argument against intelligent design.

We have a backup sugar-production line, but it is a poor one. As our glycogen dwindles, the body harvests amino acids and sends them to the liver, which turns them into glucose before forwarding the fuel to the brain. But making glucose thus is inefficient, which is probably why I was so exhausted. Were a typical person to continue in this protein-burning state, the brain would devour the body's muscles in no more than three weeks and kill the host in the process.

But that is not the faster's fate. The reason is ketone bodies, which are highly acidic compounds created when fatty acids from our fat stores are broken down for energy. The best-known ketone is acetone, as in the clear flammable liquid used to remove nail polish and scour metal surfaces before painting. Once thought a waste product, ketones are in fact fuel—and fuel that can power the brain. There is evidence the brain may even run more efficiently on ketones, perhaps because ounce for ounce they contain more energy than glucose. If so, this may help account for the heightened sense of well-being and even euphoria that some fasters describe. Ketones also blunt the hunger-producing hormone ghrelin, which is a large part of why after the first day or two, fasters no longer feel hungry. From the faster's perspective, just about the only drawback to ketones is that neither the voracious brain nor the rest of the body starts using them immediately upon exhausting glucose and glycogen. The transition to ketosis takes two or three days, and the toll extracted en route is the inefficient stopgap of burning proteins.

While my brain and body were dithering thus, other changes were occurring within me. My sense of smell, for one, grew fantastically sharp. At a street fair, I bought Elliott a bag of popcorn, and the warm odor of roasted kernels hit me as though I had shoved my snout in the bag. When we got home, Jennifer was simmering a Thai tomato soup, and I could smell every ingredient individually: the parched earth of the cumin, the fire of the chili, the mintiness of the coriander, the creamy luxury of coconut milk. I was experiencing the world as a hound or perhaps one of my underfed ancestors on the African savannah whose honed senses ensured her survival during a rough patch. Some vestigial part of me said I should be tempted by the food around me, but I wasn't in the least.

Another change took place in the blood vessels of my temples, which began pumping heartily. Previous fasts had taught me that over the next few days the throbbing would become so robust I would be able to count my pulse without putting finger to head. The first time I experienced such throbbing, I worried it portended stroke, and I wasn't calmed by the occasional wild fluttering of my heart, like a bird trying to flap its way out of a sack, which seemed to bode cardiac arrest. But my concerns proved hypochondriacal. My heart, I later learned, was merely working harder to compensate for the drop in blood pressure that fasters enjoy. In the main, the drop was harmless, but it did have one danger: if I stood up too quickly, my blood might not stand up with me. Doctors who prescribe fasting often say the greatest risk lies not where the layperson might suppose—damage to the stomach, say, or to liver or heart, which almost never happens—but in a contusion or concussion brought about by fainting. The remedy is simple: stand up in stages, pumping your legs before rising, and if you feel light-headed, sit back down immediately. I found this precept more agreeable than a daily enema and honored it punctiliously.

*　*　*

By Thursday, the fourth day of my fast, much of the odd in-my-head feeling had gone, but a moderate pain now assaulted my lower back. Some fasters believe this lumbago, a fasting commonplace, is caused by toxins dislodged from burned fats. Although most toxins are flushed out of the body via urine or sweat, some poisons, so the hypothesis goes, take up an uncomfortable residence in the lower back. Evidence to support or deny the hypothesis is scant. Dr. Françoise Wilhelmi de Toledo, research director at the world's largest fasting center, Germany's Buchinger Wilhelmi Clinic, thinks the lumbago is more probably caused by dehydration, increased acid production, or imbalanced minerals. Fasters also report coated tongues (again, sometimes thought to represent detoxification, but without much evidence) and a halitosis that fasters call ketone breath, a byproduct of powering the body on nail-polish remover. I had a bit of both, but the fur on my tongue went away after a few days, as did the sharp metallic taste on my lips. Diligent toothbrushing kept the outhouse breath in check.

At noon I went for a walk with Jennifer, who told me I was frigid, which I thought unkind, particularly as I had let her rub my lower back most of the morning. But she clarified that my hand, which she was holding, was cold—an observation never before made of a human appendage out of doors in a Tennessee August. By nightfall my feet would become cold too, and I would have to wear socks to bed. Next day I would take to wearing fleece, sometimes even outside in the muggy heat. My coldness, I surmised, was due to my lack of heat-generating digestion.

On that fourth afternoon, I went for a two-mile jog, as I had the previous three days, the pace set by my nine-year-old dog. I felt fine. Later

I tried touch football at a pace set by my seven-year-old son and nearly collapsed. Similar experiments over coming days taught me that although I could exercise moderately, even in weeping heat, for twenty, forty, even sixty minutes, just a few bursts of vigorous effort sent me gasping to the couch. Those bursts were meant to be powered by glycogen in my muscles, which I had used up days ago.

That night I weighed myself. I had not done so since starting the fast, because I wanted the satisfaction of seeing a substantial drop when finally I did. Even so, I wasn't prepared when I took to the scale and the needle stopped just shy of 151. A decline of nine pounds—more than two a day. It was hardly possible. In the first week, I had read, most male fasters lose about a pound and a half a day. (Females lose about a pound.) Two pounds a day was a rare pace, let alone more than two. I dismounted, fiddled with the scale's calibrating dial, remounted. The needle stopped at 151. I did not protest further.

At that clip, I was pleased to calculate, I would reach 135 in just one more week, but I knew I wouldn't maintain quite such a tempo. Fasters start like hares, thanks to the rapid emptying of the digestive tract and the initial loss of water, but after that they lope along. Still, if I had accelerated the first dash, it stood to reason my lope would be accelerated too. I was certain my daily exercise, which many fasters forgo, had made the difference, and since I would keep exercising, I was equally certain I would see 135 in ten or twelve days rather than the three weeks I had originally envisioned. Clearly I was a fasting prodigy.

*   *   *

To test his vow of celibacy, Gandhi slept in the nude with a nubile grand-niece. He never advanced on her, but an involuntary emission could prompt weeks of self-recrimination. I lack a grandniece, but I recalled the Mahatma's test on the day I prepared a meal for my family. On starting my fast, I had traded my traditional role of family chef for that of dishwasher. But as time passed, I missed cooking, so on Sunday, my seventh day, I made a trial of penne with olive oil and parmesan for Elliott.

I was surprised the meal aroused me not at all. The difference between preparing food and eating it was, for me, the difference between handling a bikini on the rack and handling it on the wearer. On subsequent days I made potato-leek soup, chickpea curry, and a pizza of artichoke and feta, all without yearning.

I was without yearning in other spheres too. My libido, which had been *de minimis* since Tuesday, had by the weekend become *defunctus*. I had foreseen this sorry state, another fasting commonplace, but since I was no desert father in search of the bios angelikos, it was a wound all the same. My avenues of recreation were being hedged in one by one. For paltry reparation, the throb in my temples had disappeared, my clarity of mind had returned, and my sense of well-being was once more as intact as a writer's—a sexless writer's—could be.

That evening the scale registered 146 pounds, a decline of five in the last three days, a rate only slightly less than that of my first four. My waist had shrunk from what I guessed was a pre-fast thirty-four inches—I hadn't checked in months for fear of what the horror might do to my heart—to less than thirty-two. On Monday I would search half a dozen stores for a new belt and find none. Evidently the circumference of East Tennessee Man ruled out an economy of scale for the thirty-inch belt. I finally found the right cincture in the boys' section. Over the next week I revisited the section for shirts and pants and paid cheerfully, for it is an economic fact that no one begrudges a new wardrobe so long as it is made of less fabric than the previous one.

* * *

Monday morning dawned flat, even depressive, an unexpected change from my keenness of the previous days. I felt sloth and harbored unkind thoughts toward the socialist muckraker Upton Sinclair, a faster of some ardor, who wrote of a similar stage of one of his fasts, "No phase of the experience surprised me more than the activity of my mind: I read and wrote more than I had dared to do for years before"—a terrifying thought since Sinclair wrote ninety-odd books in his ninety years.

At bedtime I weighed myself and was distressed to see the number 146, same as the night before. I stepped off the scale, checked the calibration, exhaled vigorously to unburden myself of a few ounces, and stepped back on. The needle pointed to the same spot. This was a cheat. I had swum that morning, had taken a long sweaty dog walk in the afternoon, had moved furniture in the evening in preparation for renovations—and had done all despite appalling lethargy and grievous apathy. I had known there would be days when my weight wouldn't move, that even though every day I was burning approximately half a pound of fat, some days I would retain more water, but today, when I had struggled so heroically against the oppression of fasting? I got into bed very much wanting a glass of Malbec.

Unconsciousness was long in coming. Fasters sleep less because much of what happens in sleep is the transformation of our meals into us—an irrelevance to the faster. By this point in my fast, I was sleeping only five or six hours a night and was usually grateful for the extra time to pursue the day's labors and enjoy its rewards. But after days of lassitude I preferred oblivion to another fifty pages even of Dickens.

I awoke Tuesday to the same mood and energy and at bedtime found my weight unchanged. As I debarked the accursed scale, my thoughts turned to Nanaimo bars, which consist of a bed of buttery graham cracker crumbs topped by thick blankets of custard-flavored icing and melted chocolate. After several defiantly luscious seconds, I clicked an X, trudged to bed, and pulled the comforter over my head.

*　*　*

On Wednesday, Thursday, and Friday—the tenth, eleventh, and twelfth days of my abnegation—my mood climbed somewhat from its low of earlier in the week. Life was not quite lustrous, but no longer was it gray. It helped that I had finally dropped a pound on Wednesday and kept dropping until by Friday I weighed 143.

I was truly thinning now. My cheeks took on a runner's concavity, my abdomen was approaching plumb, and my legs could have been taken for a triathlete's. One unforeseen consequence of my rediscovered thinness was

the rest of humanity suddenly looked fat to me. It was easy, of course, to
see fat in America, where most adults were overweight or obese, and easier
still in the Bible Belt, where the gut pressed hard against the buckle. Back
then, in 2009, one in three Tennessee adults was obese, and another one
in three was garden-variety overweight. (The numbers are even more dire
today.) But it was not only the overweight who looked inflated to me. The
slightest bulge of tummy, the least hint of jowl almost repulsed me now as
a sign of reckless feeding. So quickly do we forget our former selves.

Many of my acquaintances, it must be said, reciprocated my distaste,
at least on learning the reason for my atrophy. In the early going, I hadn't
advertised my fast. Like the newly expectant mother, I knew the possibility of miscarriage and didn't want a stream of condolences should my
endeavor prove stillborn. But as my labor began to show, questions grew
apace, and I had to confess.

"You're an extremist!" cried one of my brunchtime familiars—
spitting flecks of whipped cream and nearly choking on her waffle—when
apprised of my fast. After she recovered, she delivered a philippic on my
certain self-destruction that I was to hear often. I replied, purely to educate her, that if recent science was to be believed, her extreme devotion to
three meals a day, every day, might earn her a tumor. In the same altruistic
spirit, I suggested that since she had just passed forty and was getting on
in years, she might care to know that regular fasting could retard some
of the more unpleasant aspects of aging. She was sullen until her side of
bacon arrived.

Reaction to my fast seemed to correlate with the shape of the reactor.
My friend's response was typical of the plump, who proved far more hostile
than the decidedly fat. I think this was because my merely chubby friends
were perpetually tormented by the thought that if they just put in a little
more effort, they could get the damned weight off. (I had certainly felt
that way.) Having repeatedly failed, they grew first frustrated, then resentful, and some became the crabs in proverb's bucket, eager to pull down
any crab who tried to climb out. They were never happier than when an
escaped crab tumbled back in, Oprah-like, fatter than before. Nor were
they more threatened than when a crab at last escaped for good.

My friend might have reacted less violently if she had seen in my fast a way out of the bucket, but I was new to the art, defensive, and poor at explaining. In retrospect, I think she thought fasting even for a day, let alone weeks, required the same willpower that had foiled her own attempts at dieting. My proficiency at weight loss cast a judgment on her failure. The irony is that willpower plays only a bit part in prolonged fasting, and hunger none at all after the first day or two. If I had had to resist hunger's blare every day I fasted, I'd have given up before the first week was out.

The frankly obese, by contrast, were as unthreatened by my project as the slim were. I suppose this was because most of my obese friends had resigned themselves to their lot. They were like the leftists who know their hero will never ascend to the Oval Office or the Clevelanders who despair of ever again seeing a World Series trophy in their burg. They don't care for the fact, but they are certain there is little they can do about it.

*   *   *

I continued to dwindle. By the following Wednesday, the seventeenth day of my fast, the report from the bathroom was 138, three pounds from home. So near, I considered for the first time whether I might care to fast longer—say a month, or a Christly forty days, or even a couple more to out-Tanner Tanner.

I wasn't long deciding no. Endurance, even with my miserable swings of energy and mood, was not the problem. The problem was I missed eating. I wanted the sensation of food in my mouth again—the textures, the flavors, the hots and colds, the surprises, even the disappointments. I also wanted the fellowship of eating. Sitting to meals with family and friends had been sociable enough at first, but in the end it had proven an inadequate substitute for companionship, a word whose roots *com* (with) and *pan* (bread) reveal its true meaning: breaking bread with others. Not breaking bread with my intimates, I was an outsider at their rite.

Then, too, I wanted the rest of my life back. I wanted to jog more than a couple of miles. I wanted to play touch football with my son. I wanted to play touch anything with my wife. Other people wanted things of me as well. In the previous few days, some persons, maybe even one or two in my own family, had described me as irritable, even rude. On Wednesday, little Elliott, himself a bit tetchy, insulted first his mother and then his dinner, whereupon I told him, in a tone I usually reserved for the dog when he ate a whole pizza, to get out of my sight. My fast wasn't worth that price.

* * *

On Friday evening I became imbued with a mystical conviction that I had reached 135 pounds, even though I hadn't weighed myself since Wednesday's 138, and the last time I had lost three pounds in two days was more than a week ago. My faith in mysticism being what it is, I put off my rendezvous with the scale until nearly midnight, the better to wring every ounce-reducing minute from the day. When finally I stood before the machine, I offered a silent prayer to Venus, whose planet rules Libra, bearer of scales, and within whose power it not incidentally lies to bestow a pleasing form. In case the goddess was in a more Grecian than Roman mood, I appealed to Aphrodite as well. I closed my eyes, stepped up, and made sure my feet were properly placed, nothing hanging over the edge—I didn't want to look down and find an agreeable number only to discover on repositioning that it was a fraud. I opened my eyes and looked. The needle rested at 135.

This was highly promising but not, I cautioned myself, conclusive. I stepped off, recalibrated, stepped back on, wiggled around so the needle wiggled with me, and stood as still as my welling excitement would permit. The number remained—135.

Just nineteen days ago I had been a middleweight. In the interim, I had slimmed to super welterweight, welterweight, super lightweight, and now, at blessed last, lightweight. I could have KO'd Roberto Durán just then.

* * *

I was not the least surprised on Saturday morning when the scale reported 136, the first gain of my fast. During the night I had thought wantonly of food, so it was to be expected I would have added a pound. I appraised myself one last time in the full-length mirror. It revealed a stomach that would commonly be called flat, although in fact two ridges of muscle showed through my abdomen. They may have left me four cans shy of a six-pack, but I was charmed all the same. My legs were thew and sinew, my tuchus perky, and if it was true my arms were stickish and my chest boyish, I could take consolation in the fact that I was married and didn't have to be attractive to anyone.

It would have been nice to know whether my fast had done for my insides what it had done for my outsides. Had the walls of my arteries become smooth as spaghetti? Had my cells repaired mutant DNA that might otherwise have grown into a tumor? I didn't have the money to test those questions laboratorially, but not knowing had its advantages. In my ignorance, I could fantasize. I decided I had put off Alzheimer's by five years.

I breakfasted at lunch, a few hours short of twenty days. Not-withstanding my desire for mealtime companionship, I dined alone. My fast had been an essentially solitary endeavor, and it seemed fitting that my departure from it should be too. I had vigorously debated my *carte*, and particularly the *première plat*, before choosing applesauce that Jennifer had made from our backyard apple tree. I took a spoonful, and what occurred within me with my first taste was what occurred in the Starburst commercials of old, the ones in which liquid explosions of kaleidoscopic joy burst from the actors' mouths. It was an inundation. I took another spoonful, then another, each yielding the same exuberant psychedelia. I waited ten minutes to see whether my stomach would approve, and when it offered no objection, I gave it a handful of Rainier cherries. These, too, were a wonder—every one its own dessert. Thereafter, at intervals of an hour or two, I took a modest helping of fruit or vegetable, and none was less than stupendous in its savor. I capped my resurrective day with a soup of squash and ginger, though it might have been of ambrosia and nectar. My innards felt cautiously content, as when food is finally taken after an illness. By night's end I weighed a tad over 137.

The next day was a family reunion, and I could think of no way to explain to my Appalachian relatives that one of their clan was eating daintily not because he disapproved of the spread but because he was a masochist. So I moved up the food chain and ate a deviled egg. Also potato cream casserole. Also butter-fried okra. There were other coronary and gastric assailants, but they were lost to memory after a few slices of pumpkin pie. I am confident about subsuming the number six in "a few," since any rational response to pumpkin pie would be to eat ten or twelve. My stomach, however, did not respond rationally. It told me I had overdone it well before the scale said so that evening. Specifically, the scale said 140. My abdomen rumbled and gurgled for hours.

A good night's sleep quieted it, and I resumed eating with what an impartial observer might have called abandon. By Tuesday I weighed 142 pounds. At that rate, I calculated, I would weigh 940 on the one-year anniversary of my fast. I returned to clicking X's, at least on the more gluttonous of my desires, and my weight leveled. Only later would I learn how dangerous it had been to put so much food into my fasted body so quickly. Next to what Tanner sent himself, my bill of fare may have been a trifle, but it nonetheless constituted the most perilous part of my feat.

Over the next several years, whenever my girth threatened to expand, I kept it in line with short fasts and such exercise as a bum knee permitted. I did not recidivate. My weight usually stayed around 140. I felt I had unlocked a secret, and with an evangelizing spirit I wrote a long article about my fast, the response to which was gratifying. I anticipated a future in which my health continually improved with occasional fasts, but it didn't work out that way. In fact, my constitution took a turn for the calamitous. Calamity, however, brought more lessons, which have yielded the book in your hands. My loss, I hope, will be your gain.

CHAPTER 5
"THE MOST COMPLICATED CAGE"

In the thirteenth century, there appeared in the sermon of a French priest a tale that perfectly captures the tone of fasting in the Middle Ages, that dim millennium spanning the fifth to fifteenth centuries. In the tale, the monks of a certain monastery were forbidden from eating meat, a ban all the unkinder because to earn their keep, the brothers had to raise pigs that were conveyed to plates not their own. The ban, however, had an exception for hunted beasts, so one day a crafty monk snuck hounds into the pigs' enclosure and in one swift sprint converted the swine to game, thereby legalizing their consumption by the narrowest letter of the law.

Over the course of the Middle Ages, the Church's requirements to fast became so numerous and intrusive that even modest "fasts" like the meatless meals of the monastics sparked evasion. Countless Europeans quietly rebelled. "It is the nature of man," the wise medievalist Bridget Ann Henisch observed half a century ago, "to build the most complicated cage of rules and regulations in which to trap himself, and then, with equal ingenuity and zest, to bend his brain to the problem of wriggling triumphantly out again."

But there was another side to medieval fasting, for while many Christians were wriggling out of their fasts whenever and however they could, a minority were devising ever more savage ways to fast to a righteous reward. Fasting in the Middle Ages is a study of these two poles.

The gentler pole owed a great deal to the Rule of Saint Benedict. From his monastery in the Umbrian hill country in the sixth century, the merciful yet orderly Benedict dusted off the anti-ascetic arguments of earlier thinkers and instructed his monks merely to observe moderation in diet. Only during Lent, Benedict taught, was it imperative to stint on food and drink (as well as sleep, talk, and laughter). His humane principles spread throughout Western monasticism and then spilled beyond the cloister walls. What mattered during a fast, monks taught laypeople, was not the depth of one's deprivation but the degree of repentance in one's heart. They found a willing audience in the many Christians who were put off by the severity of Church fasting.

It's no small irony, then, that fasting, thus tamed, spread even more widely. In many places, to the weekly Wednesday and Friday fasts a Saturday fast was added in homage to Mary and her putative virginity. Fasts also became common before baptisms and communions, on momentous civic occasions, and in the run-up to holy days. For the pious who took fasting seriously, the burden wasn't trivial. In Siena in the High Middle Ages, Saint Martin's Fast ran from the feast of the Holy Cross on September 14 to Saint Martin's Day on November 11, after which there were just a handful of days to bulk up again before plunging into the forty-day Nativity Fast. By one scholarly reckoning, the typical medieval Christian spent no fewer than 220 and perhaps as many as 240 days a year fasting. The most devout marked fast days with only a small amount of bread, salt, and water until vespers, the evening prayers, when they would take the day's single true meal.

But for most people in most places, medieval fasting meant abstaining only from flesh and other products of animals that bred on land—land, because when the God of Genesis discovered Adam and Eve's trespass, he thundered, "Cursed is the ground for thy sake." Fish, free from damnation in their watery habitat, were licit. But because the fast days were so nearly ubiquitous, most people deeply resented even a partial fast, which is one reason Lent in the Middle Ages was kicked off by the world's biggest party, Carnival. The name derives from the Latin *carnem levare*, "the putting away of flesh"—a goodbye to meat.

The Church often turned a blind eye to evasions of fasting, particularly when the evaders wore robes. In many monasteries, the practice of feeding sick monks on fast days in the infirmary evolved until the infirmary itself was declared a fast-free zone for all monks, many of whom dined there whenever they tired of fasting, which was often. The same thing happened with the misericord, an apartment originally set aside for hearty eating during non-fasting times (its name comes from the Latin *misericordia*, "mercy") but which was transformed into a perpetually fast-free haven. In 1287, when the Archbishop of York, John Le Romeyn, called during dinnertime at the monastery at Blyth, he found the refectory, which is to say the dining hall, empty and the entire society devouring forbidden delicacies in the misericord. Six years later, the monks of Malmesbury Abbey in Wiltshire, careful to avoid such a disgrace, drew up a daily rotation under which a quarter of their number dined on meager provisions in the refectory while the other three-quarters ate with abandon elsewhere. So obstinately did monks resist fasting that the practice almost entirely disappeared from certain orders in the early Middle Ages, only to be restored by waves of austere reform in the eleventh and twelfth centuries.

How enthusiastically laypeople took to fasting depended as much on their prosperity as on their piety. During strict fasts like Lent, the wealthy may have obeyed the command to eat fish instead of meat, but they imported species so exotic and garnished them with sauces so decadent, the spirit behind the fast was utterly extinguished. More-plebeian households ate what dainties they could but were more policed, as is suggested by a Lenten law in London in 1417 that forced bakers to stop selling fine breads instead of the coarse loaves that were ecclesiastically preferred. Eventually and notoriously, the Church simply granted dispensations to whoever cared to buy their way out of fasting. Dispensations had appeared in scattered pockets since at least the eighth century and were finally pedaled by itinerant papal agents who worked like traveling salesmen, their stock a biddable salvation. The magnificent Butter Tower of Normandy's Rouen Cathedral was built at the end of the fifteenth century on the profits from dispensations to use butter on fasting days. The poor, of course, could not afford dispensations and chafed under fasting's burden. It was a deep resentment that played no small part in the rise of the Reformation.

*   *   *

In medieval Christianity, fasting became more and more the province of women and girls. Partly that was because a misogynist Church foisted it on them, but it was also because fasting was one of the few ascetic paths open to females. Males of an ascetic bent were free to deny themselves however they wished, including through that most celebrated form of medieval asceticism, mendicancy: wandering from town to town, preaching righteousness and living on alms, just as the Buddha had done fifteen hundred years earlier. The most famous Christian mendicant, Francis of Assisi, was joined on his thirteenth-century vagabonding by a crowd of disciples, but when a count's daughter renounced wealth and a propitious marriage to follow him, Francis forced her into a convent. Much the same happened to other female aspirants across Europe. Homeless meandering, they were told, was unbecoming of sacred womanhood.

Checked but not defeated, the count's daughter, who would become known as Clare of Assisi, turned to fasting. She ate nothing at all on Mondays, Wednesdays, and Fridays and very little on other days. When she became gravely ill, Francis and the bishop of Assisi, who were responsible for the spiritual upkeep of her convent, ordered her to take at least an ounce and a half of bread daily. Clare obeyed, recovered, and became an able prioress who in her later years turned away from the harsh fasting of her youth. The order she founded, the Poor Clares, survives today and like its parent Franciscanism is not known for asceticism. But as happened with Antony the Great and so many others, Clare's followers were less fascinated by her later moderation than by her early self-denial, and they held up as ideal her renunciation of wealth, her unshod feet, the ground she took for a bed, her long bouts of silence, and of course her fasting. Inspired by Clare, virgins across Europe pledged themselves to Christ, noblewomen relinquished palazzi for nunneries, wives forced vows of sexual continence on husbands, and women and girls fasted with a brutal fervor.

History calls the most illustrious of these ascetics the fasting saints. Their masochism knew few limits, for they sought through their suffering to reproduce the sacrifice of Christ and extend its redemptive power. They and many of their followers not only fasted mercilessly but thrust nettles into their breasts, rolled in broken glass, rubbed lice in their wounds, jumped into ovens, and hung themselves from gibbets, to name just the livelier of their holy entertainments. In the early fourteenth century, a nun at an Alsatian convent wrote, "In Advent and Lent, all the sisters . . . hack at themselves cruelly, hostilely lacerating their bodies until the blood flows, with all kinds of whips, so that the sound reverberates all over the monastery and rises to the ears of the Lord of hosts sweeter than all melody."

The indoctrination started frightfully young. From the age of seven to twelve, Benvenuta Bojani, who grew up in Venice in the late thirteenth century, said seventeen hundred Hail Marys and seven hundred Our Fathers every day—a hundred and fifty chants *every waking hour* for five years. From age twelve to nineteen, she wore a hairshirt she never removed, wrapped her hips so tightly with a cord that it became embedded in her skin as she grew (à la Simeon the Stylite), and doused her eyes with vinegar when sleep threatened her nighttime prayers. Each year Benvenuta made several forty-day fasts in which she alternated a day of taking bread and water with a day of eating a single niggardly item. She wrecked her body, died at the age of thirty-eight, and was beatified by the Church five hundred years later. That hers was anybody's idea of a well-lived life is as strong a condemnation of a creed as I can think of.

In all, the Church would sanctify or venerate hundreds of these women, and none was more revered than Catherine of Siena, one of two patron saints of Italy (Francis of Assisi is the other), one of five of all Europe, and for centuries held up as *the* female ideal. Born in 1347, Catherine had her first vision of Jesus at age seven and as a child secretly organized her playmates to flagellate one another with knotted ropes. She first restricted her eating when she was fifteen, pruning her menu to bread, uncooked vegetables, and water. Later she pared this meager diet to what one observer described as "nothing." She attacked her body with other asceticisms appropriate to the aspiring saint, wearing an iron chain that abraded her hips and flagellating herself in three daily bouts of ninety minutes apiece: the first for her own salvation, the second to save the living, the third to redeem the dead.

As an adult, she had no need to eat because, she said, Christ had liberated her from appetite. The circumstances were a shade unusual. The story goes that while Catherine was dressing the suppurating sores of a woman with breast cancer, she gagged at the stench, and to punish herself for her squeamishness, she collected the woman's pus in a ladle and drank it. "Never in my life," she enthused, "have I tasted any food or drink sweeter or more exquisite." That night Jesus came to her in a dream and praised her for going "far beyond what mere human nature could ever have achieved." Tenderly he pulled her head to his pierced side and let her drink the blood from his wound, after which she was relieved of her "gluttony." Never again would she need food, although she sometimes ate a little to appease worriers.

This madness seems to have appalled her wealthy family, who saw the chances for a good marriage vanishing with each new mortification—which might have been one of Catherine's motives. Certainly many other fasting saints intuited that their body was their only lever of power, and they used their asceticism to escape marriage or bully impious parents to greater devotion. Whatever Catherine's motives, her dietary and other assaults deprived her of half her weight, which could only have pleased her. Christians, she said, should have a "holy hatred" of themselves, and she condemned her body a "dung heap." Her mind was the apex creation of Philo, Paul, and Jerome, her fasting the epitome of everything that had gone off the beam in Christianity for women.

Catherine was formidably charismatic. Her innumerable lay followers believed her torments redeemed the world, and her guidance was sought by counts and countesses, kings and queens, and more than one pope. The tone she took with them was supremely, one might say shockingly, self-assured. In her letters, Pope Gregory XI was not "Your Holiness" but *Babbo*, "Daddy," and her exhortations to him—"Don't be afraid! Do something about it," "Be a courageous man for me, not a coward"—still make startling reading. Medieval women simply did not speak to men of authority in such terms. Gregory may well have been in awe of Catherine, and he certainly consulted her on matters large and small, possibly including his epochal decision to return the papacy from Avignon to Rome. He deputized her his ambassador in a dispute among unruly Tuscans, and she propagandized forcefully for his crusade of 1374.

After the eruption of the Western Schism—a nasty period of warfare among rival popes—Catherine fell into a deep depression and on New Year's Day of 1380 began a fast to expiate the sins of the Church. A month into it, she suffered a total collapse, possibly falling into a coma, and although she briefly revived, she never fully recovered. Her previous long fasts and malnutrition had probably destroyed what reserves she had. Three months later in Rome she died, only thirty-three. In her short life, and on the strength of severe fasting and force of character, she had exercised more power than almost any other woman of her era.

There was an aftermath to the story of Catherine, who in death was cleaved and sliced. Most of her ended up in Rome, a few fingers and a foot went to Venice, a rib was taken to Florence, and her head returned home to Siena. The head can still be seen today in the Basilica of Saint Dominic in all its ghoulishness, the eye sockets sunken and nose all but gone, half the teeth on walkabout, the skin yellowed and shriveled (but perhaps neither so yellow nor so shriveled as one might expect after six and a half centuries). The faithful believe these macabre relics heal. Even in death, Catherine's sacrificial body redeems.

*   *   *

The story of the fasting saints will sound familiar to many of us: the adolescent girls and young women (almost never boys or men) who rebel against family or society by asserting extreme control over their bodies, the irrationality with which they view their physique, the emaciation that tends ever to destruction. These are, of course, the traits of modern anorexia nervosa, and where detailed accounts of the saints' lives exist, we find they also shared other attributes with today's anorectics, like hyperactivity, insomnia, and euphoria. Historians call the medieval condition *anorexia mirabilis*, holy anorexia.

But while the similarities are marked, the two conditions are not the same. Each is a product of its age, the gulf between them wide. Generally speaking, the modern nervous anorectic starves herself because if thin is beautiful, skeletal must be gorgeous. The holy anorectic emaciated herself to save humankind and glorify God. Both are ill, but the modern sufferer has been made so by societal narcissism, a worship of the body beautiful and sexual allure, while the medieval sufferer was deranged by a misguided religious loathing of everything corporeal, especially the body sexual.

The harm from anorexia mirabilis, which for centuries was almost a requisite of female sanctity and thus part of the female ideal, was immense. In one study of the 261 Italian women whom the Church recognized over eight centuries as either saints, blesseds, venerables, or servants of God, more than half showed unmistakable signs of anorexia. Christianity's veneration of self-abuse may have been an understandable error of a dark age, but the modern Church's refusal to acknowledge or atone for its devotion to masochism is damning. It is, of course, of a piece with that institution's abiding misogyny.

*   *   *

Not until the great awakening of the Enlightenment would reason finally cripple ascetic fasting. The first stirrings of change were the watches that cropped up at irregular intervals to verify whether miraculous fasters were in fact miraculously fasting. One of the earliest took place in England in 1225, when Hugh of Wells, Bishop of Lincoln, appointed fifteen clergymen to observe a nun in Leicester who had supposedly lived seven years on nothing but the Host. Unfortunately for rationalism, after a fortnight Hugh's delegates deemed the fast legitimate, and Hugh gave it a bishoply thumbs-up. Watches in subsequent centuries were often equally credulous, but little by little they turned up fraud, although just as often they concluded the faster was a witch. Witches had a nefariously practical motive to fast: they needed to be light enough to fly (brooms as locomotion came later), which was the reason for the infamous municipal scales that determined whether a woman weighed less than she ought. Inquisitors often rigged the scales, but in the seventeenth century the enlightened Dutch town of Oudewater made it known that any woman who stood upon its balance would be given a document declaring her mass in correct proportion to her size. Many a frightened woman traveled to Oudewater to be certified a muggle, and visitors today can still weigh themselves in the town Heksenwaag, or Witches' Weighhouse.

As more and more purported fasting saints were exposed as frauds, they came to be seen less as religious or supernatural phenomena than psychological cases. Doctors replaced inquisitors, and many were extraordinarily compassionate. In 1573, the Dutchman Johann Weyer, personal physician to the German Duke William, gently exposed the fraudulence of a supposedly long-fasting ten-year-old named Barbara Kremers. Barbara's abstinence had been vouched for by her family and the town council of Unna, and the enraged duke was inclined to a medieval punishment for the lot of them. But Weyer convinced him the girl was too young to be held responsible, the parents were not in on the ruse, and everyone should be let off with a light reprimand. The duke eventually settled for chiding the councilors for idiocy. (Barbara, the little ingrate, later claimed her fasting had in fact been real but that Weyer had given her a potion that restored her appetite.)

By the eighteenth century, so many "miraculous" fasts had been exposed as hoaxes that the Church mostly stopped canonizing fasting saints. But not entirely. As recently as 2004, Pope John Paul II beatified the Portuguese mystic Alexandrina Maria da Costa, who was said to have lived thirteen years in the early twentieth century on no food but the Eucharist. Even today, partisans of Therese Neumann, a German mystic, occasionally lobby the Vatican for her canonization. Neumann claimed to have taken no food or liquid but the Sacrament for nearly four decades before her death in 1962, yet she was rotund, suffered from angina, and died of cardiac arrest—tokens that in ordinary mortals would suggest an overly rich diet, which may be why the Holy See has given no sign her sanctification is imminent. Apparently even the Vatican will buy only so much.

*   *   *

Not many people fasted in the Middle Ages in search of health. "A diet attempted for any reason other than spiritual improvement," Professor Henisch wrote, "and in particular for such irrelevancies as health and beauty, was nothing but a mockery." One of the mockers was the author of the late-medieval sermons known as *Jacob's Well*, who declared, "If thou faste after fysyk, . . . yet schalt thou dye for all that phisyk." But the anonymous preacher's need to say so suggested at least a few people were indeed fasting for phisyk.

They were encouraged by a vanishingly small number of thinkers, one of whom was Hildegard of Bingen, a German abbess of the twelfth century who had a scientifically inclined mind in an unscientific age. Hildegard wrote two treatises on medicine that, along with other works, earned her posthumous commendation as a Doctor of the Church, one of only four women whom Church fathers have ever deemed fit for the title. She recommended a partial fast on spelt, vegetables, and fruit as both a preventive and a restorative, although her motives were as spiritual as medical. Only modestly followed in her time, Hildegard has enjoyed a productive posterity with multiple revivals of her teachings over the last two centuries. Today several German fasting centers offer a "Hildegard Fast," sometimes amid a spa-like decadence that would have appalled the restrained abbess.

At the University of Paris, Hildegard's contemporary Alain de Lille, a theologian, also counseled fasting for health. "Fast is medicine to soul and body," he wrote. "It preserves the body from disease, the soul from sin. About its medicinal effects, earthly and heavenly philosophy agree." But Alain didn't elaborate much further, and ultimately you have to rake a pretty fine comb through the medieval literature to find more than the odd tract in praise of therapeutic fasting. That, however, was about to change, thanks to Martin Luther and a plate of sausages.

* * *

The seeds of the Reformation had been sprouting around Europe even before Luther, and widespread resentment of fasting was one of the more productive germs. In fourteenth-century England, for example, a movement known as Lollardism flourished in opposition to the corrupt priesthood and the nauseating wealth of the Church, and one way the Lollards showed their defiance was by eating meat on fast days, including during that most sacrosanct time of year, Lent. By 1517, when Luther circulated his ninety-five hesitations about Church doctrine (probably not, alas, nailing them to the church door—such are the disappointments of history), a rebellion against fasting was already well rooted.

Luther's polite theses hardly addressed fasting, but he soon became more strident and on fasting could be withering. He acknowledged that fasts were useful tools to subdue pride and lust, but he argued it was entirely up to the individual to fast or not. The Church's ubiquitous fast days and elaborate fasting rules, he said, were dictates of man, not scripture, and had become as ludicrous as the Old Testament food regulations that Jesus swept away. He denounced Rome for making people more afraid of wholesome foods like butter than real sinning and for selling indulgences that turned their fear into an unholy profit for Church fathers who didn't even believe in the sanctity of fasting: "At Rome they themselves laugh at the fasts, making us foreigners eat the oil with which they would not grease their shoes, and afterward selling us liberty to eat butter."

Luther's writings imperiled Christian fasting, but the truly telling blow was landed at a feast in Zurich during Lent of 1522, when a printer named Christoph Froschauer sat down with his workers to a plate of sausages. Haled before the city's magistrates for heresy, Froschauer pled not guilty on grounds he and his crew needed meat's nourishment for their heavy work. The magistrates replied that he should have applied for a dispensation, which the Church sometimes granted for hard labor—for a price, of course. The ruling sparked riots and street fighting, and in the end the local bishop, Ulrich Zwingli, preached one of the most important sermons of the Reformation. Zwingli agreed with Luther that the

Church had no right to ban food and that the choice to fast lay in the conscience of the individual, but he went further by declaring that fasting amounted to class warfare. The rich, he said, were hardly inconvenienced by fasting, what with their lavish dishes of exotic fish and easily obtained dispensations. But to the commoner, unable to buy the right to eat butter and forced to subsist on meager vegetables, fasting was a hardship of unsustainable proportion. Zwingli's sermon was a stake through the breast of religious fasting.

With dizzying swiftness, several Reformed Churches—the Swiss, Dutch, Scottish, Huguenot, and Puritan—abolished not only the Lenten fast but the other annual fasts and the station fasts on Wednesday, Friday, and Saturday. Some Protestant churches were less thorough. Calvinism, for instance, allowed communal fasts in times of great public distress like war. In these preservationist sects, the rules governing fasting and the fasts themselves steadily multiplied until they once again resembled the elaborately contrived Catholic practice that Luther and Zwingli rejected. In 1662, a century and a half into the Reformation, the Anglican Book of Common Prayer marked off more than half the days of the year for fasting, and only several groundswells of reform whittled them back down.

The British government put its own spin on the communal fast by secularizing it and proclaiming national days of prayer and fasting as need arose. (The idea had precedent, Charlemagne having done the same as early as 793 after a revolt by his excellently named but disrespectful son Pippin the Hunchback.) The peak of British civic fasting came in the 1640s and 1650s during and after the Civil War, when more than 130 days of what might be called crisis fasting were imposed. Afterward, such fasts were all but abandoned, but to keep the fishing fleet afloat on the sale of fast-day fish, the government continued to decree regular fast days until 1856, when the fleet fasts were finally stricken from the statute books.

The colonists from England who crossed the North Atlantic brought their fasting with them. In the earliest days of Plymouth, during a drought in 1623, the governor appointed July 16 a day of humiliation and prayer, and the rain fell in sheets. Other colonies followed suit, and over the next 130 years New Englanders observed seven hundred days of fasting and humiliation. With the American Revolution in the balance, General George Washington proclaimed May 6, 1779, a day of fasting, humiliation, and prayer, and after a string of resounding defeats to the Confederates, Abraham Lincoln called for one on April 30, 1863. The civic fast days were always shamelessly religious, usually marked with two church services and no food till late afternoon, separation of church and state be damned.

The civic fasts lingered long in America. Massachusetts didn't abolish its annual fast until 1894, and as late as the First World War President Woodrow Wilson proclaimed a national day of "public humiliation, prayer, and fasting" in which he exhorted his fellow citizens to "pray Almighty God that He may forgive our sins and shortcomings as a people and purify our hearts." Only after the Great War did civic fasting wither. There was, however, a succedaneum during the Red Scare, when jingoism against godless Communism ran high and Harry Truman signed into law an annual patriotic piety fest known as the National Day of Prayer (albeit without a call to fast), which survives today.

In Catholicism, fasting of course persisted longer. Voltaire, bridling under the French Church, issued the same complaint in the eighteenth century that Zwingli had lodged two centuries before: "The rich Papist who has five hundred francs' worth of fish on his table shall be saved, and the poor wretch dying of hunger who has eaten four sous' worth of salt pork shall be damned." But even in Voltaire's day Catholic fasting was on the wane. The Reformation had forced reforms on the Church, which tacitly acknowledged the absurdity of its fasting requirements by dropping them one by one. By the mid-twentieth century the calendars in most Catholic homes were no more blighted by ascetic fasting than those of their Protestant neighbors. After two long millennia, fasting was dead in Christendom in all but name.

* * *

But the fasting saints didn't quite vanish. Instead, between the sixteenth and eighteenth centuries, they underwent a secularization and emerged on the other side as fasting maids. Usually girls and young women, the maids only infrequently cited divine inspiration for their prolonged fasts and did not intend to inspire others to follow in their ascetic footsteps. Fame, not redemption, was their motivation. In the increasingly scientific age, they occasioned vigorous debate over how they could survive without food. Some Renaissance writers thought they lived off their own melancholic fluids, while others credited their menses, which were supposed to nourish a fetus during pregnancy and might do the same for an anatomically versatile maid. Still others thought they were sustained by tobacco smoke. One doctor in the 1820s suggested the Italian maid Anna Garbero survived her fast of two years by pulling nutrients through the air from the sister with whom she slept, which was why the sister lost weight during Anna's fast. Only occasionally did someone propose that the girls, to the extent they really did fast, lived off their own stored fat.

Despite their regular exposure as frauds, the maids persisted through the whole of the nineteenth century thanks to the clash between reason and faith. Religious minds were deeply troubled by the Enlightenment turn toward science and the scrutinous eye cast on the more outlandish claims of scripture. When rationalists declared miracles the fantasies of benighted intellects, some Christians latched on to the fasting maids as proof miracles still existed. But each new exposure of a fraudulent maid gave rationalists yet more delightful evidence that miracles had been hornswoggle all along.

The dispute culminated in tragedy in Wales in 1869. Its principal victim was Sarah Jacob, who at just twelve years old was about to become history's foremost fasting maid. Two years earlier, after a mysterious illness, Sarah supposedly stopped eating and drinking. Neither she nor her family publicized her fast, but the village vicar eventually alerted the press to the miracle, which must have been miraculous indeed, for visitors to the Jacobs' rude farmhouse—the cattle lodged at one end, the family at the other—described her as plump. Thousands made the trek, and at train time village boys hung about the station with signs on their caps reading "To the Fasting Girl."

The London medical establishment was quick to declare the fast an impossibility, which brought Christians rallying to Sarah's corner, and after many spirited aspersions, the Royal Colleges of Physicians and Surgeons dispatched four nurses from London to rigorously watch the girl. So fascinated were Britons that great crowds gathered at train stations just to get a glimpse of the nurses as they passed through to the Welsh village.

The nurses discovered almost immediately that Sarah was staining her bedclothes with urine and feces, and within days—no doubt her first without food or liquid—her health faltered. But the cold charge to the nurses from the royal collegians was not to interfere with the fast. Medicine would have its answer. As Sarah's health continued to deteriorate, she refused to admit sneaking food and drink, and her simple parents believed utterly in the miraculousness of their honest daughter. No one intervened, and after just nine days Sarah was dead, likely of thirst.

Her death was an enormous scandal on both sides of the Atlantic, with neither gullible Christianity nor indifferent Medicine flattered by the attention. This was the backdrop to the feud that erupted ten years later between the Brooklyn fasting clairvoyant Mollie Fancher and her would-be inquisitor Dr. William Hammond. Hammond had earlier been so incensed that anyone could fall for such tosh that he wrote a book called *Fasting Girls: Their Physiology and Pathology*. But the fundamentalist impulse is well fortified against reason, and belief in Fancher survived long after the controversy with Hammond was forgotten. (Henry Tanner's forty-day fast only encouraged Fancher's admirers.) In 1916, nearly four decades later, President Wilson sent Fancher, who was still claiming to live on little more than air, his regrets at being unable to attend a gala she was throwing on the fiftieth anniversary of the onset of her supernatural powers.

* * *

The resurrection of reason during the Renaissance brought the return, for the first time in a thousand years, of deep interest in therapeutic fasting. The chief revivalist was an Italian who made his fortune turning the marshes around Venice into farmlands before writing a winsome tract explaining how he had achieved lasting health and others could too. Alvise Cornaro's *Discourses on the Sober Life*, as the final edition was called, was an instant success from its first printing in 1588 and remained popular for centuries. George Washington wrote approvingly of the *Discourses* in an introduction to a 1799 edition, and at one English press in the eighteenth and nineteenth centuries the book went through fifty printings.

As a young man, Cornaro had lived high, eating and drinking with abandon, and had fallen prey to gout, arthritis, abdominal pains, and a nearly continual low fever. By thirty-five he developed "a perpetual thirst" and reacted poorly to simple sugars—telltale signs of type 2 diabetes. (According to one biographer, Cornaro may be history's first victim of diabetes whose name we know.) His doctors recommended many cures, all but one of which he tried, none with success. The one he rejected was temperance, but as he neared forty his doctors said if he didn't forsake gluttony he would surely be dead in months, and he grudgingly changed his meals from a baron's bacchanal to a pauper's pittance. To his everlasting astonishment, he felt better within days, and in less than a year every one of his former complaints disappeared.

Many a man, having achieved such a cure, would have returned to his old habits, at least to a degree, but Cornaro reasoned that if temperance had healed him, shouldn't it also maintain him in health and perhaps even add to his years? He experimented with which food and drink most agreed with his stomach and gradually removed everything that gave him grief. Yet the most striking change to his repasts was to their size. As he wrote in the *Discourses*, "I accustomed myself to the habit of never fully satisfying my appetite, either with eating or drinking, always leaving the table well able to take more." Each day he ate precisely twelve ounces of food and washed it down with fourteen ounces—about a cup and three-quarters—of young white wine. This was caloric restriction of a fairly substantial order, probably no more than 1,500 to 1,700 total calories a day, but his health went from strength to strength. He had stumbled on what he believed was a principle of well-being applicable to everyone: "to be satisfied with little . . . and to accustom ourselves to eat nothing but that which is necessary to sustain life."

He proselytized to his friends, who repaid him with the proselyte's due of indifference, and when they began dying one by one, he wrote the *Discourses* to spare others their fate. It's a jubilant and triumphal tale in which the protagonist's good health remains a wonder into his elderhood through tribulations small and large. When Cornaro was perhaps sixty, for example, his carriage overturned and he was dragged by his horses. His doctors gave him up for dead, too old to rally from his broken bones and internal wounds, but, as he wrote, "I entirely recovered—a thing, which, while fulfilling my own expectations, seemed to my doctors nothing less than miraculous." In his telling, the only time he became seriously ill was when he gave in to the worry of friends and family and upped his ration of food and drink by a few ounces a day. He recuperated from the ensuing sickness by scaling back his daily board once more.

Cornaro was hardly the first person to preach temperance for health, but what was new, as the Italian philologist Marisa Milani wrote, "is the confident and conversational way [his ideas] are expressed. And what is inspired is the way in which the author offers himself up as an indisputable example of what he believes." The *Discourses* also broke new ground by challenging the Galenic belief that the number and quality of one's years were largely determined by the strong or weak constitution one was born with. Simply by reforming one's habits, Cornaro said, even the sickliest person could live to a healthy seniority. "Cornaro is not the first to establish the end for a human life at a century or beyond," Milani wrote, "but he is the first to hold that it may be achieved by any man." It must have been quite empowering in that fatalistic age to be told you were not Fortune's plaything, that your health was to a degree in your own hands—and so much the better to hear it in a style that ran from endearing to mischievous. Here, for instance, is how Cornaro answered the most common objection to his program: "Others insist that it is far better to live ten years fewer, rather than to deprive oneself of the pleasure of gratifying the appetite. To this, I would say that men endowed with fine talents ought to prize a long life very highly. For the balance, it matters little that they do not value it; and, as they only make the world less beautiful, it is as well, perhaps, that they should die."

It's such a disarming package that we can almost forgive the old scamp for exaggerating his age. To bolster his case, Cornaro set his birthday further in the past than it really was and moved it further back with each new edition. By the time he died in 1566, he was said to have been either 102 or 104, although in fact he was no more than 83—a fine run for the era but hardly miraculous. His supposed centenarianism nonetheless stuck in the public imagination and earned him a place over the centuries as a paragon of longevity.

You will have noticed that Cornaro's philosophy of frugality did not require fasting. In fact, he referred to it only infrequently, albeit approvingly, as when he wrote, "Nature, being desirous to preserve man as long as possible, teaches him what rule to follow in time of illness; for she immediately deprives the sick of their appetite in order that they may eat but little." Nonetheless, advocates of fasting would soon adopt his idea that self-denial strengthened rather than weakened the body, and to this day his accessible, self-experimental style serves abstentious writers well. The door Cornaro swung open nearly half a millennium ago has yet to swing closed.

*   *   *

A handful of writers after Cornaro argued that to live long and vigorously, we should not only walk away from the table hungry but should now and then make a short fast. Francis Bacon, lord chancellor of England and noted expositor of empiricism (the idea that knowledge comes mainly from sensory experience), took up the refrain in his 1638 treatise *The Historie of Life and Death. With Observations Naturall and Experimentall for the Prolonging of Life*. Bacon endorsed temperance when in health and fasting when not. Writing that "sick folks can easily fast," he urged a partial fast that "makes patients very lean, by consuming the moisture of their body; which being restored again, they become strong and lusty." But he feared a healthy body could scarce endure fasting three days together, and warned, "Fasting often is bad for long life."

Increasingly, though, writers thought fasting while in health a requisite for keeping it. Sir William Temple, another English statesman and essayist, reprised antiquity's John Chrysostom when he argued "health and long life are usually blessings of the poor, not of the rich, and the fruits of temperance rather than of luxury and excess. And, indeed, if a rich man does not in many things live like a poor, he will certainly be the worse for his riches ... If he does not practice sometimes even abstinence and fasting, which is the last extreme of want and poverty ... he will certainly impair in health whilst he improves his fortunes, and lose more than he gains by the bargain." A tad ironically, these observations appeared in Temple's "Of Health and Long Life," published in 1699 after his death at the age of seventy.

Doctors weighed in too. Fasting writers today are wont to credit the sixteenth-century Swiss Paracelsus as the first modern doctor to understand fasting, but Paracelsus's views on the subject were religious and entirely conventional, and the quotation everywhere attributed to him—"Fasting is the greatest remedy, the physician within"—is another raw fiction. The first doctor of the scientific age who saw fasting for the therapy it was, was probably the Frenchman Jean Fernel, a contemporary of Paracelsus and Cornaro. As a young man, Fernel was a mathematician and astronomer, but to support his family he forsook those unprofitable pursuits and became one of France's most sought-after physicians, once treating the randy King Francis I for syphilis.

Fernel argued that fasting cured illness as well as bloodletting did—high praise for a Galenic doctor—and that in at least one respect fasting was even niftier than opening veins, "for it works gently and without any violent forcing of the body or the humors." To Fernel's eyes, fasting succeeded best against "light diseases," particularly when caught early, but even diseases "inveterate and old, it does mitigate." His ideas about why fasting worked were hopelessly entangled with Galen's humoralism, but even so, many of his observations and speculations were on the right track. He believed, for example, that when food "is either in part or in whole withdrawn from the body, so that there is want of it, then our inbred heat ... being not encumbered by the abundance of new meat, everywhere exercising its own force, grows strong." The native heat, thus strengthened, burned some tissues and turned others into substances "fit for nourishing the body . . . By these means, the whole body is eased, being disburdened as it were of its load, the breathing is made free and easy, the mind and all the senses become more ready and cheerful." This is, very roughly, what happens during a fast, as old and damaged cellular parts are broken down and either jettisoned or recycled for use in new structures.

Fernel was smart enough not to paint fasting as free of cost. He wrote, accurately enough, that "in a corrupt body, most commonly it fills the belly with ill humors: whence come gnawing of the stomach, insomnia, disturbances of the body, and giddiness or vertigo in the head . . . But those disturbed humors at last it subdues, tames, and dries out: whereupon follows great tranquility, and assuaging of diseases and many symptoms." Fasting's price, in short, was one well worth paying. Unfortunately, Fernel wrote in Latin, wasn't widely read, and today is remembered mostly for coining the term "physiology" and for giving us the earliest description of the spinal canal. Astronomers know him for the lunar crater that bears his Latinized name, Fernelius.

Not until 1719, nearly two centuries after Fernel, did an extended exposition of therapeutic fasting finally emerge—the first in fifteen hundred years and arguably the smartest thing yet written on the topic. Its author was the German Friedrich Hoffmann, one of the most widely read physicians of his time, called by admirers (a touch excitedly, it must be said) "the second Hippocrates." Hoffmann was the first professor at the medical school of the University of Halle and for a time was physician to the Prussian king Friedrich Wilhelm I. Posterity preserves him for his research into the healing powers of mineral waters and for a theory of the body that, while flawed (he thought it was a kind of hydraulic machine), nevertheless helped shove medicine off the reef of Galenic humoralism where it had so long ago run aground. Among Hoffmann's four hundred publications was a nine-volume work on how to live a long and healthy life, and in its fifth volume appeared the chapter "Introducing the Magnificent Benefits of the So-called Hunger Cure."

Given that its author had no science to go on, "Magnificent Benefits" was an impressively perceptive look at therapeutic fasting. So little had medicine progressed since antiquity that Hoffmann repeatedly and deferentially cited Hippocrates and the savvy Roman encyclopedist Aulus Cornelius Celsus (whom you may recall from chapter 3 describing primitive plastic surgery with skin grafts and calling for fasts at the onset of illness). But Hoffmann wasn't just retreading the arguments of others. He was also a discerning observer, and his guiding observation was of a piece with Cornaro's: "Indulgence in even the best and healthiest foods is a true plague for the human race." Where latter-day Cornarans like Bacon and Temple made only modest nods to fasting, Hoffmann saw fasting in Fernel's terms, as a tool to be fully embraced. He was motivated in part by a problem that had long bedeviled medical practice: when a doctor was summoned to the sickbed, the patient expected to receive medicine, which the doctor all too readily gave, even though the medicine of the day generally hurt more than helped. But Hoffmann noticed that when an ailing body was left untreated, it often healed itself and, what was more, fasting could speed the process. Unfortunately, his patients felt ill used for their fee if he directed them not to visit the apothecary but to abstain from food. What they really wanted, much like patients today, was a pill or potion that would let them keep eating as profligately as ever. "This plague is so widespread," he lamented, "that there is little hope of exterminating it."

But that didn't stop him from trying, including by singing fulsome praises of fasting. Elaborating on Fernel, he wrote, "Many grave and serious illnesses have been so happily cured [by fasting] that one is amazed at the remarkable ways which nature implements for healing; no doctor in the world would have thought of this. This is all the more praiseworthy because the fasting cure is much safer and gentler than cures with artificial herbs, which often attack and cause something completely different than you would like." Hoffmann also improved on Fernel's claim that fasting was good for "light diseases" by explaining it was most effective against ailments caused by overeating, which was why stomach troubles so often resolved with a fast. Fasting worked, he speculated, as a kind of "universal laxative, removing all excess and all unclean juices." It thinned the blood and unclogged the lymphatic channels and excretory ducts, which in turn led to cures of dropsy (edema), jaundice, and gout. Similar mechanisms were probably behind fasting's relief of skin problems, coughs, runny noses, fever ("no other remedy works so promptly and reliably for fever as fasting"), and even some nervous disorders. He also noted—marveled really—that livers and spleens long hardened by profligate living could be made soft again by fasting. Any fasting doctor today would vouch for most of his claims, and we have the science to back several of them.

Hoffmann knew people would resist so deeply counterintuitive a therapy as fasting. How often, he complained, had he seen a sick man's body command him not to eat by removing his appetite, only to have friends force food on him, which "harms the patient more than the disease itself." And sure enough, over the next two centuries, few doctors in Germany even referred to "Magnificent Benefits," let alone applied its principles, and outside Germany it was hardly referred to at all. But Hoffmann's ideas were kept on a thin life support down the years by the odd German fasting doctor, and when fasting revived in the early twentieth century, "Magnificent Benefits" was retrieved from history's dustbin and published as a pamphlet that helped turn Germany into the world's leader in therapeutic fasting—not the worst return for two hundred years of wandering in the intellectual wilderness.

Hoffmann's insightful observations about fasting were a signpost of sorts. Behind lay superstition and irrationality, ahead modernity and reason. It wasn't a clean break, but the trajectory was unmistakable, and over the next two centuries fasting would be ever more astutely observed, desacralized, and medicalized, and nowhere more so than in the New World.

CHAPTER 6

"THIS CHEAP, SIMPLE, AND VULGAR REMEDY"

Of the many and varied things that could kill an early American, one of the more common and most feared was infectious scourge. Measles, malaria, influenza, and dysentery carried off colonials by the thousand. Smallpox alone dispatched at least 130,000 during the Revolutionary War, twenty times more than were felled by British muskets. After independence, the most terrifying pestilence of them all, yellow fever, laid waste to cities up and down the eastern seaboard. Philadelphia, then the nation's capital, was literally decimated in 1793, five thousand of the city's fifty thousand inhabitants succumbing to the fever. Half the survivors fled. (There was grim justice in this: yellow fever had come to the New World with mosquitos on slave ships whose other live cargo helped the urban ports prosper.) The epidemics exposed how little physicians knew about disease, and their ignorance prompted three New York doctors to found the country's first medical journal, the *Medical Repository*, in 1797. The trio were also concerned that much of the medical theory of the day was as unmoored from reality as the Galenism it had replaced, and they intended to publish clear-eyed observations from ordinary practitioners. One such observance in the journal's second number was the first essay on therapeutic fasting in America. The weighty question its author, Edward Miller, sought to answer was whether fasting might combat various fevers, yellow or otherwise.

Miller was one of the *Repository*'s founders, and he began his appraisal with appropriate skepticism. Fasting for illness, he said, had sometimes been commended "in stronger terms than it would be proper here to repeat, and, perhaps, stronger than the reality of the case can justify." And yet given "the number, sagacity, and concurrence of the observers" and the sundry illnesses they claimed fasting healed, he proposed to give the therapy the benefit of the doubt. He hypothesized that fasting worked by the same curative mechanism that the Frenchman Jean Fernel and the German Friedrich Hoffmann had supposed, although he was apparently unaware of their writings on fasting. To eat during certain illnesses, Miller wrote, was "fraught with mischievous consequences" because food "added to the morbid stimuli" of disease. "Tottering under its present load, the system is forced to sustain new burdens," and the stomach, already taxed as the first line of defense against many pathogens, was too encumbered to fend off all of them. But "by abstinence that organ is enabled to maintain a more vigorous combat; to rally all its forces; and, finally, by dint of habit, to disarm the noxious intruder." In a novel (and, as it turned out, correct) insight, he added that although the fast itself might be potent, its curative power surely also came from the post-fast refeeding, which needed to be attended with care.

As his predecessors had, Miller praised fasting as gentler and safer than bloodletting, emetics, and purgatives and for not requiring doctors to match specific drugs to individual illnesses. (These were the days when the word *specific* was a synonym for "remedy.") Fasting, Miller said, was a *general* palliative, with "the rare advantage of being adapted to obviate the approach, or, at least, to abate the violence, of almost all acute diseases." His caution was laudable. He didn't promise fasting would cure acute illness, only that it would lessen its severity, and he made no claims for chronic diseases like cancer or tuberculosis. Still, Miller was so impressed by his survey of fasting that "if it were possible to offer to mankind a maxim of universal application to the treatment of incipient fevers," his would be *"abstain, for a proper length of time, from all aliment."* The proper length, he believed, was a few days, advice remarkably similarly to that of the Roman Methodists and the ancient encyclopedist Aulus Cornelius Celsus.

Miller's shrewdness and restraint, alas, made little impression on his medical brethren. In subsequent years almost no one referred to his essay, and he himself didn't return to the subject at any length before his death in

1812. Six years after his departure, a Quaker apothecary named Cornelius Blatchly, who had grown up fasting, wrote an essay in the *Repository* bemoaning that Miller's attempt to revive "this cheap, simple, and vulgar remedy" had been ignored, but Blatchly's elegy met the same fate. It was an inauspicious start for therapeutic fasting in America.

* * *

In the summer of 1815, nearly twenty years after Miller's essay, a young physician in Trumbull, Connecticut, had the sort of encounter with a headstrong patient that doctors have every day without sparing it a second thought but that in this case set Isaac Jennings to rethinking his entire trade. Jennings's town-and-country district was beset that summer by a fever, and the patient in question was a Mr. J. P. After confirming Mr. P.'s fever, Jennings reached for his saddlebags to retrieve medicine, but his patient stayed his hand and said he needed no specific just now, though he would let Jennings know if the fever grew worse. Jennings remonstrated with him, explaining his illness was serious, but Mr. P. was stubborn as a New England moose, and Jennings at last let him be, no doubt confident the man would send for him in a day or two.

A few days later, Jennings was riding his circuit and was taken aback to find Mr. P. hard at work in a lot. The young doctor hopped down from his horse and asked what had come of the fever. "To my surprise," Jennings wrote many years later, "I found that he had recovered entirely from his indisposition. . . . All that he had done was to keep quiet, refrain from eating while his appetite was lacking, and drinking freely of cold water as long as his febrile thirst called for it." Of the many cases of fever Jennings attended that summer, "in no instance had one recovered in so short a time, or with so mild a set of symptoms."

Mr. P.'s spiffing recuperation prompted Jennings to ask two entwined questions: Was it better *not* to treat certain illnesses than to treat them with medicines? And if so, when his medicines had previously cured patients—"for I seldom made a prescription without seeing, or fancying I saw good results: and my patients and their friends were satisfied, yea more than satisfied with my practice"—were doctor, patient, and friends fooling themselves that the medicine had chased away the sickness?

Jennings was not alone in stoking such revolutionary embers. One of his mentors, a Dr. Tisdale of Bridgeport, said to him not long after Mr. P.'s recovery, "Jennings, do you know that we don't do as much good with medicine as we have supposed that we did?"

Jennings allowed the possibility.

"Are you aware," Tisdale went on, "that we do a great deal more hurt than good with medicine?"

Jennings said he wasn't prepared to go quite so far as that.

But he would get there after another noteworthy case, seven years later, during a typhus outbreak in Derby, the seat of his new practice. Nine members of a family named French were stricken, and Mrs. French was in a desperate way, with "most distressing and alarming symptoms," like vomiting geysers whenever she ate or drank. As her condition became ominous, Jennings called on a host of medicines to calm her stomach, all in vain, which in hindsight is unsurprising since the nostrums of the day were usually ineffective unless they generated a placebo effect. Mrs. French's nurse told Jennings nothing stayed on the poor woman's stomach save cold water direct from the well, and those words determined him on an experiment. He went to a nearby spring, filled an empty medicine vial with water, and told the nurse to give Mrs. French nothing but the new elixir and as much cold well water as she wanted. When he came back that night, the nurse beamed and said, "You have at last hit upon the right medicine!" Mrs. French's stomach was becalmed, her geysers quelled, and in a few days the fever was gone.

From that moment, Jennings decided to give the same "medicine" to all of his other typhus patients. "And I had no cause to regret what some would call my temerity," he wrote, "for not one of the many cases that were under my direction that season proved fatal, though a number, to appearance, went to the border of the grave and returned."

Thereafter Jennings reduced his armamentarium to a few vials of water and bread pills that he dyed and flavored to resemble medicines. These he gave to sufferers of all kinds of disease with the advice to eat nothing and drink only water. He was more than a little uneasy applying his experiment so broadly, for, as he wrote, "I was now afloat on the broad sea of anti-medical empiricism, without chart, compass or pole-star to guide me." But time and again he and his patients landed in a safe harbor. Almost always the ill seemed to fare better under his "let-alone principle" than under his previous interventionist methods, and he concluded that mankind's long quest to conquer disease—"the combined expedition of medicine of all ages, all countries, and of all descriptions"—was in fact "the most tremendous and tragical Quixotic movement that had ever been engaged in by deluded mortals." The body, he believed, could often heal itself if medicine would only get out of the way, and when the body wasn't up to the job, the humbuggery of medicine could rarely do better.

For several years Jennings said nothing of his deception because "the public were not prepared for my views." But he was too honest a fellow to keep up the ruse indefinitely—"His uprightness and integrity commanded universal respect," Derby's town historians would write—and finally he disclosed his method to his patients. So certain was he the townsfolk would rise against him, he first arranged for another doctor to take over his practice, but the people of Derby took his benevolent subterfuge exceptionally well, and in the coming years many accepted his counsel to fast when sick.

Eventually he left Derby for Oberlin, Ohio, known then for progressive ideas about health. There he wrote lengthy books about the folly of medicine and took a turn on the board of Oberlin College and as town mayor. Like other health reformers of the time, Jennings hitched the wagon of healthy living to the horse of Christian morality. He believed a person should choose good health not for its own sake but to be a better Christian and build a stronger Christian nation. He was more on the mark when he limited his musings to the medical. Like Miller, Hoffmann, and Fernel (of whose work he was probably innocent), Jennings thought the digestive tract—that "great, extensive, and complicated nutritive apparatus"—"requires a large amount of force to convert raw material into living structure" and that mustering such a force was too much work for a sick body. By fasting, the apparatus was "put at rest, that the forces saved thereby may be transferred to the recuperative machinery."

Jennings is important as the first doctor we know of to make fasting the guiding principle of his practice, but he was no more heeded in his time than Miller, Hoffmann, or Fernel in theirs. This was curious, for the case was becoming increasingly clear that the medicine of the day did more harm than good, whereas fasting was not only safe but vastly better at ameliorating illness. One reason doctors continued to reject fasting was that although medicine had at last emerged from Galen's heavy hand, it was now moiling under a new set of ridiculous theories no less bewitching than Galenism had been.

*   *   *

On December 13, 1799, a gentleman farmer in Virginia was surveying his expansive estate on horseback when he got soaked in a dispiriting squall of snow and sleet (although one imagines he had rather the better of it than his human chattel, whose work he was overseeing). He sat dinner in damp attire and by bedtime complained of a cough, runny nose, and hoarseness. At two in the morning he awoke short of breath, clutching his chest, and soon became feverish. It was a rude start to the last day in the life of the father of the nation. George Washington was only sixty-seven and seemingly vigorous, having repaired to Mount Vernon from the White House just two years earlier.

Doctors were summoned, but as dawn arrived without them, Washington asked the overseer of his estate to bleed him. The overseer sliced open a vein in his arm and drained it of twelve to fourteen ounces of blood—a bottle of beer's worth. When the doctors, numbering three, finally arrived, they brought a variety of remedies to bear, starting with an application of Spanish fly to Washington's throat. Spanish fly was a paste made not of an airborne insect but of the Spanish fly beetle, whose dried and ground bodies raised painful blisters that supposedly drew out noxious humors like those presumed to be behind Washington's illness. Next the doctors relieved their patient of another eighteen ounces of blood, gave him an enema and a gargle of sage tea and vinegar, and then bled him twice more. In all he was bled of perhaps eighty ounces, nearly half his measure. He was further subjected to a tartar emetic (its purging action was described as "cyclonic"), wheat poultices on his neck, more Spanish fly blisters on his arms, legs, and feet, and an enlivening dose of calomel, which was simultaneously one of the period's most popular (among doctors) and most terrifying (among patients) of medicines, a compound of mercury whose side effects included bloody diarrhea and gangrene of the mouth that could cause teeth to fall out and jawbones to disintegrate. None of these therapies did the former president a bit of good, although he struggled valiantly under them.

"I die hard," he croaked to one of his doctors, "but I am not afraid to go."

A short time later he did.

Medical historians debate the nature of Washington's illness, although most think it was acute bacterial epiglottitis, a rare infection of the throat that is sometimes fatal even today. All agree, however, that his death was only hastened by his doctors' torments, especially the bloodletting. The type of care they bestowed on him was later given a name, "heroic medicine," and George Washington had just become its most famous victim.

He might have thanked a particular friend for his doctors' attentions, had he not been rendered somewhat beyond the giving of thanks. The friend was Dr. Benjamin Rush, a signer of the Declaration of Independence who had served as surgeon general under Washington in the Revolutionary War and who was perhaps the most influential physician in early America and certainly its most forceful proponent of heroic medicine. In many respects, Rush was an enlightened doctor. He helped found multiple educational institutions, including the one that became the University of Pennsylvania School of Medicine, where he taught, and he was one of the first doctors in the New World to advocate free medical care for the poor. He so pioneered the treatment of the mentally ill, and did it with such humanity, that he is generally regarded the father of American psychiatry. But he was also a devotee of "breathing a vein" and of evacuating stomach and bowels with whatever poison, guised as medicine, was required.

Heroic medicine arose in the eighteenth century from a misguided attachment to theory. Over the previous two centuries, autopsies had at last exposed Galenic humoralism for the delusion it was, but doctors still had nothing better to put in its place. To fill the void, they concocted elaborate theories, most of them nearly as potty as Galenism, and medical schools and medical journals justified their fees by spreading the theories, which was why the *Medical Repository* called for more real-world observation and less academic supposition. As the historian James Whorton has written, medical professors of the era would "hypothesize about the basic nature of disease and then deduce therapy from the resulting theory. Treatments were presumed to work because theory indicated they had to and because most patients did in fact recover." Of course, the patients recovered in spite of, not because of, the lancets and emetics their doctors inflicted on them.

Rush's pet theory held "there is but one disease in the world," which he termed "morbid excitement induced by capillary tension"—high blood pressure to us. Its cure lay in relieving the pressure, which could be done directly by emptying the veins of blood or indirectly by evacuating the stomach of food and the bowels of waste. Rush urged doctors to summon the courage to bleed patients even to unconsciousness and to slosh their innards with calomel until they drooled. Every time a patient didn't die, his ideas were vindicated.

His medicine left little room for fasting or any other cure that let nature do the healing, and he directed his students to "always treat nature in a sick room as you would a noisy dog or cat[;] drive her out at the door and lock it upon her." There could be but one hero in heroic medicine, and it would be the learned doctor, master of the latest "scientific" theory that would conquer disease. It was a terribly seductive call to arms. Young medical students, doctors of long practice, and hopeful patients were equally enchanted, with noxious consequences. "How often," one thoughtful doctor complained, was the physician "forced by patients and their friends to give medicine when it is not plainly indicated, when he would gladly watch and await the efforts of nature? This privilege is denied him; he must cure *quickly*, or *give place to a rival.*" As in Hoffmann's Germany, so in Rush's America: patients paid a doctor to act, not to counsel a three-day abstinence from food.

You didn't have to be a physician to see the cliff that heroic doctors were in danger of hurtling over. In 1807, President Thomas Jefferson cautioned a young physician about the heroic mindset: "The patient treated on the fashionable theory sometimes gets well in spite of the medicine. The medicine therefore restored him, and the young doctor receives new courage to proceed in his bold experiments on the lives of his fellow creatures." But, Jefferson suggested, "the judicious, the moral, the humane physician" should instead trust in "the salutary efforts which nature makes to re-establish the disordered functions" and not risk "conjectural experiments on a machine so complicated and so unknown as the human body, and a subject so sacred as human life." Jefferson's advice would not be heeded either.

*   *   *

Over time, though, heroism and other academic medicine generated a backlash as patients wearied not just of medicine's ineffective brutality but of its cost. Until the late eighteenth century, medicine had been a free-for-all in which just about anyone could practice, but as medical schools proliferated and theory became ascendant, doctoring became a more exclusive and costly trade, and the expense was reflected in doctors' bills. Had physicians bettered their patients' health or lengthened their years, the fees might have been tolerated, but medicine failed miserably on both counts.

The failure created an opportunity that was seized by a New Hampshire farmer named Samuel Thomson. Assessed by one admirer as "illiterate, coarse in his manners, and extremely selfish" and by another as "an old avaricious churl," Thomson hatched a school of medicine whose motto was "Every man his own physician." Like the Roman Methodists of long ago, he said his system of botanical cures could be learned in no time by any yeoman or mechanic, any teamster or housewife. In root doctoring, as the craft was popularly known, there were no fancy theories to learn, just the know-how of which plant to take for which condition. Supposedly Thomson's cures were based on tests he made, but these were grossly unscientific and proved nothing—not that the public cared. The alluring promise of self-doctoring won Thomson subscribers by the million. In 1835, the governor of Mississippi said half the citizens of his state practiced

Thomsonian medicine, and in Ohio the portion was estimated between one third and one half. But after a while people noticed the ill were about as apt to die under Thomson's system as any other, and the game unraveled entirely in 1843 when Thomson shuffled off to the interminable beyond while taking his own cure.

Thomson's lasting contribution was to have amplified doubts about medicine that cleared a path for other health reform movements, one of which, Grahamism, had an outsize influence on fasting. You are familiar with the movement's founder through the culinary delight we call the graham cracker. Born in 1794 in Suffield, Connecticut, Sylvester Graham was the seventeenth child of a septuagenarian preacher who died shortly after making his frisky genetic contribution to his son. Graham's mother was mentally ill and unable to care for her child, who was shunted from one relative to the next. A stint as a bar boy gave him a lifelong revulsion for the devil's spirits, frequent illnesses stimulated his interest in health, and he emerged from youth righteous, pinched, and not always easy to get along with. After a couple of years as an itinerant Presbyterian minister and temperance lecturer, he found his calling in the early 1830s as an evangelist of his very own gospel of health.

The main principle of Grahamism would have been recognizable to Philo: too much stimulation wrecked the body and damned the soul. Whatever felt good must, ipso facto, be the work of Satan, an unhealthful assault on that most precious of God-given gifts, the body. Graham's list of sinful stimulants was long and prudish. Even the married should shun "the convulsive paroxysms attending venereal indulgence," although people young enough to conceive were permitted an orgasm a month provided it was endured with Baptist abhorrence. His dietary proscriptions were just as severe, for he labeled iniquitous most of what Americans considered food: meat, milk, butter, condiments, spices, refined foodstuffs, and any beverage zippier than water. Even the ingestibles he allowed had to be taken in moderation because, as he wrote, "GLUTTONY and *not starvation* is the greatest of all causes of evil. . . . Excessive alimentation is the greatest dietetic error in the United States—and probably in the whole civilized world."

It was certainly true Americans were breaking new ground in gluttonous attainment, as astonished travelers rarely failed to note. In 1818, the English journalist William Cobbett wrote in amazement of the American custom at table, "You are not much *asked*, not much *pressed*, to eat and drink; but, such an abundance is spread before you, and so hearty and so cordial is your reception, that you instantly lose all restraint, and are tempted to feast whether you be hungry or not." Two decades later, another British visitor chided his hosts, "You Yankees load your stomachs as a Devonshire man does his cart, as full as it can hold, as fast as he can pitch it in with a dungfork and drive off; and then you complain that such a load of compost is too heavy for you."

In moments of grandiloquence, Graham called his cure for gluttony "The Science of Human Life," but in a simpler mood it was "proper hygiene." *Hygiene* in that era encompassed the many habits of life—from diet to sleep to exercise to dress—that contributed to health. (The word didn't assume its modern association with bodily cleanliness until after the triumph of germ theory later in the century.) According to Graham, the most hygienic of diets consisted of undressed vegetables, plain fruits, and bread of unbolted wheat that was also unleavened, for it was yeast that turned sugar into the devil's spirits. He had no science about the nutritive properties of whole grains or anything else, but he smelled something sinful in the refinements American mills were increasingly inflicting on their wheat, and he condemned the millers who "put asunder what God has joined together." His 1837 "Treatise on Bread and Bread Making" provoked Boston bakers to riot, and butchers were no happier with his claim (correct, as it turned out) that meat caused disease and premature aging. His followers had to disperse a mob that converged on one of his lectures by dropping bags of caustic lime onto their heads from the rooftop. The coarsely ground flour that Graham advocated came to be known as graham flour, from which emerged many graham products including the graham cracker. Its dryness was supposed to curb lust—something to contemplate when you bite into your next s'more.

Fasting had a small but important part to play in Graham's hygienic system. It wasn't a large part because righteous living usually prevented disease, but sometimes illness struck even the most virtuously hygienic, and fasting could speed the return to health. Graham was impressed that in victims of cholera and fever who were unable to keep down even hygienic foods, a fast could nonetheless achieve "wonderful effects." His ideas about why fasting worked were in keeping with his predecessors': when the digestive organs were rested, they "first lay hold of and remove those substances which are of least use to the economy; and hence all morbid accumulations, such as wens [boils], tumors, abcesses, etc., are rapidly diminished." Burning fat and slimming to normal proportions also helped "restore the system to the most perfectly healthy condition." One of the gratifying curiosities of the history of fasting is that nearly every writer who observed it closely—even those of otherwise muddled mind—proposed a similar mechanism that would prove correct in its essentials. This may seem unexceptional today, when the mechanism appears obvious, but we know it wasn't apparent at the time because doctor after doctor rejected it.

Graham won thousands of adherents, but in truth his hygienism was more notorious than popular. Few could abide his dietary curtailments, and scientifically minded Americans disdained hygienism's grim spiritual cast. Fortunately, more respectable figures came along and rescued the movement from an early death by rinsing it of the worst of its pietism and investing it with a bit of medical authority. The most important of these figures was the second cousin of Louisa May Alcott, the beloved author of *Little Women*. Dr. William Alcott was not nearly so well known as his cousin, but he was just as adored by those acquainted with him. Cheerful and approachable, thoughtful and open-minded, he possessed a Yale medical degree, a practice in a respectable suburb of Boston, and a gentle dignity that Sylvester Graham did not. He was also an industrious propagandist, by one count writing 108 books in his threescore years. When Graham died prematurely in 1851, at fifty-seven,* the hygienic movement became Alcott's to lead.

---

* After Graham's decease, his house in Northampton, Massachusetts, became a tavern, which would not have tickled the departed teetotaler. Today it's an eatery called Sylvester's whose owners purport to have "embraced his healthy food philosophy," but their steak-poutine breakfast and bakery case full of white-floured sin tell another story.

Alcott is often called America's first vegetarian physician, which is not quite true, but he did arrive independently and medically at many of the same conclusions Graham arrived at sanctimoniously. He observed, for example, that the healthiest of his patients seemed to be those who were least gluttonous and ate the least meat, and he filled out Graham's hygienic system with smart advice about fresh air, mildly invigorating exercise, and salubrious bathing. He also thought a little sexual congress natural, healthy, and not the most repugnant way to pass the after-dinner hours. Although not a great proponent of fasting, Alcott gave hygienism a medical imprimatur and elevated it to a modest respectability, which allowed other hygienic doctors to take fasting still further, which they sometimes did in quite splendid ways.

*   *   *

One of those doctors was Edward Kittredge, who, like Alcott, practiced in greater Boston in the middle of the century. Kittredge was an odd duck. He was a devotee of hydropathy, the pseudo-medical system that doused, flushed, steamed, froze, and otherwise subjected patients to treatment by water, and he wrote wry articles in hygienic journals under the pseudonym Noggs, probably in tribute to the bankrupt tippler in Dickens's *Nicholas Nickleby* who helped young Nicholas thwart his ruthless uncle. Read into that what you will.

He was also a fasting pioneer. Where earlier doctors fasted patients for only two or three days and only at the start of acute illness, Kittredge somehow surmised that longer fasts could help more tenacious disorders. He reported magnificent cures with fasts of up to twenty-one days, a length that apparently scandalized his colleagues. "I know very well," he wrote, "I am peculiar in my treatment of chronic disease, and many cry out 'starvation, &c.,' but I know also that I have cured hundreds of what the faculty had pronounced 'hopeless cases' by my plan, and shall not, therefore, be frightened by any bugbear from pursuing it."

Kittredge's patients were not always enthusiastic about his prescription. One ravenously hungry woman whose liver and duodenum were inflamed managed seven foodless days, improved greatly, and broke her fast against Kittredge's advice. "My rule," he wrote, "is to keep them fasting until the tongue becomes clean and the mouth tastes properly"—possibly the earliest reference to the markers that doctors would rely on over the next century in deciding when to break a fast, the idea being that once the coated tongue and foul breath returned to sweet normality, the illness behind them had been burned away. Kittredge's liver-and-duodenum patient soon relapsed, but her "good sense told her she had acted unwisely, and she readily assented to commence again her fasting, which this time lasted about seventeen days, and she then cautiously began to eat.... It is now some three months or more since that time, and she has been almost a well woman; nothing has troubled her stomach since."

The phrase "almost a well woman" was indicative of Kittredge's circumspection, which his ardor for fasting did not overrun. But as with the fasting doctors before him, neither his careful assessments nor his claims of cures won converts among clinicians. He adjudged their rejection "terribly strange."

To regular doctors, of course, it was fasting that was terribly strange. Not eating, to the conventional mind, was all too obviously an illogical depletion of vigor, the last thing a sick patient needed. More than a few physicians also saw in fasting a barbarous rejection of both God's creation and the American ingenuity that had lately yielded an endless supply of food. In his popular 1871 guide *Eating and Drinking*, the New York neurologist George Miller Beard declared that "prolonged fasting"—which he defined as skipping lunch—"is the prerogative of savages.... For the majority of Americans this mistake is a most fearful one, and has caused innumerable woes. Dyspepsia in all its phases, nervous diseases of all kinds, and death itself, are the rewards that nature is continually bestowing on those who thus refuse her bounties." Beard believed the only people who need limit their meals were "professed gluttons." For the rest, "it is far better to overeat at lunch than not to eat at all."

Fasting also found little favor among intellectuals, who couldn't stomach the moralizing that lingered around hygienism. Ralph Waldo Emerson, the ordinarily sensible essayist, mocked hygienists and other reformers for arguing "that the mischief was in our diet, that we eat and drink damnation," and his sagacious friend Oliver Wendell Holmes, the physician-poet who served as dean of Harvard Medical School, scoffed, "Some men seem to 'seek to merit *heaven*, by making earth a *hell*,' and we can readily conceive how a dyspeptic in his closet, might look a little enviously upon his sleek and oily neighbor, who sleeps well, eats well, and perchance smokes his cigar." Little surprise, then, that when science finally exposed medicine for the fraud it was, doctors, rather than turning to hygienism and fasting, embraced the new science in a myopic and self-serving way that only further drove fasting beyond the bounds of professional respectability.

* * *

In most respects, the long-overdue application of science to medicine was an undiluted good, not least for finally bleeding to death heroic medicine. Heroism persisted late into the nineteenth century because doctors, ignoring fasting, still had nothing demonstrably better to offer patients. During the Civil War, when Surgeon General William Hammond—the soon-to-be nemesis of Mollie Fancher and Henry Tanner—barred Union doctors from using the poisonous mercury compound calomel, the doctors revolted in what came to be known as the Calomel Rebellion, which ended in Hammond's dismissal and the poison's reinstatement. Even as late as the First World War, calomel was one of three active ingredients in the British Army's "Number 9" pill.

In the end, heroic medicine was undercut by two advances of the early nineteenth century: the discovery of the placebo effect, which cast the "cures" of heroic medicine in a poor light, and the emergence of statistical analysis, which showed patients in epidemics were just as likely to die under doctors' care as they were to die unattended. Little by little, doctors admitted the old way of doing things was a sham at best, a needless torture at worst. In the 1830s, after the young Oliver Wendell Holmes completed his medical training, he concluded that most of the therapies he had been taught were pointless, and he said of medications, "I firmly believe that if the whole materia medica, *as now used*, could be sunk to the bottom of the sea, it would be all the better for mankind,—and all the worse for the fishes." This sort of realization gave rise in the middle of the century to the dictum *primum non nocere*, "first do no harm." (Popularized by a Liverpool surgeon, the phrase was swiftly attributed to Hippocrates even though it was in Latin, which the Greek doctor would not have spoken.)

No medical historians have remarked the fact, but the very moment when science first revealed medicine a menace was the same in which, for the first time since antiquity, a cluster of doctors from the same culture all suggested their profession turn to fasting. It was a tantalizing chance to send medicine in a useful direction, and a few establishmentarian doctors even begged their colleagues do just that—to enlist nature as "the great agent of cure," in the phrase of the Harvard professor, doctor, and botanist Jacob Bigelow. "The amount of death and disaster in the world would be less," Bigelow maintained, "if all disease were left to itself."

But doctors were too wed to the conceit that bodies didn't cure bodies, doctors did. They spurned hygienism and fasting as "therapeutic nihilism," an unconditional surrender before the armies of disease and death. If it was true they shouldn't torment their patients with heroic measures, surely that didn't mean they should cede the field to disease. To be a doctor meant to *fight* disease, and they armed themselves with the tools and methods that science had lately devised. One of those methods was specialization, which grew out of a renewed interest in autopsies, which had led doctors to match the damaged organs of the dead—the ravaged liver of the alcoholic, the disfigured pancreas of the diabetic—with the symptoms their sick owners had shown in life. Such investigations were furthered by new tools like the stethoscope and an old tool rediscovered, the microscope, which let doctors peer inside organs while their owners yet lived. A sad consequence of these worthy endeavors was that disease came to be seen mainly as a force that preyed on specific organs rather than the entire body. Patients didn't get cancer because they ate a poor diet whose harm manifested in one person's colon, another's prostate, another's breast; they got cancer because of an unfortunate defect in their colon, prostrate, or breast. The specialization that arose from these observations gave us the form of medicine we know today, in which one doctor treats the gastrointestinal tract, another the nervous system, a third the heart. There is of course great merit in specializing, but much was also lost. In the nineteenth century, the theories that specialists devised to explain the diseases of their particular organ were hardly more accurate than the theories they replaced, and the therapies that flowed from those theories, although less immediately violent than heroic medicine, still harmed patients when they didn't kill them outright. "The mortality amongst patients did not decrease" with these changes, the historian David Wootton has written. "Instead it increased."

Specialization proved a body blow to fasting. To prescribe a fast required a holistic view, one that understood disease was often systemic and thus called for a treatment that worked on the whole organism. Doctors enamored of specialization couldn't see how starving the stomach could relieve a carbuncle on the toe, clear up a sore throat, or shrink a tumor in the groin. Medical professors, for their part, mocked as unscientific any therapy that didn't make use of the new theories on which their institutions' revenues depended. By the second half of the nineteenth century, matters stood very much where they had at century's start: the doctor who used bogus treatments that hurt his patients was lauded a man of science, while the doctor who healed his patients through fasting was a quack. Before century's end, the situation would get even worse.

* * *

To understand why, we need to take a brief look at a great war that raged within the medical fraternity across the nineteenth century, a conflict that claimed fasting as one of its many casualties. The first salvos were the century's several health reform movements, which outraged conventional doctors, none more outraging than homeopathy, the strange brew of the German physician Samuel Hahnemann. Hahnemann claimed the body could be trained to vanquish disease by introducing it to weaker, artificial versions of disease. This may sound like the solid theory of the vaccine, but where the small dose of virus in a vaccine actually teaches the immune system to make disease-fighting antibodies, the substances Hahnemann used for his cures—tree bark, viper venom, indigo, deadly nightshade—had no such capabilities. Still, in the early 1800s homeopathy was no more preposterous than most of conventional medicine, and because it was simple to teach, homeopathic doctors were soon setting up shop in every state in America and charging lower fees than conventional doctors. Other so-called irregular schools (notably the eclecticism of Henry Tanner) also made incursions on convention.

The regulars lost no time responding. Claiming to fear for their patients but in truth as much for their purses, they convinced state legislatures to pass licensing laws that required doctors hold a degree from a regular medical school or pass an exam written by regulars. The laws carried only mild penalties and often weren't enforced, but they sparked a great outcry, and by mid-century, irregulars had hounded legislators into repealing all of them. Regulars retaliated with social and financial pressures that extended even to their own members who merely associated with homeopaths. One New York doctor was expelled from his local medical society for the crime of buying sugar from a homeopathic pharmacy. A doctor in Connecticut was expelled from his society for consulting with a homeopathic doctor, his wife. And the US surgeon general was roundly condemned for helping save the secretary of state after he was stabbed (in the same plot in which Lincoln was assassinated) because he did his doctoring alongside the secretary's personal physician, a homeopath.

Only the birth of modern medical science finally brought an uneasy truce. Its birthdate can be placed with exquisite precision: March 13, 1865, the day on which Joseph Lister, a thirty-seven-year-old professor of surgery at the University of Glasgow, used the antiseptic principles of germ theory to treat a compound fracture (a broken bone that protrudes through the skin, admitting germs). Most of us know Lister today, after a fashion, from Listerine, which was first developed as a surgical antiseptic and later sold as a mouthwash. But Lister's name really deserves to be chiseled in marble next to Galileo's and Newton's, for his discovery, as he rightly if immodestly said, ranked among the greatest in the history of humankind.

Medicine would never be the same again. Before Lister, surgery was all but synonymous with death by infection, and any number of other conditions, from a popped blister to childbirth, were also frequently fatal. After Lister, the world was suddenly a lot less scary. For the first time in twenty-five hundred years, medicine had a legitimate claim to healing. New procedures were developed to take advantage of germ theory—surgery in particular flourished—and as they grew more complicated, medical education gained its first legitimacy as well. Now licensing laws made a lot more sense; no one wanted a root doctor removing her appendix. In the 1870s, regulars pushed to renew the laws and were joined by the most unlikely of allies: homeopaths and eclectics. Both sects were by then well established themselves, with their own medical colleges, scholarly journals, and professional societies, and both had developed a regular-like concern about the inroads other irregulars were making on their clientele. They seized the opportunity to join with regulars to punish the remaining orders, and one by one state legislatures brought back medical licensing, typically with separate regimes for conventional, homeopathic, and eclectic doctors. Other schools were barred altogether or sharply limited in the tasks their practitioners could perform.

The new licensing laws were a devastation to fasting. Of the three sanctioned schools, only eclecticism had any use for the hunger cure, and the eclectics were on the wane and would be all but gone by the twentieth century. Soon fasting would be left to the true outsiders of the medical field: naturopaths, chiropractors, and osteopaths. Another dark age seemed to loom over fasting.

But as we've seen, a stout little eclectic from Minnesota spared fasting that fate. The light Henry Tanner threw on the practice may have dimmed as soon as he left Clarendon Hall, but the glow was never wholly extinguished. Fasting for health was about to enjoy the greatest blossoming the world had ever seen.

CHAPTER 7

ARRESTING MY DECLINE

In the early 1980s, researchers at the National Institute on Aging conducted an exceedingly simple but majestically successful experiment on longevity. Dividing a mischief of young rats into two groups, they fed one group in the usual manner but the other only every other day. From week to week, both groups ate about the same amount because the fasting rats made up for their fast days by eating more on their feast days. In the end, the normally fed rats lived a typical lifespan for their strain, 75.5 weeks on average, but the every-other-day group lived a spectacular 138.2 weeks—fully 83 percent longer. In the 78 years of an average American life, 83 percent would come to 65 extra years. The rats had lived, in effect, 143 years.

Other trials of alternate-day fasting (ADF) followed, with results less dazzling but still formidable. In one, mice who ate every other day lived 34 percent longer than their control-group cousins, while in another they lived 40 percent longer. Researchers figured the differences were due partly to genetic variations in the strains of rodents and partly to when in their lives they started fasting. To suss out the discrepancies, an NIA team fasted three strains of mice, with subgroups in each strain starting their ADF in either adolescence, young maturity, or middle age. In general, the younger the mice began fasting, the longer they lived—as much as 27 percent longer than normally fed controls—although one poor strain that started ADF in middle age actually lived 14 percent *shorter* than the control group. Mature rodents could take heart, however, in a rosier study in which rats who started fasting in either middle age or elderhood lived, respectively, 36 percent or 14 percent longer. The studies also tended to find that those who fasted aged more slowly and had fewer cancers, less cardiovascular disease, and less diabetes—just the sort of disease-free sunset years most humans can only aspire to.

It's tempting to extrapolate from *Rattus norvegicus* and *Mus musculus* to *Homo sapiens*, to suppose, that is, that eating every other day would do a human body good. The problem is that a one-day fast is a mountain for a mouse, a molehill for us. Mice lose a quarter of their mass after just a day without food and turn feet-up after two or three, whereas even a lean human can survive a month or more fasting. To match the rodent's ADF, a human would probably need to do something more like AWF, alternate-week fasting.

Even so, when I learned about the long-lived rodents a dozen years ago, I couldn't stop wondering what ADF might do for me. Having just turned forty, I also thought of the unfortunate mice who had begun ADF in middle age and lost a few ticks of the clock for their trouble. But I reminded myself of their luckier and more numerous cousins who started fasting in midlife or even dotage and still gained what amounted to years of extra life, and healthy years at that. Would a man in midlife, at any rate this man in midlife, be more like a lucky rodent or an unlucky one? There was only one way to find out. I decided to fast every other day for a month.

* * *

I wasn't the first human to give it a go. In fact, one young nutrition researcher, Krista Varady at the University of Illinois Chicago, was busily building a career on ADF, first putting mice through their fasting paces, then people. Varady learned early that the average human rebelled at eating nothing every other day (the average lab mouse probably didn't care for it either, but its recourses for cheating were fewer), so in her human studies she used a modified ADF (mADF). On "fast" days, her volunteers ate a quarter of their normal diet, about 500 calories, while on feast days they ate as much as they liked. In one of her studies, after eight weeks of mADF, obese volunteers dropped a dozen pounds (almost all of it fat), their LDL cholesterol and triglycerides fell a respective 25 and 32 percent, and their systolic blood pressure (the top number) dropped from 124 to 116 mm Hg. Varady was agreeably surprised that on feeding days her volunteers didn't gorge themselves—they ate only about 10 or 15 percent more than normal—and that although in the early going they were hungry on fast days, hunger troubled them hardly at all after the second week. Non-obese people, per other studies, benefited from mADF in roughly the same ways the obese did. In fact, on a range of metabolic markers—blood pressure, heart rate, triglycerides, fasting glucose, fasting insulin, insulin resistance, and the inflammatory markers C-reactive protein and homocysteine— mADF delivered many of the same benefits in the short term as caloric restriction, which scientists had long ago discovered made animals live longer and healthier. Even better, mADF appeared to do all this safely, with no serious side effects or loss of lean mass or bone density.

On the other hand, it wasn't clear that modified fasting was the sole or even main reason Varady's volunteers got healthier. They might have fared well simply because they ate less overall rather than enjoying any fasting-specific metabolic improvements. But however it worked, something promising was clearly going on because other researchers were reporting good results too. In Britain, Michelle Harvie and Tony Howell, a nutritional scientist and a professor of oncology, came up with an even gentler modified fast, the 5:2 diet, which consisted of two modified-fast days a week and five days of normal eating. Harvie and Howell's volunteers, like Varady's, ended up healthier and slimmer, and thanks to a handful of popular books and TV documentaries on the diet, millions of people have tried it.

I appreciated the promise of modified ADF, particularly for those in poor health, but I confess it didn't stir me. Even a bona fide water-only ADF was a far less rigorous exercise for man than mouse, so a modified fast seemed unlikely to bring me anything like the deep gains the rodents got on their true ADF. Not that I was prepared to go as far as they did—I had no intention of fasting, say, every other week. But surely it would be no trouble to do an unmodified ADF for a month.

Well, I have seldom been more wrong. It was the most perfectly miserable month, possibly the least favorite of my life, and there have been some serious contenders.

Things started out well enough, the first fast day posing no problem. But the second, coming so soon after the first, seemed a little onerous, and by the third, my mind and stomach cried hunger and turned grumbly when I refused to appease them. After that, every fast day began with a mental judo match in which I jabbed hunger into a corner and had to throw the occasional kick across the day to keep it there. In retrospect, I'm sure the problem was the brevity of the fasts. By the end of each fast day, the hunger would finally dissipate, and I would start to feel I was getting used to fasting again and could easily have fasted much longer. But breakfast next morning broke the spell, and a day later the struggle started all over again. Since the hardest part of fasting is the transition to ketosis, it was like forever scaling a rugged acclivity without ever enjoying the ease atop the summit. I had made a Sisyphus of myself.

Worse, my fasting turned eating into a chore. On feast days I ate ravenously, downing first a bowl of cereal, then one of chili, another of curry, and a fourth of pasta before hoovering up whole bunches of grapes and bananas and sandwiches beyond count. But only the first hour of these orgies pleased me. After that, I replenished under compulsion, the chance to pack in calories before next day's fast disappearing by the hour. Incredibly, pounds were falling off me even so. I was living the fat man's fantasy, gorging all day yet losing weight—but beware what you wish for.

In the second week, my body revolted. I became lightheaded, especially on fast days, and a couple of times I nearly fainted on expeditions from one room to the next. I grew weak, and by afternoon, fasting or feasting, I was usually reduced to a hapless fragility. I thought these symptoms meant I wasn't eating enough, but even after I upped my feed and stabilized my weight, the problems continued. Some days I was so feeble I could barely sit up, and at times I doubted I could have arisen had the house caught fire. In the middle of the third week, a mysterious pain took up quarters in my kidneys, something like the discomfort of desperately needing to urinate. It persisted no matter how often I visited the toilet, and then after a couple of days it left as inexplicably as it had come. The fourth week my brain and body shut down almost as soon as I awoke. Lassitude devoured the day, and work became impossible. Two days shy of a month, I said screw it and ate a banana on a fast-day morning.

I later learned that Krista Varady had trouble getting her volunteers to stick with even a modified ADF. In a yearlong study published in 2017, 38 percent of her subjects on mADF dropped out, compared to 29 percent who ate a calorically restricted diet. Caloric restriction is notoriously hard to pull off, but apparently mADF is harder still. Varady also learned that those who persisted with mADF tended to eat diets higher in fat, presumably because of fat's satiating quality. This was concerning. We have decades of research tying higher-fat diets to an early grave and a lot of bad years before you get there, and it wasn't clear the gains her volunteers enjoyed on mADF would outweigh the harm of their fatty diets. Varady was unexpectedly nonchalant on the question. She said that on mADF's feast days you could "literally eat whatever you like," and to illustrate the point, she wolfed down a grease-soaked cheeseburger and fries at a drive-in cholesterol joint for a TV documentary. The jacket of her 2013 book *The Every Other Day Diet* gave pride of place to a pepperoni pizza and a glazed donut.

I thought this reckless. She was staking her claim to wanton eating on a very few short-term studies that had found improvements in a relative handful of biomarkers in a small number of subjects. And even in those studies, the volunteers who ate less fat were healthier. It was a giant leap from these limited data to advising the public they could eat all the Velveeta, hot dogs, and Twinkies they wanted every other day of their lives and still be protected by a modified fast. The science just didn't support it.

*   *   *

I wish I could say that after my ADF debacle I settled into a more salubrious fasting habit, but my intention outran my implementation. Now and then in the decade that followed, my fifth, I would become gripped by a fever of diligence and would fast after dinner every Sunday night till breakfast Tuesday morning, but these punctilious periods never lasted more than a few months. Mostly I fasted when my belt ran out of notches, which it did every year or two. For long spells I hardly fasted at all.

My health declined. The descent, I saw in retrospect, had actually begun in my twenties with a bit of innocent-seeming fatigue. I would sit to write, and within an hour my mind would fog over and the rest of the day would be a running skirmish with exhaustion. When I tried to nap, I could rarely sleep, and when I slept, I awoke unrefreshed. The fatigue came and went, but its trend was unmistakably expansionist, and now and then it became so overwhelming I had to abandon writing for days or weeks. A counselor posited avoidance. What in my subconscious, she asked, was driving my body to divert me from writing? I could name nothing.

My young adulthood was checkered as well with a depression that flared with the fatigue. Psychiatrists fiddled with the flavor and dose of my antidepressants to see if therein lay a cure for or the hidden cause of my lethargy, but while their recipes kept the depression somewhat in hand, they did nothing for the fatigue. By my mid-thirties, enervation overran me, and more evenings than not I slumped into a spent muddle—a no-show at chores, a dud at conversation, quick to exasperate as a father, quick to quarrel as a husband, as a friend simply unavailable.

I thought I had a fix at last when I was diagnosed with obstructive sleep apnea. My airway, I was told, was too narrow, my tongue too big—there's a joke in there somewhere—but even after a sleep doctor had me fitted with a mouthpiece that put my jaw and tongue into a well-oxygenated posture, I was still tired.

"Well, you shouldn't be," the doctor said. "You're cured."

"How can I be cured if I'm still tired?" I asked.

"You're cured because you no longer have sleep apnea when you wear the mouthpiece. You *are* wearing the mouthpiece, aren't you?"

"Yes."

"Well, keep wearing it." And she sent me away cured.

Years later, having renounced Tennessee for Colorado, thinner air forced a new round of tests, followed by new treatments: a CPAP machine to coerce my airway open further, melatonin to reset my sleep–wake clock, behavioral therapy to calm my mind, sleeping pills that I became hooked on and had a devil of a time getting off, acupuncture, yoga, exercise, and meditation. I was still exhausted. At last, my sleep doctor shrugged and said I had idiopathic hypersomnia.

"What does that mean?" I said.

"*Hypersomnia* means you're tired all the time, and *idiopathic* means we don't know why."

"What's the fix?"

"We don't have one."

I looked up *idiopathic* later. It comes from the Greek *idio*, which means "own," "personal," "private," or "peculiar," and *patheia*, which means "suffering" or "feeling." I had my own peculiar suffering. Well, almost my own. I had to share it with a few thousand Americans and tens of thousands of others around the globe. My variant was mild. Some hypersomniacs, I learned, sleep twelve, sixteen, even twenty hours a day, but their slumber, in the jargon, is nonrestorative. These poor souls almost never awake refreshed, just as I didn't from my uninvigorating naps. Nearly every waking hour, they stumble around feeling what the rest of us feel in those few moments right before sleep, when our eyelids are so heavy only toothpicks could keep them open. I endured that kind of somnambulant nightmare only a handful of hours a day. Mine was a lucky case.

Although medicine had no cure, it did have a crutch: stimulants. But on Ritalin I felt as if I were mainlining caffeine, my hands trembling, my sleep further wrecked, my irritability an ordeal for Jennifer and Elliott. My doctor switched me to modafinil, which college students know as a "smart pill" because it enables all-night studying. Though milder, it still left me over-amped with twitchy fingers and a racing mind. For years, I was greeted every morning with a choice between the poison of the disease and the poison of the drug, and no matter which I chose, I always felt I'd picked wrong. The harder these struggles became, the more my depression erupted, and in the gloom of winter I became as much a fixture in my psychiatrists' offices as the plastic plants.

I developed other disturbing conditions. The most eccentric was depersonalization disorder, in which sufferers have the bizarre and unwelcome feeling of not being part of their own bodies. Some of my depersonalized tribe describe it as an out-of-body experience, as if they're watching themselves from afar, but for me it was just the opposite. I felt as if my being had shrunk within me, my nerves stopping a half inch shy of the surface, the real me somewhere beneath. Everything above—limbs, skin, hair, eyes, ears—felt like pieces of an exoskeleton I could manipulate but couldn't really feel. It was indescribably disorienting to be folding laundry or helping Elliott with his homework and next moment find myself shriveling into my interior. Science knows neither the cause of nor the cure for depersonalization.

Toward the end of my forties, I twice had attacks I thought for sure were strokes. The left side of my face went numb, the room spun endlessly, and my muscles became so weak and uncoordinated I could barely reach the phone on the bedside table to call 911. The attacks turned out to be extravagant migraines. This surprised me because I almost never have headaches, but it turns out you can have migraines without pain. A mild clenching on the left side of my face that had come and gone over the last decade was its earliest phase. A neurologist gave me supplements that kept the major attacks at bay, but the lesser clenching was a nearly constant companion.

With these and other precedents, I wasn't the least shocked when my memory began to fail. For years I had been forgetting, without much concern, all the things middle-aged people forget: what I had for breakfast, where I put my keys, the name of my cousin's husband. But I grew anxious when I struggled to recall what I'd written that morning, the names of old friends, and whether I'd brushed my teeth five minutes earlier. One day I texted Jennifer to say I was near her office and did she want a ride home—before remembering she was three days into a conference in New Orleans. A neuropsychologist ran some tests and declared me mentally sharp for my age, which may have been true in a better-than-average kind of way, but I knew how far I'd slipped.

Throughout all of this, it never occurred to me that fasting might ease my ills. I had internalized the dichotomy, common in medicine, that segregates troubles of the brain from troubles of the body, and since fasting, so far as I knew, remedied only problems of the body, and since it was my brain that was broken, there didn't seem much in it for my woes. Moreover, fasting doctors often said their therapy worked best against diseases wrought by unhealthy eating, and I never ascribed the problems of my mind to my menu. Any number of psychiatrists and counselors had assured me, and I had agreed, that my mental defects were the yield of a rocky upbringing, a few subsequent hard knocks, and above all poor genes—whole branches of my family tree were twigged out with schizophrenics, depressives, and near-suicides. Even had someone suggested I try to fast away my mental problems, I would have said neither my twenty-day fast nor my many shorter fasts had lessened my hypersomnia or depression. Fasting, I'd have protested, was as likely to fix my mind as to regrow one of the torn ligaments in my knee.

I approached fifty in a welter of anguish and lethargy. I had run through everything on offer from conventional and alternative medicine, my career had ground to a halt, and most days the best I could hope for with family and friends was a negative good—not growling at one, not letting another down. I felt snared in a trap, and I was certain I could hear the heavy footsteps of the hunter drawing near.

* * *

In the end, it was my blubber that saved me. The three or four pounds I had habitually put on and fasted off had, over the years, become five or six, then eight or nine, then ten or twelve. The bloat mystified me, especially as I had finally heeded the avalanche of data that says eating animals and their products is terrible for us and the planet (to say nothing of what it does to them) and had become first a pescatarian, then a vegetarian, and finally a vegan.* But a healthier diet hadn't kept me trim, and once again I worried about the studies suggesting even a few podgy pounds could yield disease and early death.

* The research that ties eating plants to good health has been recounted in so many books, documentaries, and websites, it seems an unnecessary diversion to give a chapter to it here. For those who wish to know more, see Sources on Diet at the end of the book.

The holidays of 2018 were my deliverance, albeit in unlikely form. So unkind were they to my contour that I embarked the following January on a fast to quit myself of fifteen pounds. Two nights in, I ran into trouble. I was by then well accustomed to the short sleep of the faster and was unconcerned with my nightly four hours, but on that night I was assaulted by restless-limb syndrome, another gremlin of my recent years. More like gremlins, because the syndrome feels like nothing so much as a swarm of imps scurrying inside your hands and feet and demanding they get to scurrying too. Yet no matter how much I wiggled my toes, dug my fingers into the sheets, or paced the room flapping my arms, the relief was only ever slight, and sometimes the sensation grew into a pain both physical and mental. It's another disorder for which medicine has no cure and only the most ineffectual of palliatives, and there's little to be done but let it dissolve on its own, which in my case was an ordeal of hours.

By the fourth day of my fast, my nocturnal torments so exhausted me that I sometimes couldn't hold my head up during the day without using my hands, and by the fifth day I couldn't summon the stamina to floss. I decided to switch to a modified fast. I didn't have in mind the 500 daily calories favored by Krista Varady but rather the 250 used by the fasting clinics of Europe—an amount, I had learned, that was minimal enough to keep the body in a metabolic state that approximated water-only fasting. (About this state, more later.) After a few bowls of watered-down squash soup, my limbs finally rested at night and I got snatches of undisturbed sleep while still losing weight. It seemed a monumental victory, but in light of what followed, it was merest prelude.

On the sixth morning, I awoke without my usual hypersomniac's fatigue, but I attached little importance to the event. My exhaustion had always waxed and waned, with three or four unbearable days giving way to a day or two of ordinary weariness, so I gave thanks for the reprieve and thought no more of it. But the seventh day also passed without fatigue, and so did the eighth and ninth. By the tenth day of my fast, my fifth without exhaustion, I began to entertain hope something had changed. Two days later I marked my first week in years entirely free of hypersomnia. How was it possible, I wondered, to sleep half as much and feel twice as alive?

My depersonalization disappeared as well, and although winter was the worst season for my depression, and the hibernal drear that year was especially heavy, my mood slowly but unmistakably brightened. My migraine enjoyed no such remission—the clenching on the side of my face persisted—but even its grip eased a little. With each day, I became more alert, less irritable, a better contributor around the house, a more willing exerciser. Something that was coiled inside me seemed to release, and for the first time in a very long while, joy swept over me multiple times a day for no reason at all except that I was so very glad to be alive. It was a form of rebirth, and as it deepened and grew more certain, I sometimes had to break off what I was doing to wipe the tears dribbling down my cheeks.

I had changed nothing else about my life, so it was scarcely possible anything other than the fast could have been behind my revitalization. But how? And why now? Why did this fast send my disorders into remission when others hadn't? I would learn more about that later, but for the moment a new concern preoccupied me: how could I maintain my recovery once I started eating again? For the first time in my life, the thought of breaking a fast filled me with terror.

*   *   *

My exploration of what to eat took an obvious path. Since fasting doctors said the practice worked best against diseases of dietary error, I started with the premise that I'd probably been wrong to think my diet wasn't behind my disorders. It was a thought both depressing and liberating—depressing because if true, my suffering all these years was the result of what I had put in my own mouth, liberating because it might now be in my power to keep my illnesses away, provided I could figure out what to eat instead.

My search took me to the work of Dr. Alan Goldhamer, America's leading expert on fasting, whom we met in the prologue. Eight years earlier, in 2011, I had briefly interviewed Goldhamer, and as I looked back now through my notes, I saw that he'd said that although fasting could chase a lot of diseases into remission, they usually returned if the patient didn't adopt a diet of unrefined plants. He speculated this was so because for most of hominid existence, simple plants were largely what our fore-bears ate—they were gatherers and scavengers long before they mas-tered the tools and techniques to become hunters—so our bodies didn't evolve to eat the foods that make up much of the modern diet, especially highly processed sugars, flours, and oils as well as vast quantities of animal products and salt. He also said it was possible to be a vegan and still eat unhealthily, which I was pretty sure I had just demonstrated.

You may recall Goldhamer's study of hypertensive patients whose blood pressure dropped fantastically while fasting. The study, I saw on rereading now, had a catch, the one Goldhamer had told me about: the patients who maintained their incredible improvements had switched to a diet of minimally processed plants with no added salt, oil, or sugar. I had been sympathetic to Goldhamer in 2011, but the truth is I hadn't wanted to hear this part of his prescription. My article was about the breathtak-ing cures fasting could achieve, not about cures that disintegrated unless you made a lifelong change in eating. I didn't draw undue attention in the article to his unprocessed-vegan catch, and I felt both foolish and ashamed about that now.

But even a fool can learn, and after poking around in the convinc-ing science of unprocessed veganism, this one decided to make a trial of it when he broke his fast after two weeks. Out went the oily hummus on which I doted, the white-flour pasta, the store-bought crackers and bread, the boxed cereal, the jarred tomato sauce. (Once you know a little about nutrition, to read the labels of even "healthy" processed foods is to be shocked by how much salt, oil, and sugar virtually all of them contain.) I also bade farewell to the gin-and-tonics and restaurant meals. It was a lot to give up and simultaneously the smallest possible sacrifice for a shot at getting my life back.

After refeeding on applesauce and potatoes, I embarked on my new way of eating. My habitual breakfast became a giant salad of mixed greens, purple cabbage, sprouts, and tomatoes liberally garnished with avocado, berries, walnuts, and balsamic vinegar. For a second course I usually took a seedy porridge of oats, fruit, and soy milk. Lunch might be a curry of mushroom and eggplant with a side of steamed broccoli; dinner, a spicy lentil soup and a sweet potato. For dessert there were raspberry crumble, almond-millet cake, and of course pumpkin pie. Once I'd learned a few tricks of the minimally processed vegan trade—sauté with water, sweeten with dates, spice with abandon—it was surprising how delicious I could make dishes without salt, oil, sugar, or white flour.

It was also terrifying. Over every meal hovered the question "Is this the food that does me in?" and every morning I awoke panicked that the hypersomnia had returned in the night. But meal after meal, morning after morning, the disease stayed away. So did the depersonalization. My energy and mood soared, and the clenching migraines, while still a force, were clearly trending downward as well. My notes from those first months read like a page from Cinderella's diary for her night at the ball: a savoring of every ecstatic hour, with a keen awareness the clock would strike midnight and coach and gown would once more become pumpkin and rags. Surely getting rid of decades of disease—all that misery and helplessness, all those drugs and doctors—couldn't be as easy as just fasting a couple of weeks and then eating plants. It *had* to be more complicated than that. But still the clock didn't chime.

I recovered other parts of my life too. Every hypersomniac knows he shouldn't hate himself for the many things he's unable to do in his stupor, but talk to a hundred of us, and I'll wager you'll not find more than two or three who don't berate themselves prodigiously for their many failures. As I healed, I berated less, liked myself more, found a measure of patience. Others liked me better too. My memory began to rebound, and most days I could recall where I'd put my wallet, what I ate for dinner the night before, the name of my third-grade girlfriend. Cautiously, I restarted my career, and some of what I wrote was good.

I don't want to oversell this. Roses didn't fall from the heavens to line my path. But the path was now level, no longer the steep incline I had trudged up so long, and that was miracle enough. A month after breaking my fast, I was sufficiently emboldened to wean myself off my antidepressant. In the past, "going off my meds" had brought psychological collapse within months, but there was no implosion this time. Soon I was discarding other pills: the Xanax for anxiety, the Lunesta for sleep, and—with a flourish as the bottle landed in the take-to-the-pharmacy box—the modafinil for wakefulness. One day the shelf in the bathroom that held my many prescriptions was empty, soon to be colonized by a stack of hand towels that I still look on with special fondness. I hadn't felt this good since my twenties, if then.

I regretted only that the cure had been right under my nose all along and that I had lost most of a decade because I'd been too obtuse to pick up what Goldhamer had set before me. For salve, I had a lot of company. Nearly the entire medical profession for nearly the entirety of its history has been just as obtuse, and it's to this dunderheadedness, and the struggle against it, that we turn next.

CHAPTER 8

"REFUSE TO BE AN INVALID!"

In the first decades of the twentieth century, therapeutic fasting rose to a sudden and wholly unforeseen prominence, one surpassing even the frenzied heights attending Henry Tanner's fast of 1880. The ascent was largely the work of two men. One was an unassuming country doctor of sober and pious demeanor; the other, one of history's great showmen, a narcissist of unsurpassed bombast.

The country doctor was Edward Hooker Dewey. Born in northwestern Pennsylvania in 1837, he came to fasting in much the same way as that earlier Edwardian country doctor, Edward Jennings. Dewey's first inkling that medicine did as much harm as good came in a Union field hospital in Chattanooga during the Civil War, where he was dispatched after taking his medical degree from the University of Michigan. Overseeing a ward of the wounded and sick scared him plank stiff, but he later concluded "those patients were as safe, even on the first day of my care . . . as were the patients of the most experienced surgeon in the hospital," for no matter which treatment or which doctor gave it, the patients got well, or not, at about the same rate.

After the war, Dewey returned home and practiced conventionally in the town of Meadville, south of Erie. But in July of 1877, the same month Henry Tanner made his first long fast in Minneapolis, he encountered a patient who changed his life. She was a "rather well rounded" young woman already much weakened by digestive problems when she contracted typhoid. For three weeks she couldn't keep down food, water, or medicine. Eventually her thirst returned, and upon drinking she looked positively reborn, but still she had no interest in eating. Dewey heeded the message her body seemed to be sending and let her fast "until about the thirty-fifth day, when there was a call, not for the undertaker, but for food"—a sign, he believed, her body had finished its healing work. The woman's recovery so astounded Dewey that he began fasting other patients, although if they insisted on nourishment he allowed them "meat teas" and "cereal broths." Nearly all of them, he said, got well.

Seeking an explanation for how his typhoid patient had endured a fast of five weeks, he found a piece of the answer in Gerald Yeo's *Manual of Physiology*. Yeo was a professor at King's College London who reported that the typical person who starved to death lost 97 percent of his fat, 56 percent of his liver, and 30 percent of his muscle, but almost none of his brain or nervous system. Evidently the wasting body didn't eat its tissues evenly. Instead, it selected which parts to devour and spared the more crucial ones for as long as possible. Dewey recalled seeing the same phenomenon in postmortems at the Chattanooga field hospital. In men who had died of wasting sicknesses, the brain, heart, and lungs were always well preserved unless those organs had themselves been the seat of disease. It was a Eureka moment.

"Instantly," Dewey wrote, "I saw in human bodies a vast reserve of predigested food, with the brain in possession of the power so to absorb [it] . . . in the absence of food" and thus able to function, unimpaired, even as the rest of the body withered. He would find corroboration for this idea from another of his patients, a boy of four who destroyed his stomach by drinking a caustic potash. Unable to eat, the child lingered seventy-five days, his mind "clear to the last hour," the brain preserved even though the rest of his body was little more than a breathing corpse.

Dewey concluded, as his predecessors had, that in illness one needn't be "in hot haste to force food into unwilling stomachs," for to do so was to put "a tax on vital power when we need all that power to cure disease." He began fasting people fearlessly, often for weeks, sometimes months—he must have been buoyed by Tanner's foodless forty days—and began to rack up a list of victories that his previous medicines had failed to achieve. One "very much worn-out mother" with inflammatory rheumatism fasted forty-six days until her joints returned to normal and her vigor was restored. An Illinois man with a chronic catarrh of the nose and throat (an oozy blend of inflammation and mucus) whom Dewey instructed by post reported complete relief after a fast of forty-two days. A man of sixty-five who lost his appetite after a bronchial attack fasted his way back to health over two months. Stomach disorders, infirmities of the heart, and dropsy also supposedly fell to Dewey's fasts.

He seems to have been the first doctor who chanced abstinence of such great length—doubling and tripling the twenty-one days Edward Kittredge had fasted patients—but long fasts were only half of the Dewey method. He also practiced what the popular press of today would call intermittent fasting. He was his own first patient. As a younger man, before discovering prolonged fasting, he suffered from chronic indigestion and a near-ravenous hunger that left him haggard. One day a friend who had returned from Europe told him breakfast in the great capitals of the Old World was rarely more than a roll and coffee, and Dewey, thentofore a hearty-breakfast man, tried taking nothing but coffee one morning. To his amazement, he passed the forenoon in an italicized ecstasy of *"such lofty mental cheer, such energy of soul and body, such a sense of physical ease as I had not known since a young man in my later teens."* His haggardness left him, friends commented on his vitality, and soon he was urging patients to adopt what today would be called an 18:6 or 16:8 diet—taking food six or eight hours a day and fasting the other eighteen or sixteen. In Dewey's version, the largest of the day's two meals was the first, with the second kept light and eaten early so as not to burden the stomach before sleep. As we'll see later, recent science proves these principles more sound than not. Within those strictures, Dewey didn't much care what his patients ate. He believed the quantity and frequency of food, not its character, were the root of all ill—an assumption far less sound.

At the end of the nineteenth century, it verged on apostasy to tell Americans to eat less, for the stupendous Yankee appetite had only continued to balloon. But Dewey was buttressed by the cures he thought he achieved with his no-breakfast plan, some of which were apparently as impressive as those from prolonged fasting. One woman of middle years, long tormented by angina, agonies of the stomach, a rheumatism so wracking she could hardly close her hands, and severe depression, lost all of her troubles over two or three years of skipping breakfast and eating light and early. Another lady of seventy-three who had grown so deaf she could no longer hear the church bells and couldn't climb stairs without assistance got her hearing back and could walk half a mile uphill. A man in his sixties, a farmer, lost a rheumatism and chronic cough that had long discomfited him and said he was able to work harder than he had in his youth.

Beginning in 1895, Dewey set out his therapies in books that went through multiple printings on both sides of the Atlantic. The most popular was *The No-Breakfast Plan and the Fasting-Cure*, published in 1900, which found an audience not because it was especially novel—for many years, as we've seen, doctors had called for fasting and light eating—but because after Tanner's fast, the public was more receptive. It helped that Dewey was compassionate, usually avoided ridiculous claims (although he could occasionally steer himself over a logical cliff, as when he argued *every* disease was caused by overfeeding), and soaked his paeans to health in the same Christian moralism in which his fellow Americans were already well pickled. Echoing both Tertullian and Basil the Great, he argued that the discipline and fortitude acquired through fasting would improve not just the body personal but the body politic, the body religious, and of course that precious entity for which the body was but a vessel, the soul. "If you are Christians," he wrote of those who would fast, "you will become a great deal better Christians; if husbands, a great deal better husbands; if wives, a great deal better wives."

His doctrine found few friends among his regular colleagues. His local medical society demanded his resignation, and the *British Medical Journal* wrote of his fasting cures, "All that Dr. Dewey's cases prove, assuming that he was not deceived, is that neurotic zealots can go without food for long periods, but that we knew before, and there is nothing in his book to show that fasting as a panacea is other than a foolish delusion." A medical professor at the University of Pennsylvania said Dewey's patients who claimed to have walked ten miles after not eating for a month must be "falsifying" because such a feat was plainly impossible.

"Falsifiers, these fasters?" Dewey replied. "Science settles important questions by investigation, not by epithet." But in fact where fasting was concerned, men of science routinely settled for epithet.

Other minds, however, were not so closed, and among the laity the creed of Dewey and Tanner spread. Mark Twain spoke for many when he wrote in 1899, "A little starvation can really do more for the average sick man than can the best medicines and the best doctors. I do not mean a restricted diet; I mean total abstention from food for one or two days. I speak from experience; starvation has been my cold and fever doctor for fifteen years, and has accomplished a cure in all instances."

*   *   *

The narcissistic showman who propagandized for fasting like no one before or since was Bernarr Macfadden, the inimitable. Born Bernard McFadden in the Missouri Ozarks in 1868, he amended his name in adulthood to give it a whiff of what he deemed foreign sophistication. He had a childhood straight out of Dickens. His abusive father drank himself to death, and his impoverished and tubercular mother, unable to care for him, consigned him to a joyless boarding school with a skinflint headmaster who kept the pupils on starvation rations. Later he was shipped off to servitude under a heartless aunt and uncle who ran a dismal inn in Illinois.

"If there's work in him," the uncle said as he surveyed the scrawny nine-year-old, "we'll get it out."

And they did. Sixteen hours a day Macfadden scrubbed floors, washed laundry, blacked boots, helped drunks into bed, and emptied chamber pots. Only when a truancy officer came calling did he attend school. After the fleabag hostelry died, Macfadden was sold for petty cash and a scattering of produce to a farmer once described as "the stingiest son of a bitch east of the Mississippi River." The farmer kept Macfadden so poorly clothed that he got frostbite milking the cows, but he found a kind of salvation in the muscles the endless chores put on his body, and in his fitness he was building the foundations of a philosophy of health.

At twelve, he ran away to St. Louis and at last landed with kindly relatives—a family of Betsey Trotwoods to the Edward Murdstones of his past. As a teen, he bulked up with dumbbells and opened a boxing school in a stable before taking up professional wrestling as both promoter and contestant. Although only five foot six, he racked up enough victories to earn a modest fame, which allowed him to open shop as a "kinisithera-pist teacher of higher physical culture." "Kinisitherapist"—from the Greek *kinisis*, meaning "motion"—was a neologism of Macfadden's mak-ing, one of many linguistic casseroles he would cook up over the years when a marketable idea needed to be dressed up by a little Greco-Latin mangling. Among his other insufferable coinages were "physcultopathy" and "cosmotarianism." On the other hand, the verbal contrivances testi-fied to a self-taught mind not content to do things the way they'd always been done.

At his kinisitherapy studio, Macfadden debuted the slogan with which he would be identified for life: "Weakness Is a Crime—Don't Be a Criminal." He taught his pupils how to build deliciously sculpted muscles and how to eat, or rather how not to. More than a decade before Dewey published his works on fasting and skipping breakfast, Macfadden con-cluded he was stronger on two meals a day than three, and he would later whittle them to one. He also advocated prolonged fasting, which he dis-covered during a childhood bout of pneumonia. Remembering that farm animals stopped eating when sick, he tried it and thought his pneumonia improved. Like so many shrewd observers before him, he inferred that eat-ing when ill somehow interfered with the body's ability to heal itself.

St. Louis proved far too small a town for a young man of Macfadden's ambition, and shortly before the turn of the century he left for New York City with fifty dollars in his pocket, a suitcase full of dumbbells, and the new name. In New York he staged "Physical Culture Matinees" in which he flexed the rippling muscles of his fasted body, attired to advan-tage in loincloth, and chest-pressed 200-pound men who stood on his hands—proof, of a sort, that fasting strengthened rather than weakened.

To spread his philosophy of health, he wrote articles by the dozen, which were rejected by the dozen. Undaunted, in 1899 he started his own magazine, *Physical Culture*. Rarely has a periodical changed a country so quickly.

With his truncated motto "Weakness a Crime—Don't Be a Criminal" on the cover, Macfadden pitched weightlifting, exercise, and a dietary rectitude whose pillars were vegetarianism, moderation at table, and fasting. He picked up the empowering strains of earlier health reformers by arguing that "disease is not sent by divine providence," that it arose from poor diet or indolence, and through proper nourishment and exercise the unhealthy body could be restored to a "self-regulating apparatus," a "house that cleanses its own chambers." Unfortunately, proper nourishment excluded many of the staples Americans held most dear: meat, sugar, white bread ("the staff of death"), alcohol, and tobacco—much the same list of forbiddens Sylvester Graham had settled on.

Macfadden made this bitter medicine palatable with the promise of the body beautiful, photographed specimens of which, male and female, he strewed across the pages of *Physical Culture*. His models were little obscured by fabric and sometimes by no fabric at all, the generative instruments concealed by artful posing or foliage. Macfadden was refreshingly candid about all things corporal, including sex, indigestion, and bowel movements, and he ranked prudishness high on the roster of evils that physcultopathy would eliminate. Where earlier reformers like Graham urged health to subdue the wicked body, Macfadden sought health because the body was exquisite, an apex creation that gave its greatest pleasure when in optimal form. Coitus in particular was to be relished, and he instructed not just men but also—rare for his day—women in how to enjoy it. After decades of Victorian stuffiness, and years before Sigmund Freud's seminally liberating work, this was heady stuff.

Physical Culture's first print run of five thousand copies in 1899 grew to more than a hundred thousand by the end of 1900, on par with such shapers of society as *Atlantic Monthly* and *Harper's*. More than fifty million copies would be sold between the two world wars. His live exhibits of fasted bodybuilders frolicking in the nearly-altogether sold out Madison

Square Garden—five thousand people had to be turned away from one show—and earned him obscenity charges from Anthony Comstock's morality police. Convicted of mail-order obscenity, he was spared the hoosegow only after President Taft commuted his two-year sentence. His scrapes with the conservators of chastity only increased his appeal.

Millions heeded his call to exercise. Within a decade of *Physical Culture*'s founding, attendance at YMCAs around the nation tripled, and one of Macfadden's protégés, an Italian immigrant named Angelo Siciliano, was rechristened Charles Atlas and under Macfadden's relentless promotion became the twentieth century's most famous proselyte of bodybuilding until Arnold Schwarzenegger. It's not much of an exaggeration to say Macfadden single-handedly launched both the cult of the body beautiful and the era of physical fitness in which we're still living.

On the success of *Physical Culture*, Macfadden built a publishing empire whose métier was the lurid and tawdry. His *True Story*, published in 1919, was America's first confessional magazine, a sensationalist ragbag of first-person romance, celebrity gossip, and a certain elasticity with the truth. Its circulation quickly topped two million a month, and other pulp magazines followed: *True Detective*, *True Romances*, *True Marriage*, *True Love*. In 1924, he spawned a newspaper of infinite dreadfulness called the *New York Evening Graphic*, which, as one of his biographers noted, was "widely considered to be the worst newspaper in U.S. history." He and his staff also turned out dozens of bestselling books under his name, including such gems as *Macfadden's New Hair Culture* (in which baldness is fended off by vigorously pulling on one's hair) and *Strong Eyes: How Weak Eyes May Be Strengthened and Spectacles Discarded* (by squinting and otherwise scrunching the facial muscles). His empire grew so swiftly that at his Manhattan headquarters he partitioned eleven-foot-high offices vertically so that one office of five and a half feet sat atop another with a ladder running between them. (His proposal to relieve crowded New York subway trains with similar partitions found no takers.) At the peak of his powers in 1929, he employed 2,500 people who put out periodicals with a combined annual circulation of 220 million. His influence on popular culture really can't be overstated.

Among this outpouring were writings on fasting, starting with his 1900 book *Fasting, Hydropathy, and Exercise*. For those in good health, Macfadden counseled one prolonged fast a year as a kind of preventive (the same recommendation many fasting doctors give today), while for common illnesses he suggested fasts of two to seven days. For more serious diseases, fasts of up to ninety days were called for, but he preferred shorter fasts broken by periods of eating because they were safer. In the 1920 edition of *Macfadden's Encyclopedia of Physical Culture*, his ghostwriters surveyed the literature and practice of fasting and concluded it could cure or greatly ameliorate "every kind of dyspepsia and stomach troubles, . . . cancers, pneumonia, every form of skin disease, chronic headache, constipation, nervous exhaustion, low vitality, hemorrhoids, diseases of the kidneys, general debility, asthma, dropsy, various forms of liver complaint, catarrh of every kind, rheumatism, typhoid and typhus fevers, scarlet fever, and indeed practically every ill that human flesh is heir to." With the exclusion of the hyperbolic final clause, his list was more right than wrong.

Macfadden found a willing audience primed not just by the exertions of Tanner and Dewey but by the glacial creep of medical progress. Since Joseph Lister's discovery of antiseptic principles in 1865, medicine had advanced with agonizing sloth, at least so far as everyday life was concerned. Public health measures had modestly lowered the incidence of infectious disease, and diagnosis and surgery had made great strides, but doctors were hardly more adept at treating acute or chronic afflictions than they had been a century earlier. The next great medical advance—the development of sulfonamides, the first antibiotics—wouldn't come until the 1930s, so at the start of the twentieth century fasting was still as good as or better than conventional treatments for most common disorders. These were not facts that "the medical trust," as Macfadden styled them, cared to acknowledge, and he condemned their trade "the murderous science."

"Your physicians have failed you, drugs have not relieved you," he lectured his readers, "so why not cease to rely upon the judgment of others and exercise the God-given power of your own individual thought. Be a man! Be a woman!"

"Refuse to be an invalid!"

The American Medical Association countered with exposés about Macfadden's quack remedies, from which there were plenty to choose. A contender for the loopiest was a device he patented called the Peniscope, built from a glass tube, a vacuum pump, and the yearnings of middle-aged men. People fasted anyway. Newspapers at the turn of the century told of a Mrs. Emma Wacker of Lancaster, Ohio, who said she fasted away her dropsy over forty days; a Mr. Edward De Forest, the proprietor of a Turkish bath in Brooklyn, who claimed to have tamed his stomach problems with a fast of similar length; and a Dr. William S. Wilkinson of Augusta, Georgia, an uncommon regular with a mind open to fasting, who fasted fifty-seven days to chase away dyspepsia.

"Is prolonged fasting becoming a fad?" the *New York Tribune* asked in 1903.

It wasn't, but neither was it the oddity it had once been.

Macfadden tried to build institutions to perpetuate physcultopathy and fasting but without lasting success. One was a New Jersey hamlet he founded in 1905 and named, a trifle ambitiously, Physical Culture City. The metropolis-to-be was home to "no sickly prudes, no saloons, drug stores, tobacco shops or places in which one may purchase things that make for the moral undoing of man or woman." It did, however, have nudists disporting in the sunshine, to the delight of passengers on an adjacent rail line, whose seats were somewhat better filled on the side nearer the village. (At a subsequent endeavor, the Bernarr Macfadden Hotel in Dansville, New York, appreciative pilots altered their flight paths for a bird's-eye inspection of unclad sunbathers on the roof.) Physical Culture City dissolved in a chaos of dysfunction, one piece of which was that Macfadden, having tiresomely preached the sanctity of marriage, was found to be bonking his secretary. But Macfadden pressed on, championing physcultopathy through a hundred Physical Culture Clubs across the country, summer camps for schoolboys, a pair of Bernarr Macfadden Elementary Schools in suburban New York, sister colonies for undernourished boys in New Jersey and Portugal, and a military academy called Castle Heights in Lebanon, Tennessee. Benito Mussolini, whom Macfadden admired, sent forty fascist cadets to train at Castle Heights and asked the Italian king to decorate Macfadden

"Commander of the Order of the Crown of Italy." The academy endured until 1974, but the only other physcultopathic endeavor with even modest staying power was a chain of twenty Physical Culture Restaurants in New York, Philadelphia, Boston, and Chicago that served vegetarian meals for a nickel, a penny if you dined in the basement.

By the 1930s, Macfadden was easily the world's most famous health guru, but his aspirations were grander still. In 1936, he spread $100,000 in bribes to Republican officials to secure the party's presidential nomination, and when that failed, he ran for the US Senate in Florida's 1940 Democratic primary. Barnstorming the state in a plane he piloted himself, he promised to defend racial segregation, improve the "spinal musculature" of Floridians, and turn Florida into a health mecca. His campaign was a touch hampered by his being neither a Floridian nor a Democrat until a few breaths before announcing his run. After that loss, he abandoned politics and in 1944 filed papers to start his own religion. Cosmotarianism, a blend of Christianity and Macfaddenist health doctrine, was one of the shortest-lived faiths in the history of the planet. In the end, his publishing empire collapsed from mismanagement, and he died poor and alone in New Jersey—the saddest concluding words known to the craft of biography.

In his last decades, proselytizing for fasting was far from Macfadden's mind, but he had spread the gospel so broadly in his early years that other thinkers, generally of more temperate outlook, were able to pick up where he left off. One was the great polemicist Upton Sinclair.

*   *   *

Sinclair was sharper of mind than Macfadden and just as indefatigable, a true wonder of productivity. He didn't start school until the age of ten and then worked so feverishly to catch up that he overshot the mark and matriculated at the City College of New York before turning fourteen. As a law student at Columbia, he hired stenographers to keep up with the torrents of pulp fiction surging from his brain, as many as eight thousand words a day, and by the time he wrote the novel at age twenty-seven that would secure his place in history, he'd already written twenty books. That novel, of course, was *The Jungle*, which Sinclair published in 1906 to show the insupportable misery of immigrant workers in Chicago's meatpacking industry. Americans, however, were more appalled at the squalor in which their meat was prepared. Meat sales tumbled, Congress passed tougher laws for food inspection, and Sinclair lamented, "I aimed at the public's heart, and by accident I hit it in the stomach." He would go on to win the Pulitzer Prize in 1943 for his novel *Dragon's Teeth* and to lose races on the Socialist ticket for the US House and Senate and on the Democratic ticket for the governorship of California. His radical platform included such horrors as pensions to keep the elderly from starving. *Time* praised him as "a man with every gift except humor and silence"—getting it half right (he could be quite witty), above average for *Time*.

One of the books his biographers almost never mention, as if it's an embarrassment on the order of his pulp fiction, and that historians of the Progressive Era mention only to denigrate, is *The Fasting Cure*. But in fact *The Fasting Cure* is an important marker, the first prominent plea for a scientific assessment of fasting. It originally appeared in 1910 and 1911 as articles in *Cosmopolitan*, which in those days was a general interest magazine more inclined to plumb the quadrilles of the French court or the decline of the US Army than to serve up tips for sultry sex and blemish-free skin. Sinclair's first article prompted more letters to the editor, nearly all curious and favorable, than any other piece in *Cosmopolitan*'s quarter century of publishing, and the postmarks came from as far afield as Argentina, Spain, and India.

The book begins as most fasting stories do, with the author's stubborn illness. Sinclair's was a dyspepsia that evolved into a suffocating exhaustion that baffled his doctors. Unable to work for months at a time, he took the air at spas in Bermuda and the Adirondacks, underwent hydrotherapy at Michigan's renowned Battle Creek Sanitarium, practiced the rigorous food-chewing regimen known as Fletcherism, and tried every other remedy that sounded even remotely plausible. Nearly always his health improved temporarily but never lastingly, a testament to the ephemerality of the placebo effect. Over seven years, doctors, druggists, and spas relieved him of $15,000, the equivalent of nearly $500,000 today.

But in 1909 while sojourning in California he "chanced to meet a lady, whose radiant complexion and extraordinary health were a matter of remark to everyone." Together they endured a grueling horseback ascent in the Diablo Range during a wild tempest, and Sinclair was amazed to learn she managed the feat without having eaten for four days. Still more incredible, until quite recently she had spent a decade bedridden with sciatica, rheumatism, intestinal inflammation, and a chronic catarrh that left her deaf. But after a fast of eight days, "all her trouble had fallen from her."

Impressed though he was, Sinclair wasn't eager to fast himself, but when his ailments flared again, he gave it a try and was flabbergasted by the results. "Previous to the fast," he wrote, "I had had a headache every day for two or three weeks. It lasted through the first day and then disappeared— never to return." He grew stronger, his mind sharpened, and by the time he broke his fast after twelve days, most of his symptoms had vanished. Later he decided he had refed too soon, and after fasting another eight days, "every trace of my old trouble was gone. Formerly I had had to lie down for an hour or two after meals; now I could do whatever I chose. Formerly I had been dependent upon all kinds of laxative preparations; now I forgot about them. . . . I went bareheaded in the rain, I sat in cold draughts of air, and was apparently immune to colds. And, above all, I had that marvellous, abounding energy."

After his articles ran in *Cosmopolitan*, he asked people who fasted therapeutically to answer a questionnaire whose results he reported in *The Fasting Cure*. It was a small mountain of anecdotal evidence attesting to improvements in a sweeping variety of disorders: bronchitis and asthma; eczema, piles, and pruritis; nephritis and other troubles of the kidney; indigestion, constipation, and consumption of the bowels; catarrh of the head and intestines; leakage of the heart; a leg ulcerated and inflamed for fourteen years; a scrofula that had mystified doctors for five years; and on and on. In all, 109 of his respondents had fasted to treat illness, of whom 92 reported either a total cure or substantial improvement. For those who wished to investigate, Sinclair supplied names, addresses, ages, and details of their conditions. It was, in short, as diligent a compilation of case studies as a layperson of the time could have made while still holding the interest of the reading public. He hoped by his efforts "to interest some scientific men in making a real investigation." He wasn't asking scientists or anyone else to take his word that fasting worked. He was merely saying, much as Edward Miller had in the *Medical Repository* a century earlier, that such a mass of anecdotes from so many and varied people—of all ages, both sexes, from every region of the country—suggested fasting could in fact cure, and he thought researchers should investigate.

"Surely it cannot be," he wrote, "that medical men and scientists will continue for much longer to close their eyes to facts of such vital significance as this."

But most scientists did just that. Some accused Sinclair of claiming too much for fasting, and in this they were right. While most of *The Fasting Cure* has an air of judicious sensibility, Sinclair also called fasting "the key to eternal youth, the secret of perfect and permanent health" and "an automatic protection against disease" with just a few exceptions (among them "virulent diseases, such as smallpox or typhoid"). Of his friends stricken with grave illnesses, he claimed "there is not one of these people whom I could not cure if I had him alone for a couple of weeks." His overstatement was off-putting to the unconverted.

But even had Sinclair been more sober, it's hard to imagine doctors and scientists weighing his claims without prejudice. Of the seven hundred or so letters he received about his fasting articles, only two were from regular physicians, just one of whom was interested in using fasting as therapy. "Of course I realize," Sinclair wrote, "what a difficult matter it is for a medical man to face these facts about the fast. Sometimes it seems to me that we have no right to expect their help at all, and that we never will receive it. For we are asking them to destroy themselves, economically speaking." This was an early formulation of his most famous and more general maxim: "It is difficult to get a man to understand something, when his salary depends upon his not understanding it." And for a doctor to acknowledge the merits of fasting would have threatened more than his salary. To admit that the body, if left alone, could often heal itself was as good as admitting that a portion of the craft he had so laboriously learned and diligently practiced was humbug.

Many laypeople didn't care to see doctors defrocked either. An editorial writer for the *New York Times* voiced what may have been the common sentiment when he condemned Sinclair a "shallow and unscrupulous sensationalist" for provoking others to fast, and H. L. Mencken derided him "a wholesale believer in the obviously not so." The telling word was *obviously*. No science need be invoked to disprove fasting, which was all too plainly harmful. Sinclair took the rejection dryly. When his friend Arthur Brisbane, the celebrated newspaper editor and an opponent of fasting, grudgingly acknowledged that even dogs fasted when ill, Sinclair replied, "I look forward to the time when human beings may be as wise as dogs."

But while most establishmentarians were deaf to fasting, the deafness wasn't universal. The efforts of Dewey, Macfadden, Sinclair, and others were beginning to tell, and a few years after *The Fasting Cure*, scientists made their first real efforts to evaluate fasting for therapeutic use, a couple of which yielded glorious results.

* * *

Guillaume Guelpa first became intrigued by fasting when one of his medical colleagues noted that typhoid patients who lost weight recovered from the disease fairly quickly while those who maintained their weight struggled and died disproportionately. Guelpa, an Italian-born doctor practicing in Paris, hypothesized that the sick body got well by burning off the agents of disease, and if a thinned body did this better than a well-fed body, it was probably because it was unburdened by food. On experimenting, he found two to four days of fasting were enough to cure many acute illnesses, and he also observed that during fasting the intestinal flora were completely eliminated, the liver and heart shrank, blood pressure dropped, inflamed joints and muscles became less painful, and labored breathing grew easier.

Over three decades, Guelpa would fast thousands of patients, and of the many remarkable cures he reported, perhaps none were more compelling or received more notice, at least in Europe, than his cases of diabetes. In those days before the discovery of insulin, diabetes was as good as a death sentence, but as early as 1896 Guelpa found that three days of fasting and saline enemas could eliminate glycosuria, the sugar in the urine that was the leading diagnostic indicator of diabetes. (He may have been influenced by the French diabetologist Apollinaire Bouchardat, who observed half a century earlier that fasting reduced sugar in the urine.) Guelpa developed a regimen in which he fasted and purged diabetic patients for four days, fed them a diet free of meat, eggs, and alcohol for four days, and repeated the process for as many cycles as needed to reduce the patient's urinary sugar to zero. He successfully reversed scores of cases of diabetes and maintained the cures with a spare diet of fruits, vegetables, and a small amount of bread and coffee. In 1910, at a meeting of the British Medical Association, he said that although fasting a diabetic patient might seem scary, *la méthode Guelpa* "is never harmful" and could achieve a "cure of diabetes, even when accompanied by the most serious complications." The disease everyone knew to be fatal, he was declaring, needn't be. It could be reversed by simply not eating and then eating plants.

The reaction to this shocking announcement was equivocal. A diabetes specialist at St. Bartholomew's Hospital in London adjudged Guelpa brilliant but prone to exaggeration, and colleagues in France said other mechanisms, undetected by Guelpa, must be at work in his cures, if in fact they were cures. But a few doctors were more broadminded. After Guelpa lectured the British Royal Society of Medicine in 1921, the noted physician Sir William Wilcox said the Frenchman had "scarcely received in this country the praise which was his due as the father of one of the greatest advances in modern medicine." Another eminent doctor, Frederick Parkes Weber, remembered today for his work on the vascular condition Parkes Weber syndrome, urged Guelpa to write a history of how the fasting cure had been used in different countries of the world. (Would that he had.)

Like Sinclair, Guelpa believed it wouldn't be long before doctors gave fasting its due and abandoned their ineffective treatments. "The resulting benefits, for the good of society and to the great honor of our profession, will be incalculable," he wrote. "We can foresee the near disappearance of certain diseases such as diabetes and gout, the reduction in the duration of others, and the excessive rarity of their relapses."

But that halcyon future never arrived, and after his death in 1930 Guelpa and his method were almost entirely forgotten.

* * *

But before events came to that sad pass a variant of la méthode Guelpa was tried by an American endocrinologist named Frederick Madison Allen, who, however, was not so insightful as Guelpa. After a short stint as an undistinguished fellow at Harvard, Allen ran the diabetes clinic at New York's Rockefeller Institute starting in 1914. He hypothesized that a greatly reduced diet would give the pancreas (the organ overtaxed in diabetes) time to recover its proper function, and he devised a regimen in which diabetics fasted several days until their urine was free of sugar, after which they ate a vegetarian diet similar to Guelpa's but with far fewer calories. Unfortunately the Allen Plan, as it was called, failed to rehabilitate the pancreas, and the diet was so meager that the patients died of starvation or malnutrition if diabetes didn't claim them first. The only count on which the Allen Plan succeeded was buying patients several more months of life, which for a lucky few was long enough to benefit from the discovery of insulin in 1921. The most famous of these fortunate souls was Elizabeth Evans Hughes, the young daughter of Charles Evans Hughes, a Republican fixture and future chief justice of the US Supreme Court.

It's possible Allen's method failed where Guelpa's succeeded because Guelpa's repeated fasts induced repair mechanisms that Allen's single fast did not. We have little research to say, but a peer-reviewed case series from 2018 reported the reversal of type 2 diabetes in three patients who fasted twenty-four hours three times a week over several months while making dietary changes. Dr. Alan Goldhamer of the TrueNorth Health Center in California has also reported reversing cases of type 2 diabetes through prolonged fasts followed by a diet roughly similar to Guelpa's, and recent science has shown that even without a fast, a diet of minimally refined plants can greatly ameliorate or even completely reverse type 2 diabetes.

Perhaps Guelpa's regimen more closely approximated that kind of diet than Allen's did.

The discovery of insulin was a benison, as was the abandonment of the Allen Plan, but the simultaneous neglect of Guelpa's method was little short of criminal. Synthetic insulin, after all, didn't cure diabetes, which still had to be ceaselessly managed. Before her death in 1981, Elizabeth Evans Hughes gave herself an estimated 42,000 insulin injections, monitored her glucose continuously, and reported regularly to doctors. With Guelpa's treatment, she might have avoided all that or, failing a complete cure, benefited from a more subdued disease requiring thousands fewer injections. When doctors in the early part of the century were asked why they didn't care for Guelpa's method, they usually said it was too time-consuming. The time they meant was their own. The time to self-administer tens of thousands of injections, fill prescriptions, manage side effects, keep a watchful eye on blood sugar, and visit clinics was none of their concern. The companies that manufactured insulin thought their customers' time well spent too.

Today millions of diabetics are told by doctors and diabetic-advocacy groups that their disease has no cure. No doubt these authorities believe it to be so, but their ignorance is a stain on the profession that has nourished it.

*   *   *

The early twentieth century also saw the first experiments into fasting for epilepsy.* Edward Hooker Dewey reported in 1900 that he had fasted "a half dozen cases [of epilepsy], in which permanent relief seems to be assured," but the first doctor to make a systematic, if rudimentary, trial was

* To hear modern writers tell it, fasting was used against epilepsy with some regularity by the ancients, particularly Hippocrates and Jesus. But the Hippocratic Corpus says nothing about fasting to cure epilepsy (there's only a story of a boy whose seizures stopped on a day he didn't eat, with no suggestion his fast cured him), and Jesus didn't say epileptics should pray and fast, only that the *exorcist*s who wanted to drive out epileptic demons should—and the fasting part of the verse was almost certainly added later by fasting zealots. Nearly the only ancient authority to have advocated fasting for epilepsy was Erasistratus, the Greek doctor of the third century BC, mentioned in chapter 3, who said the epileptic "should maintain a regimen of constant physical labor and either fasting or minimal food."

once again Guillaume Guelpa. With his psychiatrist colleague Auguste Marie, Guelpa prescribed his regimen of fasting, purging, and vegetarian diet to twenty child and adult epileptics, most of whom had trouble sticking with the program. Even so, some improved, and two seem to have been completely cured. In a paper published in 1911, Guelpa and Marie noted the children fared better than the adults but couldn't say whether that was because they were better responders or just more easily kept on the regimen. The doctors also reported that their patients' mental acuity, dulled by their seizures or by the potassium bromide they took for them, sharpened as they fasted and did so even when the seizures continued. But European doctors were no more interested in building on Guelpa and Marie's epileptic work than they were on Guelpa's diabetic accomplishments, and Americans hardly knew of it.

By chance, though, one American doctor was fasting his own epileptics, probably in total ignorance of Guelpa and Marie. Hugh Conklin had come to Battle Creek, Michigan, in 1905 as a newly diplomated osteopath to run the osteopathic department at the short-lived Bernarr Macfadden Sanatorium. Macfadden established the outfit to rival the great Battle Creek Sanitarium of the Kellogg brothers, of breakfast cereal fame, and even developed a competing cereal, Strengtho, which flopped. So did his sanatorium after just two years. But Conklin stuck around and, mightily influenced by Macfadden, continued to fast all manner of patients. He fasted his epileptics for "as long as they are physically able to stand it," which usually came to between eighteen and twenty-five days but could be as long as sixty. If one fast didn't rid them of their fits, he refed them for a few weeks and fasted them again. And again. And sometimes a fourth time. Conklin had a reputation as a tender caregiver, but he stood with Benjamin Rush when he advised his fellow osteopaths, "Discomfort of the patient is no due consideration for discontinuance of the treatment." Unlike Guelpa, he didn't recommend any particular way of eating after his fasts, although if a patient's seizures flared once more, he found a vegan diet usually brought them under control.

Conklin reported astounding rates of success, especially in children, as Guelpa and Marie had. He estimated he cured 90 percent of his patients under ten years of age, 80 percent of those from ten to fifteen years, 65 percent from fifteen to twenty-five, 50 percent from twenty-five to forty, and very few over forty. These rates may have been overestimates based on wishful recall, but it was equally certain his cures were numerous. He was wrong, however, in his conjecture about why the therapy worked. He thought it was because fasting detoxified parts of the intestines known as Peyer's patches, which for a time were believed to secrete toxins that caused convulsions.

Because epilepsy was another disease that supposedly knew no cure and often retarded its victims dreadfully, Conklin's claims of success were as dizzying as Guelpa's were for diabetes. But the assertions of a mere osteopath were even less respected than those of the regular Guelpa, and were it not for a young patient named Henry Howland, Conklin's discovery might have left no mark on history at all. Henry's father Charles was a flourishing New York lawyer descended from *Mayflower* stock, his family tree decorated by Longfellow, Emerson, and Henry Cabot Lodge. At the age of six, Henry began seizing badly, and the medications of the day—bromides and phenobarbital—gave him no respite. Somehow the Howlands learned of Conklin's work, and in 1919, when Henry was ten, his fits by then "practically continuous," they took him to Battle Creek. Conklin fasted the boy for fifteen days, refed him for three weeks, fasted him four or five more days, refed him again, and fasted him twice more. From the second day of his first fast until two years later, when his record goes cold, he had no more seizures save for a single one when he came down with measles. The only remnant of his epilepsy appeared to be "an occasional winking of the eyes."

As it happened, little Henry had an elder cousin who was a well-regarded endocrinologist at New York's Presbyterian Hospital—the family bled blue, after all—and when he, H. Rawle Geyelin, learned of Henry's miraculous recovery, he displayed an admirable openness and decided to have a dispassionate look at the work of this osteopath from the Middle West. Geyelin met the families of two of Conklin's other patients, one who had been free of seizures for two years, the other for three years, and he was so impressed that he made a pilot trial of his own. He fasted twenty-six epileptic patients for twenty days, and twenty-two stopped seizing entirely. Most of them eventually had convulsions again, but a year after the fast two were still "without sign or symptom of epilepsy." Just as Guelpa and Marie had found, in all twenty-six of his patients the mental lassitude induced by either the seizures or anti-seizure drugs was reversed. Geyelin concluded that "when one wanted to turn a clouded mentality to a clear one it could almost always be done with fasting."

We don't know precisely why Geyelin reported so few lasting cures while Conklin reported so many, but even allowing for overexuberance in Conklin's recollections, it's possible Conklin had more success because he fasted his patients multiple times. Then again, Geyelin and Conklin might have fared more similarly than first glance suggests, because later evaluations of their work showed Geyelin freed 19 percent of 79 fasted children from seizures for the long term, while Conklin fully cured 22 percent of 127 children and adults and improved another 50 percent to some degree. If those rates don't sound extraordinary, bear in mind the epileptics Conklin and Geyelin fasted were almost always those who hadn't responded to medication. Not only were the doctors sometimes curing an incurable disease; they were curing the most incurable of the diseased, and were improving the lives of many of the rest. It was a singular breakthrough.

Geyelin gathered up much of this information—Henry Howland's recovery, the gist of Conklin's work, his own pilot study—and in 1921 presented it to a conference of the American Medical Association. The response was cautious but positive, which was itself an astonishment. For two decades doctors had been roundly ridiculing Bernarr Macfadden's fasting cure, but when cleansed of Macfadden's taint and pedaled by one of their esteemed brethren, they accepted it in a trice. It couldn't have hurt that patient zero was the scion of a Brahmin family whose vouchsafing of the cure was beyond reproof. In any event, so compelling was Geyelin's presentation that researchers at the Mayo Clinic, Johns Hopkins, Massachusetts General Hospital, and Harvard went to work almost immediately to find the mechanism behind fasting's success against epilepsy. The Hopkins researchers had a special incentive, for one of Henry Howland's uncles, John Howland, was the leading professor of pediatrics at Hopkins, and John's brother Charles—Henry's father—gave Hopkins the handsome sum of $5,000 to research the matter.

The first big discovery, however, came not from Hopkins but from Mayo. The Minnesota researchers theorized that fasting's efficacy against epilepsy might have something to do with the ketone bodies that fasters release as they burn fat. If so, it might be possible to mimic a fast by feeding patients a diet unusually high in fat—say, 90 percent. This was the birth of the ketogenic diet, the term coined by the Mayo researcher Russell Wilder. Wilder and colleagues hoped the diet would keep seizures from returning after epileptics broke their fasts and might even replace the fast altogether. In 1925, a Mayo team published the results of a trial in which thirty-seven epileptic children aged two to fourteen were put on the diet without fasting. Many became seizure-free. Those who didn't were fasted for a week, at which point all of their seizures ceased, and then were put back on the diet. In the end, nineteen of the children, 51 percent, became totally seizure-free, and thirteen of the rest had greatly reduced seizures. Only five saw little improvement in their convulsions, but even they "enjoyed a marked change in character, . . . a decrease in irritability, and an increased interest and alertness," exactly as Guelpa, Marie, and Conklin had found. Some of the children were still free of seizures up to two and a half years later, and three were able to return to a normal diet. Given that these were, again, the hardest cases—children who hadn't responded to medications—the results were outstanding.

In other studies in the 1920s and 1930s, various combinations of fasting and ketogenic diet rendered about half of patients either seizure-free or greatly improved. The most common protocol was to fast patients a few days to get them quickly into ketosis, after which they were put on a ketogenic diet for several months or years and then tapered onto a regular diet. Trials in adults were less promising, for reasons no one understood. It was as if epilepsy simply refused to be dislodged once it had sunk its roots over many years.

So far as I could find, no researchers ever put Conklin's method of repeated fasts to the test, either in adults or in unresponsive children. The epileptologists of the day accepted short fasts and the fasting-mimicking ketogenic diet but drew the line there. On rare occasion when they considered Conklin's method, they said—with little evidence—that his patients got almost all of their improvement from their first fast. They may also have thought the ketogenic diet mimicked fasting well enough to make repeated fasts redundant. (If so, they were almost certainly wrong.) A pair of Harvard researchers spoke for many in the field when they said fasting should be used only as "an emergency procedure . . . to tide the patients over a particularly difficult time" or to get them quickly into ketosis and from there to a ketogenic diet. They held, again without evidence, that prolonged fasting was simply too rigorous, even verging on dangerous: "We do not share the enthusiasm of those who . . . look on fasting as a beneficial rejuvenating experience."

Nevertheless, a minor medical miracle was unfolding. The research quickly filtered down to practice, and conventional doctors around the country turned to fasting and a fasting-mimicking diet to treat the disease—a first in modern medicine. By 1930, less than a decade after Geyelin introduced Conklin's work to his regular colleagues, the standard text on epilepsy by a leading Harvard professor gave just one brief chapter to medication and fully half the book to administering the fasting-mimicking ketogenic diet. Over the next decade every textbook on epilepsy sang the praises of fasting and the ketogenic diet, but none credited its progenitor, the much-mocked Bernarr Macfadden.

Fasting's heyday didn't last long. In 1938, a new anti-seizure drug with fewer side effects than its predecessors, diphenylhydantoin (DPH), was introduced. Other drugs followed, and fasting and the ketogenic diet soon fell out of favor, just as the Guelpa method had for diabetes when insulin was discovered. The new anticonvulsants were easier to administer than fasting and a special diet and were lavishly promoted by the manufacturers they enriched. They also scratched a psychological itch, for they were the fruit of an exciting new understanding about the workings of neurotransmitters. In an age reverential of technological advance, nothing so pedestrian as fasting stood a chance against a pill that had sprung from the deciphering of a piece of nature's code. By 1960, just two decades after the introduction of DPH, the advice on epilepsy in the standard textbooks had entirely reversed. Now the leading work from Harvard gave just a single paragraph to fasting and the ketogenic diet, its author flatly declaring, "For most patients, young and old, drug therapy is the kingpin of treatment." For "patients," substitute "doctors."

Just as insulin was no cure for the diabetic, anticonvulsants didn't heal the epileptic. They only kept her seizures at bay. And although the side effects of the new drugs were less severe than those of the previous generation, they were far from harmless (DPH commonly caused agitation, drowsiness, constipation, and nausea) and had to be taken for life. But doctors soon stopped telling patients about fasting and the ketogenic diet and eventually forgot about the treatment themselves. Generations of epileptics whose fits might have been cured or lessened by fasting never got the chance.

For decades, the fasting-and-ketogenic regimen survived only at a few specialty clinics, which by the 1980s were winnowed to one, Johns Hopkins. That, however, would be enough. Charles Howland's grant of $5,000 would eventually pay the greatest of dividends by sparking a rebirth of fasting that would bring relief to thousands.

CHAPTER 9

"TRUTH THOUGH THE HEAVENS FALL"

Henry Tanner may have been the father of modern fasting, and Bernarr Macfadden its grand impresario, but no one in America did more to put fasting on a sound footing, to sort through and synthesize what had come before while adding a new store of discriminating observations, than Herbert Macgolfin Shelton. A careful practitioner and prolific writer (some would say too prolific), Shelton was instrumental in keeping fasting alive in the United States in the long decades after Macfaddenism ebbed away.

Shelton was born in 1895 on a farm outside Dallas and discovered Macfadden's *Physical Culture* at the age of fifteen. Drawn first to the illustrated brawn, he was finally captivated by the tales of rejuvenation through fasting and eating plants. After making an informal study of the "drugless healers" of the past century, he enrolled in a Chicago venture of Macfadden's known variously as the College of Physcultopathy or the College of Drugless Physicians, which offered a degree it wishfully described as a doctorate of physcultopathy. Shelton would long admire Macfadden—he and his wife Ida named their first child Bernarr—but he was clear-eyed enough to see the curriculum was a shoddy jumble, and he left to study at the American School of Naturopathy and the American School of Chiropractic. He also trained at several sanatoriums, one run by an MD partial to natural cures, another by one of the founders of naturopathy, another by an osteopath, and yet another by a homeopath. In the end he observed, as Edward Hooker Dewey had, that no matter which doctors from which schools were doing the treating, the patients seemed to get well at about the same rate. Most doctoring, it seemed to Shelton, amounted to interfering with the work of the body, and he concluded the physician's proper role was to support the body as it healed itself.

Settling in New York, he ghostwrote articles and books for Macfadden, including a health column for the frightful *New York Evening Graphic*. He was fired from that job after a piece he wrote about the dangers of smoking angered the paper's tobacco advertisers. He had greater success with his small medical practice, although he was careful never to call it that. "I never cured anyone in my life," he told his patients. "I only direct and educate the health seeker in understanding how to supply the normal conditions of life under which the body carries forward its self-healing process with the greatest efficiency."

Shelton's view of disease can be distilled to a few principles. Most of what was called acute disease, he held, was not in fact disease but the body's response to it and shouldn't be interrupted. "*In treating an acute disease,*" he wrote, employing the italics he often favored for reasons known only to himself, "the first rule to learn is: DON'T DO IT." To his eyes, a patient recovered best when her body dispensed with illness as evolution taught it to do. Eating only impeded the process, and fasting nearly always shortened it. Shelton's patients with typhoid fever, for example, usually got well after eight to twelve days of fasting compared to three weeks on food, and "the courses of measles, scarlet fever and pneumonia are correspondingly shortened." He treated chronic disease in much the same manner, although experience taught him that fasting wasn't strictly necessary. A reduced, hygienic diet and ample rest often brought a cure, albeit much more slowly than a fast. In any illness, chronic or acute, the most important thing was to stop doing whatever had caused it—usually, to Shelton's mind, eating meat or processed foods, drinking alcohol, smoking, or overworking. When those errors were corrected, patients usually improved, but they stayed well only if they adopted a diet of fruits, vegetables, a little dairy, and nothing heavily refined—no white flour, white rice, sugar, salt, or alcohol.

Over his long career, Shelton would expand on these principles in dozens of books under his own name, a cascade of millions of words, almost none copyrighted because he thought the knowledge of how to achieve good health was the rightful property of humankind and should be freely available to all. He loathed being edited, which left much of his Galenic outpouring unreadably prolix. But for readers with patience and stamina, the reward of his oeuvre was a discerning assessment of the body's ability to heal itself and a demonstration of the folly of conventional medicine.

His New York practice brought him many examples of that folly. A young woman from White Plains came to him with a lump the size of a billiard ball in her left breast. For months she had put off consulting doctors for fear the growth would be pronounced cancer—this was the era of the radical, disfiguring, and often-pointless mastectomy—and when at last she sought counsel, four regular doctors indeed independently diagnosed cancer and urged a mastectomy. Shelton's examination suggested only a severely enlarged gland, and he recommended a fast. Three foodless days later, the woman returned to his office, over the moon. Her lump was entirely gone, never to reappear in the thirteen years Shelton remained in contact with her. None of the four conventional doctors, she told him, had bothered with a biopsy. "Each man," he wrote, "advised an operation upon the basis of a wild guess."

In another instructive case, a man came to Shelton with a large abdominal tumor that *had* been biopsied and diagnosed as giant cell sarcoma, which at the time was thought to be a cancer. The tumor disappeared in seven days of fasting. "Of course he didn't have cancer, but he did have a diagnosis," Shelton wrote, and conventional medicine would later agree that giant cell tumors weren't cancerous. It was characteristic of Shelton that even when he could have claimed a cure of cancer through fasting, he claimed misdiagnosis instead. He was an empiricist guided by what he observed, and he never saw fasting cure cancer. "I have seen cancerous growths greatly reduce in size during a fast," he wrote, "but I *have never seen one totally eliminated. And in some cases, cancerous tumors persist in growing." In cancers of the pancreas and liver, he even thought fasting might hasten death. (The going belief among fasting doctors today is that fasting can send liquiform cancers like lymphoma into remission and might slow the growth of certain solid cancers but is unlikely to eliminate them entirely.)

Regular doctors who had given up their patients for lost never asked, when they came back healed, how Shelton had remedied the unremediable. They seemed to write off his cures as spontaneous remissions, just as the doctors of Ivonne Vielman, from the prologue, would decades later. The damning word that regulars used to dismiss Shelton was *unscientific*. Medicine, as they saw it, was a practice built on an understanding of mechanisms, the stuff of laboratories and white coats, while Shelton's therapies, arising from his and others' observations, belonged with the root doctoring of the last century. It was a curious obtuseness. Much of conventional medicine had sprung from astute observation—Edward Jenner's vaccine, Joseph Lister's antiseptics, and the fasted epileptics of H. Rawle Geyelin come to mind. But the origins of Jenner's and Lister's discoveries were long forgotten, and Geyelin was a worthy of the American Medical Association, no outsider to the orthodox clique like Shelton.

Shelton wore his outsiderdom like a badge. "I am not 'scientific' and in the present state of 'science' I would be a fool if I were," he wrote. "I'd rather be right than to be 'scientific.'" Another time he moderately opined, "*Science* stubbornly clings to its errors, and resists all effort to correct these. Once an alleged fact has been well established, no matter how erroneous it is, all the gates of hell shall not prevail against it." Never mind that gates don't prevail against anything—he was right that *Science* wasn't budging.

*   *   *

Worse, it was coming for him. In 1927, police seized him at his New York office for practicing medicine without a license. (His licenses were in naturopathy and chiropractic.) "I never prescribed drugs to anyone in my life!" he protested, but a judge ruled his examination of a client and prescription of a diet, for which he received payment, constituted the practice of medicine and fined him a hundred dollars. Lacking money for an appellate attorney, he paid. He was certain his outspokenness about the malpractice

of "the medical trust" had put him in the law's crosshairs, and he was probably right. Regulars across the country were stepping up their fight against
irregulars, and a common tactic was to enlist the aid of friendly prosecutors
to harass the unorthodox. Some of the prosecuted were indeed quacks (as,
of course, were some of the regulars). One fasting "doctor," Linda Burfield
Hazzard of Washington, even intentionally starved several patients to
death and helped herself to their jewels and assets. But the prosecution of
cautious practitioners like Shelton suggested a motive having little to do
with concern for patients.

A month after his first arrest, Shelton was jailed and fined again, and
three months later once again. Following the second arrest, Governor
Franklin Roosevelt supposedly said, "Shelton can stay in jail the rest of his
life." Whether he uttered the words or no, it was obvious Shelton would
have no peace in New York, and in 1928 he uprooted his family for San
Antonio, where he opened Shelton's Health School in a two-story frame
house, his family on the first floor, patients on the second. It speaks to
the man's contrarianism that even in flight from persecution he set up his
fasting-and-vegetable shop deep in the heart of longhorn steer country.

Shelton kept his fees low, sometimes treated for free those who
couldn't pay, sometimes didn't charge those who didn't improve under
his care, and sometimes adopted a "pay only if you're satisfied" policy. His
books and occasional itinerant lectures attracted a loyal following, as did
his policy during lectures of staying until every last question was answered,
which could take up to seven hours. Sometimes the talks ended in hand-
cuffs. At an address in Milwaukee in 1932, he was arrested for pedaling
medical advice, and three years later he was cuffed again in New York for
practicing medicine without a license. "I wouldn't practice medicine if
I *had* a license!" he retorted, but the judge gave him a month at Rikers
Island. He fasted the duration and wrote most of his next book.

America's few other fasting doctors, most of them steeped in Shelton's
hygienic writings, were thoroughly harried and hounded in this period
as well. The naturopath and chiropractor Gerald Benesh was twice convicted in Ohio for practicing medicine without a license, and the second
conviction, in 1952, came with a $1,000 fine and three-month sentence

to the Toledo Workhouse. A New York naturopath named Christopher Gian-Cursio was arrested once in Buffalo and three times in Rochester and served a full year in Rikers following a 1947 conviction. By one count, Gian-Cursio was tried no fewer than eight times in his career.

In 1948, the embattled practitioners banded together to form the American Natural Hygiene Society, and their chief work sometimes seemed to be scaring up money for the families of colleagues hauled off to prison. Their most ambitious act was the purchase, in 1975, of land outside San Antonio for a College of Natural Hygiene, but this proved a fever dream. No campus ever arose from the scrubland. The forces of *Science* had all but subdued fasting.

* * *

And yet for all that, Shelton's little health "school" thrived. It migrated to successively larger dwellings, eight in all, and in 1959 Shelton built his grandest edifice yet on a low rise he called Mount Hygeia, for the Greek goddess of health. Its construction was supported by a $50,000 grant from Charles Elmer Doolin, founder of the Frito Company, who had taken the cure under Shelton and no doubt had amends to make to health and gastronomy. The new building wasn't much, a two-story box with a stingy porch grafted onto the front, but it overlooked pleasant country and had beds for forty.

Shelton's ceaseless publishing carried his teachings far beyond San Antonio. A monthly he started in 1939, *Dr. Shelton's Hygienic Review*, ran for more than four decades (at a loss because he refused to take advertising that, as he put it, did violence to his principles), and the most famous of his thirty books, the atypically edited and concise *Fasting Can Save Your Life*, sold half a million copies. A pair of Europe's pioneering fasting hygienists, Albert Mosséri in France and Keki Sidhwa in Britain, got their start after reading Shelton's work—Mosséri coming across it in his native Egypt, Sidhwa in his native India. Among Shelton's other correspondents were George Bernard Shaw and Helen Keller, and Gandhi was so impressed that he asked Shelton to come to India for six years to spread the nature cure.

Shelton was inclined to a two-year sojourn, but the Second World War intervened, and Gandhi's assassination in 1948 ended the opportunity.* In 1956, the American Vegetarian Party made Shelton their presidential nominee, an honor he neither sought nor, he said, had the qualifications for because as a vegetarian he didn't fish, as a hygienist he didn't smoke, and "I never learned how to play golf."

By the time he opened the Frito building on Mount Hygeia in 1959, Shelton had supervised more than thirty thousand fasts, and many of the cures he claimed make for stirring reading. One was of a thirty-nine-year-old woman who had suffered from Parkinson's disease for six years. She lost her tremors after a fast of thirty days, only to see them return when she refed. Shelton fasted her fourteen more days, and again the tremors disappeared only to reappear with food, albeit weaker than before. After another fourteen days of fasting, they disappeared for good and never recurred in the decade Shelton was in touch with her. Her progressive improvement with repeated fasts was typical of his Parkinson's patients, but, he wrote, "full recovery is not the normal rule. The majority of fasters make sufficient progress to become useful again, but retain part of the tremor."

A thirty-eight-year-old optometrist came to Shelton with multiple sclerosis so advanced that leading neurologists told him there was nothing to do but prepare for the end. He had given up his practice and was so debilitated he had to be carried inside Shelton's school. He fasted two weeks, spent five more weeks on a diet of fruits and vegetables, and improved enough to walk out of the building under his own power. "He was not a well man at the end of seven weeks," wrote Shelton, who would have preferred his patient to have fasted serially. "It is too much to expect a full recovery in such a short time. But he had made such great improvement that he felt justified in returning home and getting back to work." This, Shelton said, was "a mistake that the sick frequently make," for repeated fasts almost always secured a deeper healing and a more stable remission.

---

* The origins of political fasting go back to the Middle Ages but didn't take wing until the early twentieth century with the hunger strikes of British suffragettes, then Irish Republicans, and later Gandhi. It's no coincidence the strikers were all battling British oppression—each movement learned from the last—but it's mere conjecture that British cuisine had something to do with their form of protest.

Shelton never saw fasting reverse a case of multiple sclerosis completely, but his patients always came to him in the desperate late stages of the disease, and he wondered whether early MS might be reversed by fasting.

A bacteriologist who had been slowly crippled by arthritis, joint by painful joint across twenty-eight years, arrived in San Antonio "a twisted and distorted man walking with the aid of crutch and cane, in a much stooped position. He was unable to turn his head from side to side, and in constant pain." When Shelton told him it would take at least two years to get better, the man said, "I have taken twenty-eight years already. What are two more?" He fasted thirty-six days, ate a hygienic diet, then made a second long fast and several short ones. It took not two but four years, but in the end "his spine is almost straight, the use of his arms and legs is normal, he can turn his head, he walks in a nearly upright position, he does not use cane or crutch, he has no pain, he looks the 'picture of health,' and he works like a slave. He has remained in excellent health with no recurrence of pain or swelling for a period of seven years."

Shelton didn't hesitate to fast the aged. One of his more successful elder patients was an impotent seventy-year-old who arrived with an enlarged prostate, chronically congested sinuses, a six-year deafness in one ear, and an asthma of thirteen years for which he had been hospitalized five times. When Shelton told him he would have to discontinue his medications, he said, "But what shall I do if I have an attack of asthma?"

"You will grit your teeth and clench your fists and suffer through it," Shelton replied.

The man submitted, and his asthma went away almost immediately, as commonly happened with Shelton's asthmatics. Gradually his sinuses stopped flowing and his prostate shrank to nearly normal size. On the twenty-fifth day, he asked if he might break his fast, and Shelton answered it was his choice but it would be premature. The man fasted on, regained his hearing after thirty-six days, and by the time he broke the fast on the forty-second day was no longer impotent.

There were other successes against the disorders of venery. One man's syphilis disappeared after a fast of sixteen days and stayed away for the thirty years Shelton was in contact with him. Another man with gonorrhea who suffered pain, fever, and a weeping discharge whenever he went off penicillin was freed of all those symptoms after a fast of twelve days. A woman of thirty years and no libido fasted twenty-seven days, ate a hygienic diet for two months, and was once again appropriately libidinous. Her opposite, a nymphomaniac of forty-nine years, lost her uncontrollable sexual cravings after a sixteen-day fast and thereafter enjoyed a normal urge to copulate.

The recoveries go on and on. A forty-one-year-old who had had seven operations for recurring nasal polyps finally got rid of them, apparently for life, after twenty-four days of fasting. A young seaman with retinitis pigmentosa who came to Shelton with only fifteen percent of his vision fasted seventy, forty, and twenty-one days, fully recovered, and became the first mate on a Great Lakes vessel. Shelton also claimed reversals of colitis and amoebic dysentery, gallstones and hay fever, eczema and psoriasis, chronic urticaria (an allergic skin rash), bronchitis and fistula, migraine and neuritis, tic douloureux (a facial pain), varicose ulcers, gastric ulcers, duodenal ulcers, pellagra (a nutritional deficiency), glaucoma and epithelioma (an abnormal growth of the skin), acidosis and epilepsy, rapid heartbeat, slow heartbeat, hearts that skipped beats, endocarditis (an inflammation of the lining of the heart), Reynaud's disease (poor blood flow in the extremities), and locomotor ataxia (an inability to control movements).

His scores of anecdotes were consistent, credible, and ultimately overwhelming, yet over half a century not once did a man or woman of science give this tower of evidence the slightest public consideration. Late in his life, Shelton took a philosophical view of the neglect, writing that "as between my work and that of the 'science of medicine' and the 'science of dietetics,' I'll await the verdict of time with calmness and without fear." He wouldn't live long enough to see the verdict rendered in his favor. In his own time, cruel silence was his reward.

*   *   *

Also persecution. Although for most of his career the authorities of Texas only mildly molested him, in 1963 an investigator from the State Board of Medical Examiners posed as a patient with a stomach ulcer, and when Shelton recommended a fast of several weeks, he was prosecuted for practicing without a license. He seems to have been exonerated (the record has grown murky), but his acquittal set him back $1,500 in attorney's fees, nearly $15,000 in today's money, a lot for him.

Matters soon took a turn for the worse on multiple fronts. In the 1960s, he began to show signs of Parkinson's disease, which he believed was a consequence of his relentless work schedule, and neither fasting nor hygienic living reversed it. He turned over day-to-day operations of the clinic to a protégé, a chiropractor named Virginia Vetrano. She ran the school without event for a few years, but between 1973 and 1978 something went off the rails and four of her patients died. Shelton had apparently lost only three fasters in half a century, an unexceptional record for a doctor with desperately sick inpatients, but Vetrano's four deaths in five years bespoke rank malpractice. In one of the fatal cases, she inexplicably limited the man's water intake to no more than two cups a day, a violation of a cardinal rule known to every fasting doctor: keep your patients hydrated. She probably did something similar to the other unfortunates because they died not of starvation but of conditions like cardiac arrest, likely brought on by severe dehydration. Vetrano was no murderess in the mold of Linda Burfield Hazzard, just a cavalier and slow-witted practitioner who repeatedly mistook the signs of someone dying before her eyes for a routine fasting crisis.

The widow of one victim sued Shelton and Vetrano and was awarded $873,000, and after the family of another victim won a smaller judgment, the clinic was shuttered. Among the last acts of Shelton's life were declaring bankruptcy and signing over Mount Hygeia to one of the aggrieved families. He died in 1985, just shy of his ninetieth birthday. On his tombstone was etched one of his *cris de cœur*: "Let us have the truth though the heavens fall."

His decision to hand over his clinic and his good name to an incompetent was a failure as stupendous as it was perplexing, for he had often written of the need to carefully supervise fasters, and he knew well that the missteps of a fasting doctor would not be lightly punished. With the fall of his clinic, fasting, already demeaned and defamed in America, was further discredited. His story would prove a cautionary tale for the country's next great practitioner of fasting as he tried to nurse the craft back to respectability.

CHAPTER 10

A GENTLE DEPRIVATION, 1

In 2012, after publishing my article about my twenty-day fast, I received a call from Françoise Wilhelmi de Toledo, who, along with her husband Raimund, ran the Buchinger Wilhelmi Clinic in the south of Germany. Theirs was one of the world's oldest fasting clinics, the present campus founded in 1953 but with earlier iterations going back to 1920, and it was also the most famous. Wilhelmi de Toledo said a nice thing or two about my article—always the right way to begin an acquaintance with a writer—and then gently mocked my refusal to let anything other than water pass my lips. It was she who told me I could have stayed in a fasted state even while consuming up to 250 calories a day, which is what the patients in her clinic routinely did.

"Where were you when I needed you, Françoise?" I said.

She extended an invitation to visit, but an opportunity didn't present itself until 2019, when I had the good fortune to be living in Barcelona, a mere hop from Buchinger Wilhelmi. As it happened, moving to Barcelona had also given me cause for a fast. When Jennifer and I arrived in Spain that August (Elliott having decamped for college), I seemed the very personification of health. In the seven months since my healing fast in January, my hypersomnia and other ills had stayed in blessed remission, and I had been a dynamo of energy, swashbuckling through the endless paperwork to obtain visas for self, wife, and dog, finishing a pair of built-in bookcases I had earlier abandoned as too draining, trading blows with double-dealing roofers, cobbling together the proposal for this book, and packing away all our possessions so the family renting our house would have somewhere to put their socks. Clean living, it seemed, had kept my demons in their chamber.

But days after arriving in Spain, the familiar fatigue crept in. I hoped it was just the transitory harvest of overdoing things and then hurling my body across eight time zones, but the exhaustion only deepened, the days took on the old gauzy texture, and my migraines, which had nearly disappeared, returned with renewed tenacity. Once more an unseen wraith was tugging me into an enervating undertow. I tried a couple of short fasts, but they helped for only a few days at a time. It was all too terrifying and, I thought with affecting pity, rather hard on someone of such righteous habit.

Having read Shelton and other fasting doctors, I knew some chronic diseases simply didn't go away with a single prolonged fast, and I suspected my January therapy had more subdued than vanquished my demons. They must have been licking their wounds, sharpening their claws, and awaiting the right moment to bushwhack me again. Somewhere over the Atlantic they had pounced. I decided a concerted response was called for. It was time to fast at Buchinger Wilhelmi.

That, however, was not a decision for the financially faint. Basic rooms at the clinic ran nearly $300 a night, and although I was to learn that wasn't high for what you got, a stay of two weeks was all my budget would bear. Fasts at Buchinger Wilhelmi were preceded by a preparatory day of gentle eating and followed by multiple days of refeeding, so a two-week stay meant nine days of fasting, which I feared wouldn't be enough to nip the hypersomnia. When Shelton's patients lacked time or money for longer fasts, he recommended fasting sequentially. I tried that now, fasting in Barcelona for five days on water, giving myself a week to refeed, and then packing every warm piece of clothing I'd brought to Spain and heading off on a brisk November morning for the Alpine Foreland.

* * *

Otto Buchinger was a doctor in the German navy when he came down with the strep throat that would change the history of fasting. The year was 1917, and the infection passed without event, but a few weeks later he developed rheumatic fever, a condition in which the body, reacting errantly to lingering streptococcal bacteria, turns upon itself. The fever invaded Buchinger's heart, inflamed his liver, nervous system, and joints, and came so close to killing him that his colleagues called his wife to his bedside to say her goodbyes. He survived but with a liver that barely functioned, a weak heart, and nerves and joints so fraught that at times he could get about only with crutches or a wheelchair.

In 1918, near the end of the First World War, Buchinger was discharged from service an invalid and sent to one of the military convalescent homes to which he had discharged so many patients himself. He grew only more enfeebled. The prospect before him, at the age of forty, was that of a declining state pensioner with a wife and four children in a war-ravaged state too poor to spare more than a few pfennigs for its infirm citizens. It was a cruel comedown for a man who only a few years earlier had been in the fullness of life, the doctor to Crown Prince Adalbert. The prince, a keen hunter, had appreciated Buchinger's skill as both marksman and medic, and Buchinger had chaperoned him on state visits to the grandest courts of Asia, Africa, and Europe. In his travels, Buchinger had seen many rheumatic cases like his own, and he expected his wife would be burying him sooner rather than later.

But one day he learned of a doctor in Freiburg who was taking on cases as hopeless as his and achieving the most remarkable cures. The doctor, Gustav Riedlin, had learned about fasting from a fencing partner who saw it practiced in the America of Edward Hooker Dewey and Bernarr Macfadden. In 1919, Buchinger put himself under Riedlin's care and fasted nineteen days on water and tea, with results no less than astounding. The inflammation in his joints and nerves vanished entirely, and even before he completed his fast he was once more walking like a young man. His heart again ticked as regularly as a Jura timepiece, and his liver, so far as the diagnostic tools of the day could discern, thrummed like the busy factory it was designed to be.

Like other gravely ill patients who experienced extraordinary cures through fasting, Buchinger was by turns amazed and baffled. How was it that none of his other colleagues knew about this cure? Why were there no courses on fasting in medical school, no mention of it at conferences? Buchinger was one of the rare conventional doctors receptive to the idea that fasting might be as powerful as, maybe even more powerful than, the methods in which he had been trained. He gathered what information he could and learned that fasting had been resurrected in Germany largely as it had in America, as a result of the publicity attending Henry Tanner's forty-day fast in New York. But just as in America, fasting didn't find its footing in Germany until the turn of the twentieth century. In 1901, a Bavarian doctor named Adolf Mayer published a small book called *Fasting Cures, Wonder Cures*, in which he wrote, just a little overheatedly, "But whatever the essence and kind of illness, in whatever place it appears—the most rational therapy is certainly a very energetic cure of thirst and fasting." Mayer admitted his preferred type of fasting—dry fasting, or fasting without water—seemed to many "peculiar, strange, unnatural," but because there were so many dreadful illnesses that medicine couldn't fix, "any method that can cure them, however excessive and strange it seems, is justified." Dry fasting would prove a bridge too far for most Germans, and it fell to Buchinger's rescuer Gustav Riedlin and another doctor, Siegfried Möller, to advance the more palatable method of fasting with water.

Möller had two great influences. One was Dewey, whose book *The No-Breakfast Plan and the Fasting-Cure* came to Germany thanks to the untimely decease, in 1898, of Dewey's first wife. Hardly had Dewey got fitted for his widower's weeds than he took another bride (thirty years his junior, the hound), and she, Kathe, having been born in Germany, translated his writings into her native tongue. Möller struck up a correspondence with Dewey, who told him, among much else, that against the grimmest illnesses long fasts often triumphed where short fasts were defeated and that he had successfully fasted two patients for sixty-five days and another for seventy-five. Möller's other great influence was the French doctor Guillaume Guelpa, who, as we saw in chapter 8, used a series of short fasts and vegetarian diet to cure diabetes and epilepsy.

In 1926, seven years after fasting with Riedlin, Buchinger's gallbladder mutinied, and he fasted under Möller in hope of calming it. His gallbladder's revolt may have been a lingering consequence of an intemperate youth, for he had once been a heavy drinker (also a dueler, and he had the *schmiss*, the intentional saber gash on the cheek, to prove it). He fasted twenty-eight days at Möller's sanatorium in Dresden, possibly with a small amount of food (by one report, Möller allowed his patients white wine and cookies), and his gallbladder was pacified, never to trouble him again. The success of his two prolonged fasts and of others he heard and read about convinced Buchinger of their superiority over short fasts, but he wasn't dogmatic. For people who couldn't or wouldn't undergo longer deprivations, he thought serial short fasts served a purpose, which pleased me.

Riedlin and Möller were only the most prominent of Germany's early fasting doctors. In the first few decades of the twentieth century, the country had more doctors with fasting practices—for the most part, regular physicians, not naturopaths or other irregulars—than the United States would the entire century. They proliferated in part because of a German social movement of the late nineteenth and early twentieth centuries called *Lebensreform*, or Life Reform. Lebensreformers were the original hippies. They preached back-to-naturism and argued for shedding all that was toxic or confining about society. They took woodsy exercise in the sunshine far from cities choked with smoke and soot, and they abandoned corsets, stiff collars, and sometimes the rest of their attire. More than one forester, stumbling into a glade, had his day enlivened by their naked dancing. The Lebensreformers replaced rigid sexual mores with permissiveness—an early form of free love—and supplanted refined and elaborately prepared foods with raw vegetables, fruits, and whole grains. They had no patience with inflexible medical doctrine and protested the worst of medicine's brutalities, like the vivisection of animals. Eventually some Lebensreformers moved to California, where they deeply influenced the seekers who became America's hippies in the 1960s.

Buchinger was too prudish to be a Lebensreformer proper, but he was a seeker at heart and embraced much of the movement's health program, as did several other doctors who believed establishment physicians knew far less than they pretended and should have the humility to accept therapies that didn't arise from laboratories or medical schools. This was fertile ground for fasting, but World War I nearly spoiled the field by leaving many Germans hungry and malnourished. Yet in 1920, not two years after the Armistice of Compiègne and just one year after his first long fast with Riedlin, an undeterred Buchinger opened the Dr. Otto Buchinger Cure Home in the Hessian town of Witzenhausen.

His first patients were dubious of the cure home's cure. If going without food was so healthful, they demanded, why were so many hungry Germans sick? Buchinger explained that surviving on half rations was not the same as fasting—it was malnourishment. Only when a patient abstained from food completely or nearly completely did the body heal itself. He was selling furnaces to Bedouins, but if ever a man was equipped to do so, it was Otto Buchinger. Not only did he have his own potent tale of salvation through fasting, but he was immensely charismatic and was invested with the authority of a conventional doctor and a decorated military officer. He also had experience pushing contrary truths. Although he had started his military career a hard-drinking rake, he later decided alcoholism was ruining the navy and became one of the country's leading advocates for temperance. A shriller voice would have made a legion of enemies, but Buchinger's tone was more concerned than condemning, and he remained popular enough with his besotted fellows that they only gently poked fun at him as "Dr. Fachinger," after a mineral water by that name. It was like being called Dr. Perrier.

Buchinger failed to convince the admiralty to give up spirits, but he persuaded his patients to forgo food. He quickly filled the rooms in the spacious house that did double duty as clinic and family home and soon was stashing patients in rented rooms all around Witzenhausen. Later he bought a proper sanatorium, which he also swiftly outgrew. Without intending it, he had just taken the first steps toward making himself history's most successful fasting doctor and Germany the fasting center of the world.

* * *

Arriving at the Buchinger Wilhelmi Clinic under cover of darkness, I was ushered to the dining room, a tastefully appointed space overlooking an uninspired parking garage. The other guests had already eaten, so I dined alone, simply and excellently, on a salad, fruit, and cooked vegetables. Each table bore little name cards, so I could see my companion tomorrow would be one Jeffrey Pidge.* The clinic purported to nourish not just the body through fasting but the spirit through revitalizing activities and a supportive community. To foster communal esprit, fasters were given small nudges, one of which was assigned seating at meals on feeding days. After passing dinner in speculation about Pidge's identity (I settled on either a Melbourne shipping magnate or manager of the top-grossing Ladbrokes in Blackpool), I was shown to my room by an energetic young woman with dyed red hair who explained the house rules and gave me an agreement to sign. I swore to be a lovely addition to the clinic who wouldn't smoke, drink alcohol, wear perfume (because fasters have heightened smell), or use a phone anywhere on the grounds outside my room.

"Anywhere," she said with great cheer, "means *any*where": the waiting room outside the nurse's station, the walkways between buildings, even the balcony of my own room. In fact, if I was going to make a phone call in my room, would I be pleased to ensure the doors and window were tightly shut? And if I saw anyone breaking any of the numerous rules, would I be pleased to tell the staff?

Being enlisted as a narc from my first minutes at the clinic was not as awkward as you might think. After three months in Spain, whose winsome citizens treat their magnificent country as an open-air ashtray—depositing cigarette butts on every street, beach, public garden, private garden, kindergarten, and maternity ward—I promised with unbecoming glee to stool on any miscreant who dared cross my newly empowered path. I only just held off asking whether my new friend and her colleagues would be open to a little extraterritorial policing in Catalonia.

The next morning I awoke to what I can only call a $4,000 view of Lake Constance. The near shoreline rose steeply from the lake, which

* I have changed the names and some identifying characteristics of patients to protect their privacy. The names of staff are real.

had been gouged out by a retreating glacier, and the clinic, a few hundred meters up the hill, had a commanding vista. It was especially splendid this morning because the Alps, far beyond the water, consented to emerge from the clouds that usually obscured them in autumn. Françoise Wilhelmi de Toledo had told me many people preferred to fast in fall and winter because the days were more ethereal and conducive to reflection, and Otto Buchinger had written that for fasters autumn was "the most contemplative season. And even richer in beauty than all the others, at least for artists and poets, who seek meaning and mature depth more than brilliance and youth." I would find this was true enough, but after two or three successive days of not seeing our nearest and to me dearest of stars, I would also learn to appreciate every minute of sunlight I was treated to. The opposing lakeshore was serene, dotted with a few small settlements separated by kilometers of undeveloped field and forest. The bucolic emptiness, I would find as the days passed, contributed mightily to the peaceful feeling that descended on me with my fast. So did the gentle larches outside my balcony for which my dormitory, Villa Larix, had been named.

I headed to breakfast to start what the clinic called the digestive-rest day, a break for my innards from the hard work of digesting before they began the hard work of healing. The digestive-rest day was a big change for most guests: three vegan meals of fruits and vegetables with few oils, no added sugars, and little salt. It differed from my normal diet only in its paucity—600 calories, a third or a quarter of my usual 2,000 to 2,500—and in having oil and salt. For the typical American who consumed a prodigious 3,000 calories a day of processed, animalic fare, it would have been quite a settling in.

Breakfast was unseasonably fresh fruit carved into a diversity of geometric shapes, and as I was halfway through this delicious 200-calorie repast, Mr. Pidge showed up. He turned out to be neither an Australian tycoon of the seas nor a Lancashire gambling impresario but a quiet little Shropshire native who had recently started phasing out his consulting business in London in preparation for retirement. On my questioning, he said shyly that he and the missus had just relocated to the Scottish Lowlands, which they deemed more suited to the tranquility of advancing age. He

quietly added, on my further inquiry, that he had just completed a fast of
ten days. This was his second visit to the clinic, and he was on his second
day of refeeding. He seemed calmly appreciative of the food, but then he
was probably calmly appreciative of most things in life. Had he been four
years old, he would have been a welcome guest at any table since he spoke
only when spoken to and with a minimum of syllables. We passed long
periods in silence.

When I remarked that he hadn't managed to convince his wife to join
him, he pondered this noiselessly for so long I wasn't sure he'd heard me,
but finally he said meekly, "My wife and I are both introverts."

"You don't say?" I said, but he didn't smile.

Whole minutes later he added, "No, she did not want to come. Not
at first anyway. But as my visit drew nearer, she changed her mind, and she
is coming in a few months." He spoke slowly, without colloquialisms or
contractions, and after several long moments added, "I think it is good that
we are here separately because there are a lot of emotions and psychological events which can come up during a fast and which may perhaps be best
dealt with singularly."

And with that outpouring, he observed the rest of the meal quiet as a
mouse in cheese. When I had scooped every last morsel out of the skins of
my fruit (for only a fool leaves edibles on his plate when a fast looms) and
was taking my leave, I asked what kind of consultancy he ran.

"Personnel and human resources."

*   *   *

Among an impressive flurry of documents I had been given in the previous
night's orientation was a two-pager headed "Therapyschedule." It had me
down for no fewer than eight appointments today. Three were related to
a study of toxins that Wilhelmi de Toledo, in her capacity as the clinic's
director of research, was overseeing and in which I was participating. (She
and her husband had recently handed over the direction of the clinic to
their son, Leo Wilhelmi.) The clinic was taking the blood and urine of a
hundred guests, and the hair of a subset of us, to see if fasting would rid

us of heavy metals like mercury and lead and of agricultural pesticides like arsenic and glyphosate. On my way to breakfast, I had surrendered a quantity of blood that seemed more appropriate to the deathbed of George Washington than to a fasting clinic, but when I asked the technician how much she was taking (I wasn't watching because doing so has sometimes provoked arresting changes in my state of consciousness), she said, "About thirty milliliters"—one-tenth of a can of Coca-Cola. It is good to get your humiliations over early in the day.

After breakfast, another technician came to my room to teach me, without demonstration, how to pee in a cup and on a strip of paper that would show how many ketone bodies I was producing, the number of which I was to record. She was followed by a pair of hair harvesters. Although my blood and urine would show how much I had detoxed (or not) during my fast, there remained the question of whether I would continue to detox as my body rebuilt itself afterward. This would be determined from a sample of hair I mailed to a lab a month after I'd gone back to Barcelona, which would be compared to the sample harvested now. The clinic paid for the analysis of blood and urine but not of hair, which was ambitiously priced at €400. I figured Elliott, who has his mother's intelligence, was bright enough to do without textbooks for a semester.

The polite young harvesters, one man and one woman, asked where I'd like my hair taken from. "Vee can do it on your heed," the man said, "but zen you vill have a hole. Beetter on zee body."

I removed my shirt, and his eyes lit up. Once, on assignment in the Peruvian Andes, I had to change shirts in the middle of a hike, and from behind me a guide had shrieked, "*¡Eres un mono!*" You're a monkey! The fingers of my German hair harvester twitched with eager anticipation in his tiny scissors—he was accustomed to tamer pastures. He set to work, frolicking among the tufts of my back while his assistant, who bore a tiny cardboard balance on which the clipped hair was weighed, tried to look anywhere but at me. After removing a hectare of carefully weighed mange, the harvester declared himself satisfied; his assistant, by facial expression, declared herself relieved. My back itched for the next two days, a cross I bore for science.

Next was a tour of the surprisingly expansive clinic. Nine or ten substantial buildings housed guest rooms, doctor's offices, a gym, a yoga studio, a demonstration kitchen, and lecture halls of varying size. They were packed up and down several acres of hillside with an outdoor tennis court and a thermal pool tucked among them. The architecture was mid-century European, the angles crisp, the vibe clean. It didn't feel crowded, only agreeably dense. Just beyond the clinic's borders the pleasant suburban precincts of the town of Überlingen hemmed us in on all sides, again not disagreeably.

Lunch followed. Mr. Pidge was not in attendance—perhaps he was dealing singularly with an emotion or psychological event—but at the table next to ours sat Charles Grupniak. Charles was a onetime corporate lawyer from Surrey who had seen the error of his impecunious ways and had since gone where the real money was: managing investments. Business was so good, he said, his principal client had to move to Monaco.

"Had to?" I asked

"Had to."

"How come?"

"I made him too much money. Monaco's a tax haven, you know. He couldn't afford all the taxes he'd have to pay in the UK."

And all this time I had thought the rich were taxed because, having more, they could afford to pay. I felt a species of enlightenment.

"How much money are we talking about?" I asked.

"He's worth two hundred and fifty million dollars right now, and if I manage his assets right, he'll be worth another hundred and fifty million in four or five years."

Charles was starting his fast the following morning, same as me. With tax-dodging as an opening, I was afraid he was the kind of chap you didn't want to meet early in one of these affairs, the type who would keep telling you how well he had done in coal derivatives for some asshole in Birmingham who'd made his first billion in child trafficking. But while Charles certainly had that side to him, he also turned out to be charming and curious on many subjects that had nothing to do with turning the merely rich into the salaciously rich. He was a first-timer to Buchinger

Wilhelmi and had come because of an elaborate bet with a friend. The previous summer, the friend had asked over swordfish in Miami how he was getting on with his goal of losing weight. At that point Charles had just started trying to rein in his eating and drinking and had lost only a kilo or two, which left a lot to go. His target was ninety kilograms, just under two hundred pounds.

"Right, here's what we'll do," the friend had said. "You get down to ninety by next first March, and I'll take you to the best restaurant in London for a ten-course dinner and the best wines money can buy."

That sounded good to Charles, but before he could agree, his friend said, "Now, what's your waist size?"

"Thirty-six."

"Thirty-six. Right, now you're going to have to wear a pair of thirty-four trousers to this dinner. And I'm going to buy them and bring them, and you'll have to get into them. Now, how's your exercise plan coming?"

"Sometimes I jog twice a week," Charles said, "and I want to get to where I can run a 5K."

"A 5K? Five measly K? *Anyone* can run a 5K. Christ, anyone can run *10K*. No, what you're going to do is run a 10K, and you're going to do it in under an hour."

His friend tried to heap on additional conditions, but Charles drew the line after the sixty-minute 10K. They shook hands on the deal four months ago, and in the time since, Charles had clearly gotten used to telling the story with an endearing self-deprecation. I couldn't have been the first listener to give his body a furtive once-over and then try to wipe a dubious look from my face. Onto the front of his average-sized frame was a very substantial bulge that ran from sternum to waist, as if he were hiding a baby in a sling under his shirt. His friend, he later told me, called the protrusion just that: his body baby. This particular contour, I would soon see, was the most common among the male patrons of Buchinger Wilhelmi, just as its heavy-hipped analog was the norm among female guests. There were svelte fasters too, but not many, and a few who were so enormous your heart went out to them as they negotiated the stairs around the hilly campus. Most of the guests, though, like Charles, had merely added a pound or two a year starting in their twenties until one day at forty or sixty they found themselves thirty-five pounds heftier than they should have been. They were borderline obese or just over the border, and they had come to make sure they stayed on or returned to the right side of the frontier.

"I'm not getting rid of all this in the ten days I'm here," Charles told me as he patted the baby, perhaps having detected doubt in my eyes. "I'm just hoping the six days of fasting will set me on my way. I need to do more, but who has the time?"

"And how's the running going?" I asked.

"I can do 5K in thirty-seven minutes," he said. "I hope to get it down to half an hour before March. Then on race day, I'll just have to do it twice back to back."

I suggested endurance didn't really work that way, but he shrugged as if to say it was as much as he could do.

"Not to doubt your capabilities," I continued, "but in the unlikely event you don't meet the terms of the bet, what do you have to give your friend?"

"A large donation to the charity of his choice. And if I win," he added in a flight of fantasy, "in addition to taking me to dinner, he has to donate to the charity of my choice."

"What charities have you chosen?"

"He's going to make me give to a trust for obesity," he said, chuckling. "He likes to wind me up."

Charles didn't say what charity he had picked, and I didn't ask. It was an appealingly good-hearted bet, and I didn't want to ruin my rosy view of it by hearing his choice was the Royal Andorran Trust for the Refinement of Tax Dodging.

*   *   *

After lunch I was examined by Mrs. Dr. Lischka, not to be confused with her husband, Mr. Dr. Lischka, also of the clinic. Mrs. Doctor was trim, poised, and attired every inch in white from her sleek tennis shoes to her sleeker cropped hair, technically blond. At Buchinger Wilhelmi, all of the doctors and nurses were dressed just as immaculately and snowily, as was the clinic itself: the interior walls were whitewashed, the furnishings in the guest rooms were of white laminate and blond wood, the beds had crisp white linens, and the guests, nearly all white themselves, shuffled up and down the halls in fluffy white bathrobes and white slippers. The bleach bill must have been staggering.

Mrs. Doctor was the chief physician, responsible for overseeing the nine doctors on staff and a much larger pride of nurses and for ensuring the likes of me didn't die on her watch. She took the usual readings and sat me down for that rarest of treats in a doctor's office: the unhurried chat. I had hoped she would enlighten me about fasting's effects on my idiopathic hypersomnia, but in her decades of experience she hadn't come across a single case of it—the typical fate of the sufferer of a rare disease. She was not without hope, however. The migraines I was experiencing might be due to a deficiency of vitamins or minerals, and it was possible the same played a part in the hypersomnia. She ordered some tests of the blood her colleague had syringed out of me (which, however, revealed nothing out of order) and told me in the meantime to relax and submit myself to several adjunct therapies the clinic had found helpful for migraine and fatigue. From the clinic's 162-page therapy catalog, Mrs. Doctor proposed several of the twoscore varieties of massage on offer. I was happy she didn't recommend leeching, also among the offerings, although I was subsequently stunned to learn that peer-reviewed research in journals like *Annals of the Rheumatic Diseases* and *Annals of Internal Medicine* supported the use of leeches for osteoarthritis and other woes of the joints. In the end we settled on four vocabulary-expanding massage treatments: myoreflex therapy, craniosacral therapy, manual lymphatic drainage, and Ayurvedic massage.

Next I proceeded to a session with a therapyplanner, which sounded like an app but proved to be a human who scheduled my massages and other treatments, after which I met with a nurse to talk about still more aspects of my fast. She said I was to drink bottled water by the troughload and lie down when tired. Not until five o'clock was I able to repair to my room for a few minutes of the clinic's much-heralded rest. In her book *Therapeutic Fasting*, Wilhelmi de Toledo had written, "Allow yourself to enjoy serenity during the fast. Avoid all stressors and let the rush of every-day life fade."

"Sure, Françoise," I thought, "just as soon as you let me."

At the dinner hour, Mr. Pidge appeared, or at least the sitting and chewing parts of him did. He left the talking part in his room and proceeded to introvert his way through the meal with such doggedness in the face of my gentle inquiries that I eventually left him in peace. Thanks to him, however, I was enjoying my own psychological event singularly. In the past I have sometimes thought myself perilously introverted, deficient in several of the smoothing graces of amiable society. But beside Mr. Pidge I felt the very master of conversation, and I was finally able to complete a conjecture for which I've long sought a conclusion both plausible and profitable. The conjecture was: "If this writing career doesn't work out, I can always—." I could now add the conclusion: "—consult in personnel and human resources in Britain."

*　　*　　*

Otto Buchinger's clinic in Witzenhausen survived interwar hunger and poverty, but it almost didn't outlast the Nazis. After his discharge from the navy, he became a Quaker and a pacifist, and when the brown shirts in town hailed der Führer, he took to saying, "*My* Führer is Jesus Christ." The Nazis removed his crucifixes from the clinic's walls and replaced them with photos of *their* Führer and replaced the nuns who served as his nurses with "brown sisters"—attendants faithful to the Nazi regime. By 1936, Buchinger had had enough of the master race and moved his clinic to Bad Pyrmont, a spa town in Lower Saxony that was a seat of German Quakerism with a local government less sympathetic to Nazism. The new clinic featured such luxuries as electric lighting and a bathroom on every floor and quickly became an even bigger success than the previous clinic. Partly this was because Buchinger had just published his landmark *Das Heilfasten* (*The Fasting Cure*), which became Europe's bestselling book about fasting, never out of print across thirty-two editions and translated into several languages, although not English. Once more his sanatorium overflowed, and he rented so many rooms around town for the spillover that the municipal council capped him at just under two hundred beds. Bad Pyrmont was a posh resort, and its burghers didn't care to have the town known as the starvation spa.

Buchinger's insubordination to the Nazis eventually caught up with him. On the eve of the Second World War he was brought to court in Munich on a charge of disloyalty, the penalty for which was losing his medical license. The grounds were a letter he had sent to a Jewish patient that ended up in the pages of the Nazi magazine *Der Stürmer* (*The Striker*). Buchinger told his patient the Nazis had pressed him to stop treating Jews and that, although it pained him both as a human being and as a doctor to say so, he must advise him not to come to the clinic because he couldn't guarantee his safety. Fortunately, Buchinger had allies in positions of authority from his military days and through their intervention was acquitted at trial. But in his boldness he had risked more than his license. His wife Else was half-Jewish, her father one of that particularly despised class of Hebrew bankers, and after the war the family discovered her name on a list of candidates for the death camps. Had her husband angered the wrong people or the war lasted longer, Else might have been one of the Reich's millions of victims.

Most of Buchinger's beds were commandeered during the war for wounded soldiers, but afterward the clinic returned to fasting and thrived once more, for Buchinger had hit on a formula so winning he almost couldn't fail. Its cornerstone was making fasting gentle, even pleasurable. Although he had learned to fast on water with Riedlin, in his own clinic he used a modified fast of the kind I benefited from in chapter 7. Two or three hundred calories a day in thin broths and diluted juices spared his patients the fatigue and nausea, the hunger pangs and headaches that are common to water-only fasting. The slight nourishment also gave his patients the strength for walks in nature, which Buchinger, the old Lebensreform confederate, thought an essential part of the cure. In this he differed from the American hygienists, who protected their fasters as carefully as truffles in a gift box, only rarely allowing them anything so exerting as an outdoor stroll. Buchinger introduced other softening touches. From the pad in his office he dispensed not prescriptions but the poems of Goethe and Rilke, and in the evenings he lectured, answered questions, played music on a phonograph (Beethoven was his obsession), or read poetry. Although he was a somewhat reserved man, in an era when so many physicians held themselves icily aloof his willingness to engage with patients as fellow humans was a welcome gift.

His personal touch, of course, would have counted for little had his patients not also healed, and heal they did. His daughter Maria, who would become the face of the clinic after his death, once asked him, "What should we tell people who want to know what fasting can cure?"

"Better to ask me what fasting can't cure," he returned. "It's only a few illnesses: tuberculosis, hyperthyroidism, advanced cancer, one or two other diseases. In all other cases, and especially chronic illnesses, it's worth trying a fast."

Still, some illnesses proved more susceptible to his method than others. Arthritis, for example, frequently disappeared entirely, especially if the sufferer fasted early in the disease, although even elders long gnarled and deformed usually improved at least a little. Gout, which is arthritis caused by an excess of uric acid, often vanished but only after repeated fasts and only if the patient was able to endure painful excretions of salty urates. Asthma fell to fasting too, but if a strong allergy was behind it, it typically receded only enough for the asthmatic to get through allergy season without medication or misery. Skin disorders yielded, in Buchinger's words, "almost without exception to every prolonged fast, with regressions in peeling, inflammation, and itching, as well as psoriasis and chronic eczema." The cure, however, could be long in coming. Psoriasis, for instance, usually went away only after two or three prolonged fasts spread over a year or two.

Buchinger regularly saw gallstones and kidney stones disintegrate on fasts, and two-thirds of his patients with gastritis, enteritis, and unruly intestinal flora also found relief. The one-third who didn't were a continual mystery to him. He reasoned that digestive problems ought to heal when the digestive tract was rested, but he never found a way to help this recalcitrant third, and he was candid about his failure, even acknowledging that in rare cases fasting could make the condition worse. One of his patients with hyperacidic gastritis became hematemetic while fasting—that is, he vomited blood. Heart patients, by contrast, almost always fared superbly, no matter how advanced their disease. "After a few days of fasting," he wrote, "sufferers of angina who before had to stop every 100 meters dare to cover 2,000 meters without attacks or spasms. And after a week they're undertaking walks of an hour at a good pace."

Buchinger also found, as Guillaume Guelpa had, that fasting improved or cured type 2 diabetes, especially when caught early. The same went for disorders of the liver, even in daunting cases like cirrhosis, but the healing was often unpleasant because, as Buchinger wrote, "of no other organ does fasting demand so much as it does of the liver." His migraine cases, I was selfishly interested to read, had an odd fasting signature: the headaches often disappeared but just as often came back after the fast with such vengeance as to drive the patient to bed. Later the pain eased again and left the sufferer with fewer and less severe migraines. Goiter (an unsightly swelling of the neck from an enlarged thyroid gland) improved on a fast of about three weeks, and periodontal disease cleared up so well—the swollen gums deflating, the teeth seeming to strengthen—that dentists sometimes asked their patients what on earth they had done to bring about so wonderful a change.

Many of Buchinger's cures were unexpected even to him, including three successes with glaucoma. One patient, fasting at an early stage of the disease, was cured completely, while the other two fasted much later in the disease and merely improved. Since one of glaucoma's causes is too much pressure on the optic nerve, they may have benefited from the drop in blood pressure that occurs during a fast.*

Buchinger insisted that fasting not only cured disease but prevented it, and he believed the healthiest of his more than thirty thousand patients were the ones who fasted regularly. He assumed (correctly, as we'll see) that

---

* Buchinger wasn't the only doctor to report improved eyesight through fasting. Edward Hooker Dewey told of an oculist whose vision after prolonged fasting was "7 degrees stronger" than before and of a young woman who discarded her glasses of thirteen years after a long fast. In 1912, a man who fasted thirty-one days in a laboratory of the Carnegie Institution could see twice as far as previously, and Herbert Shelton wrote that "restoration of good vision, in errors of refraction, is not at all uncommon."

the same repair mechanism that healed disease could head it off before it formed, and for many of his patients fasting provided a springboard to healthier habits. "Whoever doesn't turn the fast into a portal to a new world of eating, drinking, and purer life," he wrote, "hasn't appreciated this cure for what it is. The faster who returns home must be a new individual who reforms his life."

But for all his enthusiasm, Buchinger didn't paper over fasting's failures. Like Shelton, he never saw it cure cancer, and he thought it was useless as well against diphtheria, ulcers of the stomach and duodenum, malnourishment, tuberculosis, debility of the heart following scarlet fever, and Graves' disease (an autoimmune disorder of the thyroid). He also stressed that fasting wouldn't cure aging. The elderly could and should fast, but no one should pretend it would restore lost youth. Old age, he said, was a disease without cure.

His career wasn't free from error—he dabbled far too long in homeopathy, for one thing—but his achievement was formidable nonetheless. Unlike Shelton, he built a durable clinic, and when he threw out the cloudy bathwater of conventional medicine, with its unnecessary pills and harmful procedures, he kept the baby. In his therapeutics there was a place for the well-timed antibiotic, the widely used vaccine, the cautiously administered lumpectomy. He insisted, however, that the doctor's first reflex be to help the body heal itself, that conventional medicine be the second, not first, line of defense. It seemed to me an eminently sensible unification of natural and conventional therapies, and the only pity was that a century after he fasted his first patient, Buchinger's ideas were accepted by only a minority of doctors even in Germany. His creed had spread, but not far.

* * *

My fast began my second morning at the clinic. It was inaugurated, as were all the days of my visit, by a check-in with a nurse, preceded by a spirited half hour of group dynamics and mental gymnastics as a dozen robed and slippered fasters waited in a jumble outside her door and tried to keep straight who had arrived when so as not to get pipped by a johnny-come-lately. When it was my turn, I learned I had dropped from yesterday's 140 pounds to 138.5, even having eaten three modest meals. I couldn't have cared less about the weight, but to the extent it represented the start of my body tearing itself down to rid me of my odd ailments, I was gratified.

I hurried off to stretching and movement classes that left me limbered, invigorated, and charmed by the teacher's ability to demonstrate poses while instructing in German, French, and English. I returned to my room feeling well prepared for the first big event of the fasting calendar, an ordeal my fellow guests referred to as The Salts—always uppercased when spoken. The most traumatized used all caps.

Otto Buchinger believed fasting was a wonder of biology in every respect save one: the human body had never figured out how to properly eliminate its fasting bowels. When a faster stops stuffing food into his digestive tract, the food already there has less incentive to proceed to the exit. It lingers. According to Buchinger and his heirs, this lingering causes people to remain hungry longer, as if their bodies were demanding more fodder to push the food through the canal. Another and graver problem is that the dawdling food rots, and to this putrefaction are added oozy secretions and dead cells from the intestinal lining that we're constantly sloughing off in a process of renewal. (They make up an imposing share of our feces.) Buchinger got rid of both the hunger and the unsavory intestinal stew with a simple purgative.

I wasn't convinced it was needed. Although there's no denying muck idles in the fasting gut, there's also no data to say it's harmful, and it seemed to me if fair Nature had favored us with a mechanism like fasting, she would probably have found a way to evacuate the waste more promptly if it was going to hurt us. Most fasting doctors in the United States, relying on a similar logic, don't recommended intestinal cleanses. Then again, Nature couldn't have foreseen that a gut would hold half a bag of Doritos, yesterday's bloodwurst, a bacon donut, two dozen pesticides, and enough heavy metals to file a mining claim. Such contents might explain why Buchinger's patients, after purging, frequently lost not only their hunger but also their rheumatic aches, nerve pains, and headaches.

Ultimately I decided I had come to the clinic because the Buchinger Wilhelmi family, having overseen a quarter-million fasts in the last seven decades, might know a thing or two I didn't, so I buzzed the nurse from my room, told her I was ready for The Salts, and said a silent prayer to their patron saint, Johann Glauber, for an easy trial. Glauber was a half-German, half-Dutch, wholly self-taught apothecary with a kindly reputation (he may have given free care to the poor) and a taste for experimentation. Four centuries ago, he made the exhilarating discovery that a form of sodium sulfate had potent laxative properties, and in my mind's eye he is forever making abrupt but gleeful sprints to the outdoor privy. At a time when purging was still one of the main treatments for illness, he prospered off his discovery, which he named *sal mirabile*, "miraculous salt," but which posterity was generous enough to rechristen Glauber's salt.

The molecules of Glauber's salt are too large to be absorbed through the intestinal lining, so when you swallow them they remain in your gut. If you then drink large amounts of water, the water molecules will bind to the salts and won't be absorbed by the intestines, which will bloat up as if you had eaten an enormous meal. Your bowels will proceed to evacuate everything inside them, and you will be left with a tract free of rot, a belly free of hunger, and just possibly a body free of one or two other discomforts. Some modern fasting doctors have been even more enamored of Glauber's salt than Buchinger and his descendants. Guillaume Guelpa, that prolific purger, once serially fasted a middle-aged painter for eighty days across five months, the fasts interspersed with seventy gut-blasting purges of Glauber's salt. The painter slimmed from 192 to 132 pounds and must have had the slickest viscera in France. (Buchinger respected Guelpa's on-off fasting but wasn't convinced it did any better than a continuous fast.)

At dinner the night before my encounter with The Salts, I had attempted to engage Mr. Pidge by asking what they were like. He made a disagreeable face, took a shallow, little-bird breath, and offered his most impassioned statement of our acquaintance.

"The experience is *frightfully* perturbing," he said before returning with a shudder to his plate.

Presently an attendant arrived in my room bearing a tray with a half-liter carafe of warmed water mixed with an ounce of Glauber's salt, and a smaller carafe of very diluted raspberry-lemon juice. Mrs. Dr. Lischka had instructed me to wash down the salts, which she said would be bitter, with chasers of the sweet juice. I did as told and found the juice wasn't really needed. The salts just tasted like Alka-Seltzer without the satisfying fizz.

Before I was even one-third through the salt carafe, my stomach took on a Thanksgiving-afternoon roundness and expressed the confusion usual to that day about why my brain, supposedly in charge of my mouth, kept allowing more stuff to be put into it. I got a queasy, trembly feeling at the back of my jaw as though I might throw it all up—clearly my gut "brain" knew better than my head brain that these molecules didn't belong in my intestines and was calling for a reprieve. But I yielded to the higher authority of Mrs. Doctor and drank on.

I had read accounts of fasters who said, in language considerably more florid than Mr. Pidge's, to expect a firehose of excreta. But my first movement, which came half an hour after my first sip, was thoroughly normal in every respect save the reek—it smelled like something belched out of a sulfur pot at Yellowstone. A helpful "what to expect" video from the clinic had advised far worse to come. In fact, it said I might become so volcanic, I should remain in my room for several hours and under no condition stray farther than a quick dash from a commode until three or four eruptions had occurred. I sat on my bed and read and drank a kettle of tea. Nothing happened. An hour passed, and I downed glass after glass of water, as Mrs. Doctor had advised, but still nothing. Another hour went by, and then another. I consulted Otto, who had written, "Usually 4 to 7 stools are produced soon afterward, the last ones being entirely liquid," but I produced neither solid nor liquid.

As I ruminated on my unproductivity, it occurred to me that my diet of plants, loaded with fiber, might have made the Glauber's salt less necessary. Fiber moves nosh swiftly through the GI tract, and mine may have been comparatively unclogged to begin with, hence my single expulsion. Other guests, if their diets were as bereft of fiber as those of most

Westerners, may have been more in need, their packed colons requiring repeated gushers to clear.

When I reached five hours without further action, I went to see the nurse. It was a glorious fall day, and I was eager to go on the afternoon hike after missing yesterday's outing because of my many appointments. I hoped the nurse would tell me whether I was having a weird delayed response to the salts that would put me at risk, if I went hiking, of finding myself two miles up a Bodensee hillside with something foul trickling down my leg. The nurse, a sweet thirtysomething whose English was basic but far better than my pidgin German, had trouble understanding my concern.

"You have had no movement?" she said the third time I explained.

"I've had one," I said. "But just a small one. Not explosive either." I helpfully pantomimed, with rousing sound effects, the sort of movement I had expected. "Is that OK? Can I still go on the hike?"

"Well, since you have not moved—"

"I've moved," I said, but she wasn't hearing me.

"—then we could do an enema."

Enemas were the other half of the Buchinger bowel-clearing regimen. Like everyone else, I was scheduled to get one every other day during my fast, starting two days after the Glauber's salt, and I was in no hurry to move up my date with the irrigation tube. I tried another tack.

"I was thinking that maybe vegans—you know, people who eat only plants, with a lot of fiber—don't have much poop stuck in their bowels. Maybe one movement is all that happens when we take The Salts."

"You are vegan?" she said, her eyes wide, her tone wonderstruck—the very tone I would have used had someone told me they were a flat-earther or a Miley Cyrus fan.

"I am vegan."

"You do not eat meat?"

"Wouldn't be much of a vegan if I did, now would I?"

But she was too intrigued by the novel specimen in front of her to be sidetracked with frivolity.

"You do not eat fish?"

"No."

"Not poultry?"

"Not a feather."

"Not eggs?"

"Nope."

"Not milk?"

"Not from a cow."

She regarded me with a look of deepest pity, then said, "We can do an enema."

Now pause with me a moment. Here was a woman who saw dozens of fasters every day, a substantial portion of whom she was helping through the Great Salt March. If she had been at her post even as little as a year, she had helped hundreds of patients, and if she had been there a few years, thousands. But not once, it seemed, had she been presented with the possibility that someone's bowels might not need salt-based cleansing because their diet kept them spit-polish clean already. This fact was remarkable in itself. Even more remarkable to me, and not a little disheartening, was that when presented with such a medical novelty—presented, that is, with a possible clue why her patients were made so miserable by the salts and how they might avoid the misery—she did not say, "But this is incredible, *mein Liebling*! What is this magic eating way you do that keeps so clean your intestines? I must share it with others." Even in a place as enlightened as Buchinger Wilhelmi, the friendly young nurse was like most of the nurses and doctors I had seen in a long career frequenting them. She had a job to do: take my pulse, make sure I wasn't getting dehydrated, answer basic questions, move on to the next patient. Care and cheer were her stock in trade, not curiosity.

I told her we could wait and see about the enema. I went back to my room, laced on my hiking shoes, and went on the hike, which proved intestinally mundane. My bowels didn't move again until the next day, and when they did, the output was altogether unexceptional.

*   *   *

If there is a finer thing to do on a crisp November afternoon than to walk the leaf-strewn hills around Lake Constance, I can't think what it is. The grass on the hike was of the lushest green, the trees clung to the last of their fall colors, and the line of the Alps, marching along the far side of the lake, made the vista almost gaspingly picturesque. Fifty of us, split into smaller troupes by pace, tromped manfully up bluffs and womanfully into dales and non-binarily across high plateaus. We passed through fallow vineyards and over little rills on gently decaying wooden footbridges, now and again stumbling onto a small bedroom community of such well-kept loveliness that I never stopped imagining myself sitting in a comfy chair at one of the cottage windows with a cup of hot tea between my palms and on my lap a fine book by a handsomely paid writer of modest renown but luminous insight. I walked an hour before I saw my first piece of litter—a sentence impossible to write on any part of the Iberian Peninsula.

Old Otto held that "the cure of the body and the health of the spirit are so interdependent, the one so utterly conditioned on the other, that even a child couldn't miss the fact," and he believed the outdoors was where the spirit soared. In his time, long before the clinic's calendar was crowded with water gymnastics and art therapy sessions, fasters hiked twice a day, with the fittest hikers covering four miles in the morning and six in the afternoon. One modest hike per day suffices for his inheritors, although its commencement is regulated by the same punctual standard to which Buchinger himself adhered. A *New York Times* correspondent once showed up for a 6 a.m. hike at one minute past the hour and had nothing to show for her early rising but the lingering smell of diesel from the bus that ferried hikers to the trailhead. (I thought this karma for the *Times*'s food coverage, which ought to be arraigned for battery on behalf of every American stomach.)

We hikers fell in and out of conversation, and I got to talking with a Swiss mother of three teens, a very thin woman who had come to the clinic not, as most other fasters had, to lose weight but because of a crushing fatigue of mysterious origin. Her doctors had dismissed her complaint as neurotic, but a naturopath said she might be a victim of "electrosmog," which she described as pollution from electromagnetic fields. The naturopath suggested she sleep under a special net that dampened the fields. She did, and her fatigue lifted, but she came to the clinic anyway because she had already put down a deposit she didn't want to lose.

When I suggested it was just as well she had come, because the fast might help her health generally, she looked at me quizzically. When I explained that fasting repaired damage at a cellular level, thereby preventing diseases, she said, "But a fast can really do that?"

This surprised me. I'd have thought anyone who signed on for a ten-day fast in hope of curing a rare disorder would have known about both the preventive and curative power of fasting, but she didn't, and she was by no means the only one in the dark. In fact, the more people I talked to, the more it became clear most of them had no clue about fasting's reparative work. This was perhaps not shocking among those who'd come only to lose weight, but their reluctance to believe me even after I told them about the research never failed to surprise me. It was especially odd because we were greeted each morning with bite-size video tutorials, many of which discussed fasting's restorative effects, and every guestroom in the clinic had a copy of Wilhelmi de Toledo's *Therapeutic Fasting*, which explained in one of four languages how fasting replaced damaged and diseased cells with healthy new ones. Either the fasters weren't watching and reading, or the message was just too counterintuitive to digest.

The most extraordinary case was Morgan, a rotund and jocund Scotsman in his seventies who was wrapping up an illustrious career as a physician, researcher, and professor of medicine. Morgan held appointments at two European universities, one not far from the clinic, the other in the British Isles, and he had once run a national science foundation. He could speak engagingly about recent breakthroughs in cancer treatment, and he had many wise and sad things to say about medicine's narrow focus on treating instead of preventing disease. One night he told a group of us that he had tried decades ago to start a preventive medicine center at a teaching hospital.

"Would you like to know what my colleagues told me?" he said with a disbelieving shake of the head. "They said, 'Morgan, dear boy, what are you doing? Don't you realize if you keep the patients from getting sick, you're going to take away all our customers?' And they forced me out."

But when the conversation turned to fasting, Morgan's knowledge was worse than elementary. He told me, for instance, that I had no need to fast because I was slender, and when I replied that fasting might just keep me from getting cancer or having a stroke, his face was pure bewilderment. When someone asked his opinion, as a man of medicine, how long a human could survive without food or water, he said without hesitation no more than ninety days without food or three without water. On the first count, he was shy of the record, which had been set half a century earlier, by a mere 292 days, and on the second count he would have been right only if he'd exchanged days for weeks. Morgan was on his fifth visit to the clinic in twenty years, each stay lasting a month. That someone of his inquisitiveness and learning and his experience fasting could have understood it so poorly floored me.

Not all physicians were as ill-informed. A middle-aged Danish doctor of nuclear medicine who was on his seventh visit to the clinic and who single-handedly raised the couture of our hikes by tramping in a tweed jacket said he was quietly educating his patients about fasting: "They come to me obese and say, 'Doctor, I've got a thyroid problem.' I say, 'You don't have a thyroid problem. You've overeaten. And there are ways to lose the weight without taking an unnecessary thyroid supplement.'"

But he was a rarity, and in the end I concluded that among the clinic's many impressive successes, educating its patients about fasting's mechanisms wasn't at the top. It made for somber reflection about whether a therapy so paradoxical could ever be accepted by a wider public.

*   *   *

My days at the clinic settled into one of the pleasantest routines I have ever kept. After skirmishing in the queue for the morning checkup and being gently invigorated by an hour of yoga and stretching in the gym, I would return to my room, and soon one of the tea fairies, as I came to think of them, would appear with a tray bearing a teapot, a mug, and a small saucer so robustly filled with honey that the first time I saw it I exclaimed, "You've got to be kidding me."

"Excuse me?" said the tea fairy *du jour*.

"It's just—well, that's a lot of honey for someone who's fasting."

"You do not have to take it if it does not please you."

But I took it, and it pleased me. I even licked the saucer it came in.* It was hard to believe I wouldn't be bumped out of ketosis at least temporarily by what I estimated was two tablespoons of sugar—120 calories' worth, half my day's allotment. (A clinic info sheet claimed it was only a tablespoon, but it never looked so miserly as that. I always imagined a kitchen fairy, a cheery plump one endued with great pity for the poor starvers in her care, ladling an extra tablespoon into the saucers while the fairy superior's back was turned.) I also worried the sugar would stimulate my appetite for more, which is precisely what happened within a few minutes the first time I lapped it up. But the hunger passed nearly as quickly as it came, and on subsequent days I wasn't hungry at all after taking the honey. Ketones blunt hunger, and I suppose as I went deeper into ketosis they, or something else, simply overpowered the nectar. In any case, I noticed no ill effects in the long run, and my ketone-measuring pee strip the next morning confirmed I was steadily progressing into ketosis. Once I fully arrived there, on my fourth fasting morning, I remained, daily honey or no.

Among the guests, the undisputed favorite of the daily rituals was the hot-liver nap. In the late morning, while we were out doing warrior poses or rambling through barren cornfields, liver fairies tucked boiler-hot bladders of water under the blankets of our beds. When we repaired to our rooms after lunch, we snuggled into our toasty beds, pushed buttons for the nurses' station, and someone arrived shortly to swaddle us in a thin cotton wrap that held the water bottle snugly against our liver. For an hour we lay on our backs feeling as cozy as dogs in ThunderShirts. More than one guest analogized to being a babe at mother's breast.

---

* A vegan eating honey? Well, not routinely, but yes. I've yet to see a convincing argument that ethically produced honey more than mildly inconveniences bees, the earth, or, if eaten only occasionally, human health.

The idea behind the heat was that it supported the cleansing and detoxifying work of our livers. There was little research either to support or refute the claim, but it felt undeniably divine, every bit as relaxing as a hot bath but with less fuss. After an hour, when we unswaddled ourselves, a tea fairy appeared with another tray, this one bearing not honey but a couple of wedges of lemon, which were nearly as delicious.

The rest of our day consisted of a lunch and dinner of broth with our fellow fasters, meditation workshops, healthy-cooking seminars, and in the evening a lecture, concert, or film. Each day was a bounty of well-measured delights meant to uplift that hard-to-define part of us that Wilhelmi de Toledo called the spirit. I don't believe in the spirit, but mine felt magnificent all the same—more magnificent, in fact, than during any prior fast. It wasn't hard to see why thousands of people every year paid to deprive themselves at Buchinger Wilhelmi. The clinic made fasting feel like no deprivation at all.

CHAPTER 11

"WHAT'S CONSIDERED TOO DIFFICULT?"

One of the more astounding aspects of the 143-year-old rats, the ones from chapter 7 who, when fasted every other day, lived 83 percent longer, was that it took until the 1980s to create them. It was astounding because scientists had known for half a century, in a general sort of way, that fasted animals lived longer and more healthily, but almost no one tried to put that knowledge to more specific and profitable use.

The first researcher to skirt the edges of fasting for longevity was Charles Manning Child, a zoologist at the University of Chicago who in 1915 noticed that when he fasted and refed flatworms, they became "indistinguishable from young, growing animals in appearance and behavior, . . . [and] their general behavior indicates very clearly that they have become physiologically young during the course of reduction." Eight years later, Sergius Morgulis of the University of Nebraska observed that although the cells and nuclei of fasted animals shrank, they did so without functional impairment, and upon refeeding they grew the way cells did in embryos and young animals. The cells appeared, in short, to have been rejuvenated. At the same time, Margarete Kunde of the University of Chicago was remarking the obvious but often overlooked fact that when a dog was fasted to nearly half its weight and then refed, "approximately one-half of the restored body is made up of new protoplasm. In this there is rejuvenescence." (*Protoplasm* was a catch-all term for the stuff that makes up most of a cell.) She was right, of course: each time an animal builds new tissues after a fast, it conjures up a mass of fresh, youthful-seeming organelles, which suggests fasting is indeed a form of partial rejuvenescence.

In the late 1920s, an Australian researcher at the University of Adelaide with the lavish name Thorburn Brailsford Robertson took the field to the next logical step. Previous investigators had observed that the cells of animals were capable of dividing only a limited number of times and that the ravages of age increased as organisms neared the limit, after which death followed. Since cells seemed to divide only when their nuclei grew to a certain size, Robertson wondered whether slowing their nuclear growth would cause them to divide later and, if so, whether aging itself would be slowed. Given the rejuvenation that researchers like Child, Morgulis, and Kunde observed in fasted animals, Robertson tested his idea by fasting albino mice two consecutive days each week. Sure enough, their nuclei grew more slowly and they lived modestly longer, about the equivalent of four extra years in humans. Unfortunately, Robertson's controls were flawed, which made his results questionable, and before he could experiment further he died of influenza at just forty-five years old. Time would prove wrong some of his ideas about fasting, cellular division, and aging, but his basic premise—that by slowing growth, fasting could keep animals young longer—was essentially correct. Unfortunately, poor Robertson's bad luck continued posthumously, and his findings were published in the obscure *Australian Journal of Experimental Biology and Medical Science*, where they were noticed by hardly anyone.

The next consequential effort to extend life through fasting came from one of the more curious odd couples in modern science. The senior partner was Anton Julius Carlson, a stern, Swedish-born professor at the University of Chicago who was described by *Time* as "a rugged old man with a brick-red face and . . . a lifelong worship of cold hard facts." His junior, Frederick Hoelzel, was a German-born autodidact who lacked a college degree but had a penchant for dietary experimentation. Hoelzel once fasted forty-two days, and he made a small fortune with a noncaloric but allegedly tasty bread that filled the stomach while leaving the figure trim. When the stock market crash of 1929 wiped out his riches, he turned himself over to Carlson as a human guinea pig in return for a bed in Carlson's lab, where he gained a reputation for eating indigestibles: glass beads, nuts and bolts, rubber tubing taken spaghetti fashion with pasta sauce. Most of these delicacies passed through him without event, but a half cup of talcum powder that turned to paste in his intestines nearly killed him. His health couldn't have been helped by the frequent X-rays with which Carlson marked the progress of the oddments through his gastrointestinal tract. In 1933, when Hoelzel was forty-six, a reporter wrote, "His hands are like those of an invalid, white, blue-lined and bony, his Adam's apple stands out from a scrawny neck, and his skin is colorless except for a network of fine blue lines."

But Hoelzel wasn't just a human lab animal. He taught himself to become a researcher and co-authored numerous papers with Carlson, including a series of studies published between 1946 and 1948 that picked up where the unfortunate T. Brailsford Robertson left off. In those experiments, Carlson and Hoelzel fasted groups of recently weaned rats either every other day, every third day, or every fourth day and found that the more the rats fasted, the longer they tended to live. They didn't become 143-year-olds, but one coterie of every-other-day eaters lived 25 percent longer—an extra twenty human years—and they were also healthier. Among the females, 37 percent of the control rats developed breast cancer, but only 7 percent of the every-other-day fasters did, which came to just one rat. And while the tumors of the controls emerged in middle age and grew to nearly half a pound, the tumor in the one fasting rat appeared shortly before her death and weighed less than an ounce. Carlson and Hoelzel speculated that the more the rats fasted, the more they burned up defective organelles and cells that would have turned into cancer had the rats been eating.

Spare a minute for this monumental finding. What Carlson and Hoelzel had just demonstrated was that in one mammalian species—a species whose basic biochemistry shared countless similarities with our own—regular fasting not only gave the equivalent of two extra decades of life; it also conferred health and very nearly eliminated one of the most dreaded of all diseases. Had a drug achieved this result, we would hail the names of Carlson and Hoelzel alongside that of Alexander Fleming, penicillin's discoverer. But since you've made it this far in the narrative, you won't be surprised to learn that no scientist who read their well-circulated papers (two of them appeared in the prominent *Journal of Nutrition*) dropped what they were doing and asked, "So how do we test this wonder treatment in humans?"

Part of the blame, it must be said, rested with Carlson and Hoelzel, who didn't trumpet their finding, apparently because they were concerned about the stunted size of their long-lived, every-other-day fasters. You and I might trade a few inches in height for a longer and healthier life, but in the 1940s to be tall and strapping was to be vigorous, so Carlson and Hoelzel drew attention not to the every-other-day fasters but to the every-third-day fasters, who were full sized. Those rats, however, didn't live nearly as long, and they got far more cancer, so were hardly cause for scientific titillation. Only researchers who closely scrutinized Carlson and Hoelzel's tabulated data would have seen the promise in the alternate-day fasters.

Two other forces conspired to turn scientific interest not just from Carlson and Hoelzel's discovery but from fasting for longevity generally. One was the mild popularity of caloric restriction. Although not many researchers in that era thought the study of longevity would yield actionable results, the few who did tended to restrict their curiosity to the practice of simply eating less. As early as 1917, researchers had shown that animals lived longer when they were underfed, provided they got adequate nutrients, and in 1934 and 1935 the Cornell professor Clive McCay and his graduate student Mary Crowell demonstrated in a pair of famous papers that feeding rats a calorically restricted but nutritionally complete diet increased their lifespan by 70 percent. McCay was said to have been inspired by reading our friend Alvise Cornaro's *Discourses on the Sober Life*, and like Cornaro, he had a certain charisma and knew how to use the media. Thanks to McCay's promotion, the story of his outstandingly long-lived rats seeped into the fringes of public consciousness and monopolized the small amount of scientific interest in extending lifespan. A dozen years later, most scientists in the field probably saw Carlson and Hoelzel's research as little more than an elaboration on McCay and Crowell—and a not especially enticing elaboration at that, since eating less was thought to be easier than fasting. The irony is that exactly the opposite is true. But few scientists knew or recalled that thousands of people had fasted with relatively little discomfort in the Macfadden era.

The other force that turned scientists away from fasting was a trial by Ancel Keys known as the Minnesota Starvation Experiment. Keys was the University of Minnesota professor who created the US Army's K-ration and later rose to fame as the popularizer of the Mediterranean diet. During the Second World War, with malnourishment pervasive around the globe, US officials wanted to know more about the disorder and how to care for its victims. Keys recruited thirty-six young conscientious objectors, most of them Quakers, Mennonites, and Brethren, and cut their diet in half for six months with results that ran from grim to macabre. Wracked with hunger, the men grew irritable, fatigued, and depressed. They lost a quarter of their weight and all of their sex drive and fantasized endlessly about food. Several became deeply unsound of mind. One chopped off three fingers with an axe and then couldn't quite articulate why he thought that was the best way to leave the trial. After Keys published his results in 1948, scientific interest in fasting for longevity all but disappeared. No one wanted to go through *that* for a chance at longer life, never mind *that* wasn't what fasting was like at all.

Not until 1973, a quarter century after Carlson and Hoelzel, did anyone return to fasting for longevity, and even then the experimenter wasn't much interested in fasting. Don Kendrick was a professor of psychology at the University of Hull in England, and what he really wanted to know was whether stroking his rats' backs would make them live longer. It didn't, but for comparison he fasted another group of rats on two nonconsecutive days each week, and they lived 17 percent longer. His finding revived interest in fasting for longevity, and the ensuing tests culminated in the NIA's 1982 study that created the 143-year-old rats.

But although fasting stood still in the lab after the Minnesota Starvation Experiment, several desperate clinicians resorted to it to combat a problem that was proving no less vexatious than, and nearly as unsolvable as, aging.

* * *

In June of 1965, a Scotsman of twenty-seven years and thirty-two and a half stone, which is to say 456 pounds, presented himself at the University of Dundee's Department of Medicine with the desire to lose weight. The fellows of the department, thinking so dire a case might call for dire measures, suggested that not eating for a short period might help him control his appetite. They did not intend a prolonged fast.

The Scotsman, known in the annals of science only as A. B. but to his familiars as Angus Barbieri, agreed to the fast, and the fellows hospitalized him as a precaution. For several days he took water and a daily vitamin pill. His vital signs were normal. He said he felt fine, even better than fine, and that nothing that passed for food in Scotland tempted him. He asked if he might continue his fast at home, and the doctors, thinking of no reason he shouldn't, released him on condition he return for periodic tests of his urine and blood. The checkups weren't intended to make sure he wasn't sneaking food, but they had that incidental effect. One week disappeared into the next, taking with it, on par, six of Barbieri's pounds. His checkups showed he had less sugar in his blood than a normal man, but he was not hypoglycemic, and his movements and thinking were unimpaired.

Summer turned to fall, and fall to winter, but Barbieri continued vigorous. During the fourth and fifth months, the fellows thought it prudent to supplement his daily vitamin with potassium, but that was all. With each new month, they were less certain the fast should continue, but they could find no reason to halt it, and anyway Barbieri was so determined to reach his target of 180 pounds he probably wouldn't have heard of stopping. He celebrated a year without food with a glass of water. Seventeen days later, 276 pounds the lesser, he reached his mark. He ate, but not from hunger.

His case was reported in the *Postgraduate Medical Journal* in 1973, and the *Guinness Book of World Records* cited him for "Most Weight Lost," although Guinness later removed the honor for fear of inspiring unsupervised imitators. "Heaviest Weight Dangled from a Swallowed Sword" remains.

Barbieri was merely the most stunning exemplar of a tiny renaissance in the study of fasting in humans—specifically, in obese humans, whom researchers had had little success helping. The revival began with a paper published in 1959 by a doctor in Atlanta who fasted his obese patients and found the therapy worked—always. The physics of calories-in, calories-out brooked no failure. Moreover, people who were put on the zero-calorie diet, as it was called, weren't driven half-mad by hunger the way ordinary dieters were. The scientific journals of the 1960s and 1970s are speckled with tales of astonishing losses of Barbieri-like magnitude. A twenty-year-old woman from New South Wales fasted off half of her 312 pounds in eight months. A thirty-year-old Glaswegian slimmed, also in eight months, from 281 to 137 pounds. Another Scot of sixty-one years fasted ten days, ate ten days, fasted ten more, and so on for a year and a half until he lost 213 of his 441 pounds.

Unfortunately, most of the subjects eventually put the weight back on, just as normal dieters did. In retrospect, this is hardly surprising since they generally ate the same kinds of things in the same kinds of quantities they'd eaten before their fasts. (Researchers were less certain then than now that what people ate, as opposed to how much they exercised or which genes they inherited, made them obese.) The reinflation of the zero-calorie dieters convinced most researchers that fasting for obesity was a bust, but their conclusion was premature. Clinicians who gave their fasters counseling and taught them how to plan a healthier diet reported they kept quite a bit of the weight off. So did fasters who made occasional maintenance fasts of a day or two when their weight ticked up—precisely my approach. Regrettably, there were very few long-term follow-ups to see if these tactics worked three, five, or ten years out.

Such follow-ups might not have mattered anyway, at least not to doctors, who showed little interest in supervising prolonged fasts or doing the post-fast hand-holding to keep their patients trim. Their view of fasting wasn't helped by the death of a handful of the obese fasters, the circumstances of which are as instructive as they were tragic. The researchers who supervised the fatal fasts had no experience in the practice and didn't consult fasting doctors like Herbert Shelton or Otto Buchinger who might have helped them avoid several grave errors. One of those errors was fasting people with severe contraindications like advanced heart failure. Another was letting fasters take metabolism-altering substances like caffeinated drinks and prescription drugs, whose effects on the fasted body are far stronger than on the fed body. The researchers also gave their fasters vitamins and minerals, which might sound advisable but is in fact malign on a water-only fast. One way a wise doctor ensures her fasters are in good health is by monitoring various markers in the blood and urine. If a faster has a precipitous fall in, say, potassium, the doctor knows to break the fast to keep the patient's heart, kidneys, and other organs from suffering. A supplement that artificially elevates potassium can mask the stresses that would otherwise have caused potassium to fall, but the doctor, seeing only normal potassium, thinks all is well and continues the fast even as the faster struggles internally.

Recent research suggests the supplements used in the obesity studies were unnecessary because the fasting body conserves its essential vitamins and minerals instead of using them up or excreting them in the urine and feces. This explains why if a faster and an eater both go three months without vitamin C, the eater will get scurvy while the faster won't. The fasting body takes the absence of food to mean no more vitamin C is on the way and preserves its stores, but the fed body expects vitamin C to arrive as usual, so uses and excretes its stock. The same thing happens with thiamine and the disease of its deficiency, beriberi. Some fasting doctors speculate that supplements throw off the fasting body's delicate nutrient-conservation system because nothing in evolution prepared us to get tiny doses of vitamins and minerals when we're otherwise not eating. When those doses arrive, some part of the confused fasting body apparently takes their presence to mean it's eating again and starts dumping rather than conserving vitamins and minerals.

The harm from that dump might be a long time showing. Even the fasters in the obesity studies who seemed to have enjoyed good health may have suffered organ damage that was masked by supplements or drugs. Angus Barbieri might have been such a case. Initially, he seemed the embodiment of health. Five years after his fast, having added just sixteen pounds to his slenderized 180, he was the uncommon obese faster who did not recidivate. But his success didn't last, and over the years he regained much of what he had lost. In 1991, at the distressingly young age of fifty-one, he died of gastrointestinal bleeding, congestive heart failure, and obesity. We'll never know whether his heart failed because its muscle was weakened by an overlong fast, the damage hidden by supplements. The opposite is also quite possible—that his fast left his heart in fine fettle, maybe even better than before, and he simply ate his way back to cardiovascular trauma. But even before Barbieri met his sad fate, conventional doctors looked at the fatalities of the 1960s and 1970s and decided fasting was unsafe, and in one sense they were right: fasting under a doctor inexperienced in the art was a poor risk, especially for unhealthy patients.

The story of fasting for obesity had a sequel, one even more sorrowful than the first installment. A few obesity researchers didn't want to give up on fasting and turned to modified fasts as a safer bet. Unfortunately, their preferred "fast" was a diet of liquid protein, which they adopted from a misguided fear that the fasting body burned too much protein, thereby putting muscles, including the heart, at risk of withering. In fact, although the body briefly burns a bit of protein as it switches from eating to fasting, once the faster enters ketosis, protein is mostly conserved. Even the small amount the body continues to burn may be aged or damaged, in which case getting rid of it and replacing it during refeeding is almost certainly healthy.

The "protein-sparing fast," as the diet was sometimes called, prospered because of a unique advantage it had over water fasting: it required the purchase of a product that a corporation could advertise and sell. This was a 300-calorie-a-day protein drink, foul of taste but deliciously priced (for the manufacturer) at what would be nearly ten dollars in today's money. Thirty calories to the dollar was profitable indeed, a rate that would see a Qdoba burrito selling for thirty bucks. Advertising propelled the protein-sparing fast to a swift popularity, and the most widely read book about it, *The Last Chance Diet* by the osteopath Robert Linn, sold more than 2.5 million copies in the late 1970s.

What last-chance dieters didn't know was that by slurping down great gobs of protein—up to 100 grams a day, more than double what most people need—with virtually no carbohydrates or fats, they were throwing off their bodies' exquisite fasting metabolism, just as the obese fasters had done with their supplements. Ultimately their disoriented bodies broke down far more protein than they would have on a water fast, with grievous damage to their hearts. It couldn't have helped that the diet's protein was of the poorest quality, typically extracted from the ground-up ears of livestock. The supplement Robert Linn hawked was made first of cowhide, later of pigskin.

Some of the liquid-protein dieters lost fantastic amounts of weight— one man shed 321 pounds in a single year—but here and there people started dropping dead of cardiac arrest as they refed. Autopsies showed their damaged hearts couldn't handle the strain of digesting and processing food again. In all, nearly sixty dieters, most of them young and generally healthy, died before the protein supplements were pulled from stores. Congress and European parliaments held scathing hearings, aggrieved families brought litigation, and reporters rightly castigated the diet's reckless propagators. Many journalists, however, located the root of the problem not in an unproven semi-fast on pigskin but in fasting, full stop. It was one more dark hour for the oldest cure in the world.

* * *

The few researchers who continued to look into fasting for health labored in deepest obscurity. The exception who proved the rule was an immunologist at Oslo's National Hospital named Jens Kjeldsen-Kragh, who for a brief period in the 1990s, almost without trying, became the world's most important fasting researcher. Between 1979 and 1988, a handful of other Scandinavian investigators undertook small, mostly uncontrolled studies that suggested fasting and a vegetarian diet could relieve the devastating pain of rheumatoid arthritis, the autoimmune disease in which the body attacks the linings of its own joints. Conventional medicine didn't then and doesn't now have a cure, only the promise of slightly slowing the miserable deterioration of sufferers through drugs whose side effects are alarming. The Scandinavian studies were the first to lend scientific confirmation to the observations of Herbert Shelton and Otto Buchinger that fasting could often reverse autoimmune diseases, including rheumatoid arthritis. (Buchinger himself, you'll recall, cured his own rheumatic disorder with fasting.) Conventional doctors almost entirely ignored the Scandinavian research, but it was so promising, and other treatments were so ineffective, that money was raised for a larger trial. Kjeldsen-Kragh, a conventional doctor with expertise in rheumatology but little in fasting, agreed to lead the experiment—to his great benefit, because its dazzling results landed in *The Lancet*, one of the world's most prestigious medical journals.

In the trial, fifty-three subjects with rheumatoid arthritis were divided into two groups and sent for a month to either a health farm or a convalescent home and then completed the rest of the trial at their own homes. The group at the health farm did a modified Buchinger-style fast of seven to ten days, after which they ate a vegan diet low in allergens for three and a half months before switching to a lactovegetarian diet. The group that started at the rest home ate normally throughout. Both groups were assessed at regular intervals for a year.

Just four weeks into the study, the fasting-and-vegan group was improved on nearly every measure of arthritis the researchers checked: number of swollen joints, number of tender joints, degree of tenderness, duration of morning stiffness, grip strength, overall pain, and levels of inflammatory markers like red blood cell sedimentation rate, C-reactive protein, and white blood cell count. After a year, they maintained nearly all of these gains, were in better overall health than before the trial, and lost an average of nine pounds.

The control group also had less overall pain at first but didn't do as well on other markers, and their modest improvements disappeared as soon as they left the rest home. After a year, they were in more pain than before the trial, and on nearly every other metric, including their own assessment of their health, they had badly deteriorated—the usual course of the disease.

The contrast could not have been sharper, the placement of the results in *The Lancet* could not have been better, and one might have thought—if one knew little of the history of fasting—that fasting's future looked bright. But again almost no one paid attention. No rheumatologist canceled his patients' appointments and packed them off to fasting clinics; no rheumatology association suggested the standard of care be amended to put fasting at the top of the list. Kjeldsen-Kragh got a few more papers out of the study and then went back to immunology, never to do fasting research again. All the same, that the editors of *The Lancet* had published rather than ridiculed his results suggested change, however halting, was afoot.

It has, alas, been quite slow footed. For years there were almost no other studies on fasting for autoimmune disease, and only in the last decade have a few researchers finally returned to the field. Their results, though preliminary, are scintillating. In one trial, when mice with multiple sclerosis (the disease in which the body strips its own nerves of their insulating sheaths) were fasted, they had less nerve damage and performed better on motor and mental tests. Even better—and this is truly sensational—in 20 percent of the mice the MS was completely reversed. To all appearances, fasting cured them. It's a finding worthy of headlines that have yet to be written. In pilot trials in humans, patients with MS who fasted intermittently or ate a fasting-mimicking diet reported fewer symptoms and a better quality of life in as little as two months. Were I the sufferer of an autoimmune disease like MS or rheumatoid arthritis, I imagine I would spend my days oscillating between joy over the work finally being done and fury that scientists had so long and so inexplicably—so *unscientifically*—ignored a promise all too visible.

*   *   *

Fasting enjoyed one other spectacular revival at the end of the last century, and it came about thanks entirely to a Hollywood director and his wife, Jim and Nancy Abrahams. In 1993, their son Charlie began having seizures on his first birthday and was soon convulsing up to a hundred times a day. A profusion of medications had almost no effect, and Charlie stopped growing—physically, cognitively, and behaviorally. After consulting five pediatric neurologists, the Abrahamses elected brain surgery, but it, too, failed to slow the seizures. Nor did Charlie find relief from a pair of homeopathic doctors or, all else having come to naught, a faith healer. Charlie's many doctors all said he was headed for mental and physical retardation.

Nine months into this hell, while rooting around the stacks of a medical library, Jim Abrahams came across a volume on childhood epilepsy by a pediatric neurologist who ran the epilepsy clinic at Johns Hopkins in Baltimore. Deep within John Freeman's book, all but buried under a barrage of advice about drugs and surgeries, were three pages discussing a protocol that Hopkins doctors had been using on epileptic children for most of the century: they fasted the children briefly and then fed them a high-fat diet, and many either stopped seizing completely or had far fewer seizures.

Jim Abrahams didn't know it, but Freeman and his colleague, a dietitian named Millicent Kelly, were very nearly the world's sole remaining practitioners of fasting and the ketogenic diet for epilepsy. They weren't exactly overwhelmed with customers. Some years the clinic that had once fasted and dieted many scores of children a year now administered the therapy to no more than ten. Freeman had tried to get the word out about the Hopkins protocol, but neurologists around the country roundly dismissed him, and publisher after publisher rejected a book he proposed on it. Some of the publishers said they feared parents would fast their children at home unsupervised. So Freeman had settled for the three pages in his more general book on epilepsy. Those three pages, however, were enough.

Not that Jim and Nancy Abrahams did anything useful with Freeman's information at first. His protocol sounded too far-fetched, and none of the five specialists in pediatric epilepsy they had consulted had so much as mentioned it, so what were the odds it was effective or even safe? Still, the next time Jim Abrahams saw Charlie's primary neurologist, he said they were down to two leads and asked which they should pursue: Dr. Freeman in Baltimore or an herbalist who worked out of a strip mall in Houston.

"Flip a coin," the neurologist replied. "Neither will probably work."

The Abrahamses flipped a coin and flew to Houston, but after a month of scented teas improved Charlie not a bit, they boarded a plane to Baltimore. Nearly two years old, Charlie weighed just sixteen pounds. The protocol Freeman and Kelly put him on was a little different from the one Hopkins doctors had used in the past. As recently as the 1960s, Hopkins patients were fasted until they lost 10 percent of their body weight and then transitioned to a ketogenic diet that was 80 percent fat. Freeman kept the diet much the same, but he thought a prolonged fast inhumane and shortened it to between twenty-four and forty-eight hours, just enough to get the child into ketosis. On the second day of Charlie's fast, his seizures stopped, and they remained quiescent when he was moved to the ketogenic diet. Almost immediately he began to develop normally again, and two years after his first visit to Hopkins, he was slowly weaned off the diet. His seizures never returned, and he grew to adulthood as healthy as his brother and sister.

The Abrahamses were by turns thrilled and dismayed. Their child had been devastated by thousands of seizures, they and their insurers had run through $100,000 in treatments, and not once had a doctor mentioned this long-proven, altogether effective, utterly safe treatment. The neurologist who suggested flipping a coin would later say he had known all along the Hopkins protocol had been proven sound; in fact, he was a friend of Dr. Freeman. But he had declined to tell the Abrahamses any of that because Charlie hadn't yet exhausted all "medical approaches"— that is, hadn't tried every possible drug and procedure. Until he had, the neurologist saw no point in bothering with anything so kooky as a nutritional therapy, which, whatever else it was, wasn't "medical." It is as damning a summary of conventional medicine as a conventional doctor has ever uttered.

The Abrahamses decided to overhaul this sorry landscape. They created the Charlie Foundation to Help Cure Pediatric Epilepsy and produced a series of videos about the ketogenic diet that the foundation sent, gratis, to tens of thousands of families and nearly every pediatric neurologist in the country. The foundation also sponsored conferences, trained hundreds of doctors and dietitians to administer the fast and diet, and gave Freeman the money to publish the ketogenic book that publishers had rejected. Jim Abrahams directed a TV movie, . . . *First Do No Harm*, in which Meryl Streep played a mother who defied her benighted doctors to take her epileptic son to Hopkins, where he was cured. After NBC's *Dateline* aired an episode about Charlie and the ketogenic diet in 1994, the tiny staff at the Hopkins center was suddenly fielding thousands of calls a month. Doctors who had long said they used anticonvulsant drugs because nobody wanted to mess with fasting and diet hadn't considered the screamingly obvious facts that drugs don't work for nearly 40 percent of epileptics and even when they do, some parents think it worth seeing if a brief fast and a temporary diet might rid their child of the disease rather than damning him to a life of medication with serious side effects.

Nudged by the Charlie Foundation, researchers returned to the Hopkins protocol and largely confirmed what doctors had reported decades ago: a little under half the children they fasted and put on a ketogenic diet became free of seizures, and another third greatly improved. These were exceptional numbers for patients who had already failed one or more drugs. "You've already peeled off the easiest cases," one neurologist explained. "It's like running a one-hundred-yard dash with a weight chained to your leg." In 2008, British researchers published the first randomized, controlled trial of the ketogenic diet for epilepsy (fasting wasn't part of the study), in which 145 children who had failed at least two medications did either three months of the ketogenic diet followed by three months of their usual treatment, or the reverse. On the keto diet, their seizures dropped an average of nearly 40 percent, and some of them ended up virtually or entirely seizure-free. On their normal diet, their seizures *increased* nearly 40 percent. On this and other evidence, it's a wonder neurologists are even allowed to prescribe drugs to child epileptics without first trying the Hopkins protocol.

Scientists are still working out the mechanisms by which fasting and the ketogenic diet counter seizures. The ketone beta-hydroxybutyrate (BHB) almost certainly plays a part, but its precise nature is a mystery. It could have to do with the way BHB stimulates a neurotransmitter called gamma-aminobutyric acid, GABA, which inhibits some of the brain's overexcited transmissions. Or it might be related to how BHB stimulates better functioning of neuronal mitochondria, the power plants of brain cells. There may also be roles for the gut microbiome, whose composition is improved by fasting, and for inflammatory cytokines, which decrease with fasting. We are likely many years from knowing.

We also still have no idea about the relative importance of fasting versus the ketogenic diet. Would more patients be freed of seizures if they fasted a couple of weeks instead of a couple of days? What if they made repeated fasts in the style of Hugh Conklin, the doctor at Bernarr Macfadden's sanatorium? Sadly, most scientists seem to be of Dr. Freeman's opinion that fasts are essentially inhumane and have declined to explore these vital questions. In some ways, we are just as much in the dark as our forebears a century ago.

The Abrahamses' efforts may have brought fasting and the ketogenic diet to doctors' notice, but the majority of physicians still want nothing to do with it. In 2005, more than a decade into the Charlie Foundation's work, a survey of eighty-eight leading pediatric neurologists revealed that not one used the Hopkins protocol as a first-line treatment, only 36 percent used it with any frequency, and even they did so only after numerous drugs had failed. The other 64 percent, asked why they either rarely or never used the protocol—even when every other treatment had met with defeat—said it was just too difficult for patients and doctors.

That complaint, Jim Abrahams said, is "one of the things that pisses me off the most. . . . When you're holding your kid while he has hundreds of seizures a day, and then you find out doctors aren't giving you all the information because they think 'it's too difficult'—where in medical school did they teach a course on what's considered too difficult for the parents of a critically ill child?"

Abrahams had no illusions matters would change soon. The incentives, he said, were all wrong. "It's not in the form of a pill, it can't be administered with a scalpel, and the only people who profit from the ketogenic diet are the patients." Why would a neurologist care about something so irrelevant to his lucrative practice as that?

* * *

For scientists, however, there is more cause for hope. In the 1980s and 1990s, a new generation of researchers took a look at the incomparable 143-year-old rats, at Kjeldsen-Kragh's startling success with rheumatoid arthritis, and at the salvation of Charlie Abrahams, and thought there might be something to this fasting business after all. Little by little, they have begun piecing together the mechanisms of fasting, and their discoveries make clear it can both prevent and heal disease.

It has long been known, as I mentioned in chapter 4, that after a fasting body uses up all its glucose from the last meal, it will convert glycogen stores in the liver and muscle to glucose and run on those for a few more hours. Once the glycogen dwindles, the body resorts to fat, which is broken first into fatty acids and then into ketones, which start to appear in the blood between eight and fourteen hours after the last calories are consumed—sooner if the glycogen in the liver is exhausted through exercise. (Running for an hour can make ketones appear in a faster's blood in just four hours.) For the first twelve or so hours after ketones appear, they remain at quite low levels, but then they increase dramatically. The increase is a sign the body is making the metabolic switch from running on glucose, which is the hallmark of fed metabolism, to running on ketones, the hallmark of fasting metabolism. The switch takes another one to two days to complete, and as the body makes the transition, it turns proteins into glucose to run the brain and other organs. Once the body is in ketosis, this catabolism of protein tapers off.*

Researchers used to wonder whether fasting made people healthier simply by making them lose weight, but it's now clear that going through the metabolic switch and running for a time in fasting mode is behind most of the gains. Burning ketones is one reason. Ketones, as you may recall from chapter 4, can deliver energy more efficiently than glucose. In

---

* If the body runs too low on fat, it will return to burning proteins, including vital proteins like cardiac muscle. This change represents another metabolic switch: from fasting to starvation. Even slender people typically take a month or more to reach starvation, and the average padded American would take months.

one experiment, rat hearts suffused with the ketone BHB contracted more strongly and used less oxygen than when running on glucose—essentially doing the same work with less effort. BHB also induces reactions in the brains of mice and humans that generate new neurons and new connections between existing neurons. But running on ketones is not the only and probably not the most important reason fasting makes us healthier, which is why people who try to mimic fasting by taking ketone supplements are disappointed. It's also one reason why, unless you suffer from one of a few grave conditions like epilepsy, eating a high-fat ketogenic diet offers more peril than promise.

Fasting also improves our health by making us less inflamed. Inflammation may sound trivial, the mild problem of the stubbed toe, but at a cellular level it's a sinister contributor to a vast number of maladies, and it worsens as we age. Allergies, arthritis, asthma, cancer, cardiovascular disease, celiac disease, dementia, diabetes, irritable bowel syndrome, kidney disease, and non-alcoholic fatty liver disease are all, to one degree or another, inflammatory diseases. Even short fasts reduce inflammatory agents like interleukins, C-reactive protein, and tumor necrosis factor, and long fasts subdue them still more. Less inflammation means not just less disease but also less metabolic exhaustion because our cells aren't constantly struggling to fight inflammation. The benefits of this metabolic rest show up in all kinds of ways. Fasting mice, for example, learn and remember better than normally fed mice in part because fasting downregulates the inflammatory interleukins in their brains.

Fasting also generates antioxidants that neutralize reactive oxygen species (ROS), the byproducts thrown off when cells metabolize oxygen. ROS have a bad reputation, but in the right amount they help cells receive and transmit signals. If, however, we eat a bad diet, smoke, drink alcohol, become too stressed, or don't get enough sleep or exercise, we can generate too many ROS, which can damage our DNA and other cellular parts. The antioxidants created by fasting will mop up some of the excess ROS and spare us a portion of the damage.

Recent research has also proven that fasters are more sensitive to the hormone insulin, another inestimable benefit. Each time we eat, glucose from our food is transported through the bloodstream to cells all over our bodies. The cells are protected by what amount to locked gates, and the keys that turn the locks to let the glucose in are molecules of insulin, which the pancreas releases with each meal. A fatty diet can gum up the locks, in which case the keys won't work as well. In this state, called insulin insensitivity, glucose lingers in the arteries where it can damage arterial walls, and over time the damage can turn into atherosclerosis and a horde of other ills. Insulin insensitivity also makes the pancreas work harder as it tries to produce more insulin—more keys to try in the gummed-up locks. When the situation grows desperate, we call it diabetes. (Contrary to wide belief, type 2 diabetes, the most prevalent kind, is caused neither by too little insulin nor by eating too much sugar but by eating too many animal fats and vegetable oils, which make the cellular locks malfunction—which is why a low-fat vegan diet can reverse diabetes.) When Guillaume Guelpa reversed diabetes through fasting, it was almost certainly because his diabetics became more sensitive to insulin. Even in a non-diabetic body, when fasting induces greater sensitivity to insulin, the results are healthier arteries and a rested pancreas.

Researchers have also discovered that fasting intensifies one of the most ingenious and advantageous of all cellular processes: autophagy, whose name comes from the Greek roots meaning "eating the self." Our cells are forever trying to prolong their useful lives by repairing worn-out parts, but when a part becomes too damaged to fix, it's either discarded or recycled. Autophagy is the recycling process. In autophagy, the cell envelops the spent part in a kind of vat (known as the autophagosomal membrane), which it builds for the purpose and into which it pours acid. Once the part is dissolved, its broken-down components are sent elsewhere to become the building blocks of new parts. Autophagy goes on all the time but usually only at a very low level because our cells are too busy doing other chores, above all processing nutrients from our food. If we go without food long enough, cells take advantage of the break to do more recycling. Herbert Shelton, not incidentally, predicted fasting's role in autophagy as long ago as 1950. "When once we have learned that the body is able to rip its structures to pieces," he wrote, "and re-use and re-arrange their constituents to match and fit its organs, we are prepared to understand how fasting so quickly brings about a rejuvenation of the body."

Autophagy declines with age and harmful habits, and since the decline contributes to diseases of elderhood like dementia, boosting autophagy seems likely to head off or lessen their severity. In one promising experiment, a team at the University of Florida fasted mice with Charcot-Marie-Tooth disease, which robs nerves of their ability to conduct electricity properly and turns even simple motor tasks like walking into an ordeal. After fasting every other day for five months, the CMT mice enjoyed a marked uptick in autophagy and, apparently in consequence, had healthier nerves and were more adept at exercises like balancing on a rotating drum and maintaining their grip on a steel ring.

Fasting also stimulates the repair of DNA, which is no small thing since our DNA is the set of instructions that guides the work of our body. Our cells repair DNA routinely but, again, only at a modest clip because of their other duties. Fasting accelerates the clip. In a simple but telling experiment at Germany's Albstadt-Sigmaringen University, scientists drew blood cells from volunteers before, during, and after a partial fast of three weeks, then damaged the cells' DNA with ultraviolet radiation. The cells of some volunteers had trouble repairing the irradiated DNA before their fasts, but during and after the fasts the cells of those same volunteers became much more skilled at fixing the damage.

Fasting has also been shown to improve the gut microbiome, whose immense contribution to our health we're only beginning to appreciate. The microbiome is the two to five pounds of microorganisms, chiefly bacteria, that are our constant intestinal companions. The best of them help us digest food, make vitamins we can't do without, regulate our immune system, and protect us against their nastier, disease-causing bacterial cousins. The worst of them repay our hospitality by contributing to, or possibly causing outright, obesity, leaky gut, heart attacks, colorectal cancer, lupus, rheumatoid arthritis, and much else of a disagreeable and sometimes terminal nature. Which bacteria thrive depends largely on what we feed them. The healthy bacteria flourish on minimally processed plants, apparently because they adore nothing so much as plant fiber. The unhealthy bacteria revel in meat, dairy, alcohol, and refined sugars. Fasting wipes out the vast majority of both good and bad bacteria, which gives us a chance to start fresh. If we refeed on plants, we stimulate the good bacteria to recolonize our gut and crowd out the bad bacteria, which is surely one reason many fasting doctors have found that the patients who do best after fasting are those who eat plants.

Refeeding after fasting has been less studied than fasting itself, but there are hints it may be just as important to health. We now know, for example, that refeeding activates stem cells, those life-giving progenitors of other cells. When Charles Manning Child, Sergius Morgulis, and Margarete Kunde said a century ago that the cells of their fasted worms and dogs looked rejuvenated upon refeeding, they were onto something.

Investigators have also discovered that the more we fast, the better we become at many of the above processes. Repeat fasters make the switch from fed metabolism to fasting metabolism more quickly and with less effort than first-time fasters, and their cells go about some of the repairs and recycling more efficiently during and after the fast. (This may explain why although my fasting initially did nothing for my hypersomnia and other disorders, repeated fasting tamed them.) Scientists have multiple names to capture aspects of this phenomenon—adaptive stress response, hormesis, preconditioning, cellular stress resistance—but I like to think of it as the exercise principle. If you've never exercised before, your lungs and muscles will protest at your first jog around the block, but jog each day for a week, and your body will eventually do the work without complaint. In time you'll be able to jog a few blocks, then a mile, then three miles, all with less discomfort than that first burdensome block. In the long term your body will also perform more efficiently when not jogging. Fasting works much the same way. One study found that although animals make fewer antioxidants as they age, the rate of loss was slower in those who fasted regularly, even in the periods when they were eating. In other studies, when animals were subjected to the traumas of surgery, extreme heat, acute inflammation, or radiation, the ones who had previously fasted were better at making repairs than the ones who hadn't.

Research into fasting is still a niche field, the work of just a fistful of scientists, but they have uncovered a lot in a short time. As good science so often does, their discoveries have raised as many questions as they've answered. No question is more pressing than how we might use our new knowledge to protect ourselves from disease, and the most exciting answer to emerge so far has come against one of the most ungovernable diseases of all—cancer.

CHAPTER 12

"A CRAZY IDEA WITH NO RELEVANCE"

In the early 1990s, a graduate student at the University of California at Los Angeles named Valter Longo waded into the backwater that was the study of aging and, after splashing around ineffectually for a spell, decided he and his colleagues were going about their work all wrong. At the time, the field of lifespan extension was still one of the more disparaged domains of the sciences. If there was a consensus about aging among researchers, it was that our genes largely determined our years, and we couldn't do much about our genes. We might shorten our allotted span through bad behavior like smoking, or extend it a few years with exercise and a good diet, but nothing we did would push back the inevitable date with the undertaker by a decade or two.

Only a few scientists disagreed with this view strongly enough to stake a career on it. Carrying forward the work on caloric restriction by Clive McCay and colleagues, they had shown that eating less, provided nutrition was adequate, bestowed better health and substantially longer life on virtually every kind of lab animal: worms, flies, snails, fish, crabs, dogs, monkeys. One of the more prominent researchers in the field was an iconoclast named Roy Walford, in whose UCLA lab Valter Longo worked. Walford had marked his graduation from medical school in 1948 by casing the roulette wheels of Las Vegas and Reno, and upon discovering each wheel favored certain numbers over others, took the houses for enough cash to buy a yacht and sail the Caribbean for a year. (After *Life* and *Time* sketched his exploits, casinos took to shuffling the wheels around their parlors.) Walford once spent a sabbatical walking and hitchhiking across Africa, and another walking across India in a loincloth, stopping now and then to take the rectal temperature of yogis. Holy men, it turns out, *are* more chill than the rest of us.

When Longo first went to the Walford lab in 1992, it had no Walford. He was holed up for two years in the Arizona desert as the chief medical officer of Biosphere 2, three acres of interconnected glass structures meant to simulate a space colony. (Biosphere 1 was Earth.) When the terranauts, as the eight researchers inside Biosphere 2 styled themselves, had trouble growing enough food, Walford took the opportunity to conduct the first long-term experiment of caloric restriction in humans. The results were fantastic: the researchers' blood pressure, cholesterol, triglycerides, insulin, and blood sugar all reverted to levels not seen since adolescence. But the price was a mammoth hunger and plummeting morale, and when the terranauts at last emerged from their glass cage, they were a hangry and dispirited bunch. Few of them chose to restrict their diets back in Biosphere 1, no matter the benefits of caloric restriction.

Longo respected Walford's work, but he thought his mentor and other scientists of his generation had erred in studying longevity at the level of the whole organism to the neglect of figuring out which mechanisms inside the organism made it live shorter or longer. He decided to search for the mechanisms in hope of discovering that manipulating a molecule here or a process there could extend the lifespan or healthspan of animals, including humans. Scientists often start their mechanistic hunts in mice, but so little was known about aging that even a mouse, with its thousands of processes that might influence longevity, seemed hopelessly complicated to Longo. Like-minded young colleagues were turning to simpler organisms like worms and flies, but to Longo's mind even these were too intricate, and he decided to go all the way back to one of creation's less embellished organisms: *Saccharomyces cerevisiae*—budding yeast to scientists, baker's yeast to cooks, brewer's yeast to tipplers. The beer-loving equivalent of "oenophile" is "cerevisaphile."

The drawback to Longo's approach was that humans and yeast didn't seem to have a lot in common. Yeast aren't even animals; they're fungi.

They consist of just one cell to our tens of trillions, they live a couple of weeks to our fourscore years, and science has yet to record the yeast that died of Alzheimer's, cancer, or a broken heart. To many scientists, it seemed almost too obvious to point out that the genes controlling aging had to be specific to each species, which was why a toddler could live to eighty-four but a turtle only to forty-four and a terrier to fourteen. A lot has happened in the billion years since we and yeast last shared an ancestor.

On the other hand, that we did share an ancestor means to this day we still have thousands of the same genes. Longo suspected some of those genes must be among the most fundamental of all, maybe the very genes that enabled life and in some way guided the growth and senescence of our most distant predecessors. Perhaps the work of those genes hadn't changed all that much over the last thousand thousand thousand years, either in us or in our yeast cousins. Or if it had, maybe it had in similar ways in both of us. We had both, after all, had to survive in the same tumultuous environment, and we had both succeeded marvelously where millions of other species failed. The more Longo thought about it, the likelier it seemed humans and yeast might still age in ways governed by similar mechanisms, and he ignored the naysayers who told him he was wasting his time.

Longo's individualism was perhaps nourished by the unconventional path he took to science. As a teenager, he left his native Genoa to play rock and roll in Chicago and wound up enrolling in the renowned jazz studies program at the University of North Texas. In his sophomore year, he was told that to fulfill his major he would have to direct a marching band. The marching band is a cultural institution not held in the same regard in the Italian littoral of Longo's upbringing as it is in the American Whataburger Belt of his college days. The morning after he learned of the requirement, he marched into the registrar's office and changed his major to biochemistry. He continued, however, to play guitar in a touring band well into his PhD years and even signed a development contract with Interscope Records, the artistic home of Eminem, Snoop Dogg, and Nine Inch Nails. Today, having crossed the frontier of fifty, his mop of dark hair and futon eyes would still do the lead guitarist of a boy band good service.

Longo eventually parted company with Walford and his organismal research and moved down the hall to a lab whose scientists were more amenable to his search for basic mechanisms. Discoveries came quick. In an early experiment, he fed yeast once, then fed them no more, and they lived up to twice as long as normally fed yeast. This was as exciting as it was unexpected. It was one thing to nearly double the lifespan of a mouse by restricting his diet or fasting him every other day. It was another altogether to feed a creature in its youth, take away its food forever, and cause it to live twice as long. How in the world, Longo wondered, had this extreme form of fasting delayed the aging of his yeast?

Before he tried to answer that question, he ran the same experiment in bacteria, which turned into Methuselahs just as his starved yeast did. This was even more arresting because bacteria are prokaryotes, a form of life even simpler than yeast. Yeast, like you, me, and every other animal and plant, are eukaryotes. (The cells of prokaryotes lack the pride-inducing nuclei and complex organelles we eukaryotes have.) If fasting could radically extend longevity in not just two species but two entirely different kingdoms of life, Longo was looking at a phenomenon that might indeed go back to life's origins.

Returning to his fasted yeast, he studied which genes might be responsible for their longevity. Genes are short strands of DNA that we can think of as little packets of instructions telling cells, or parts of cells, to do specific tasks. Each gene is itself turned on or off by molecules and processes collectively known as a gene-regulatory pathway. When a yeast ingests glucose, for example, the glucose is sensed by certain pathways, which turn on specific genes, whose instructions direct the yeast to burn the glucose for fuel. (The byproduct of that combustion is appreciated by boozers the world over: alcohol.)

When Longo began his work, scientists already knew that yeast genes in families called RAS and PKA were activated when glucose arrived and were deactivated when the glucose was burned up. Longo found clues suggesting that when the RAS and PKA families were deactivated, other processes downstream were switched on or off, which seemed to cause his yeast to live longer. To test whether this was so, he acquired mutant yeast with various RAS and PKA genes knocked out and fed them abundantly. If he was right that the deactivation of one or more of those genes made his fasters live twice as long, then some of his mutant yeast, lacking one of the genes in those families, should also live twice as long no matter how much he fed them.

And that is exactly what happened. His mutant yeast lacking a gene known as *ras2** lived doubly long regardless of how much glucose they ingested. Longo had just identified the first gene regulating how yeast age. In fact, he had just identified one of the first genes regulating how any organism aged.

Over the next few years Longo mapped out the entire RAS-PKA pathway. He learned that when yeast burned up all their glucose, *ras2* was switched off, which caused a chain reaction that switched on two proteins known as Msn2 and Msn4. "Msn" is short for "Messenger," but Msn2 and 4 proved far more than mere messengers. They had at their command hundreds of genes responsible for protecting yeast from damage and for repairing what damage they sustained. When Longo subjected his yeast to freezing temperatures, Msn2 and 4 moved into the yeast's nuclei and told enzymes there to make a sugar called trehalose, which in turn stimulated antifreeze proteins to keep the yeast from icing over. When he subjected yeast to extreme heat, Msn2 and 4 put an end to normal protein production and ordered the creation of special heat-shock proteins, which helped other proteins to fold correctly and stay that way rather than unfolding and malfunctioning, as they tend to do at high temperature. When he bathed his yeast in hydrogen peroxide, which wrought oxidative havoc on DNA and other components, Msn2 and 4 ordered the creation of antioxidants to neutralize the damage. The two messenger proteins went about this sort of work constantly, but when Longo fasted his yeast, they did it far more vigorously and the damage was repaired much more quickly. It was this ability to protect and repair, regulated by the RAS-PKA pathway, itself regulated

---

* Scientists distinguish genes from families of genes and their regulatory pathways, all of which typically share the same name, by italicizing the names of genes but not of their families or pathways.

by the presence or absence of glucose, that allowed fasted yeast to live twice as long as their fed kin. Longo knew he had found something big.

But not many of his colleagues agreed. They thought he had found a one-off, an anti-aging pathway that might work in lowlife like yeast but that had no bearing on higher organisms. Leading journals declined to publish his findings, and he had to content himself with turning his work into his doctoral thesis and a couple of articles in minor journals that for several years were mostly ignored. But he kept at it and expanded his search. He figured even an organism as simple as yeast, with its six thousand genes (humans have about twenty thousand), must have more longevity pathways, so he subjected billions of yeast to various stressors and examined the genes of the ones that lived the longest.

"The idea was if they're protected against everything we throw at them, they're going to be also protected against aging," he said. And if they were protected against aging, it was likely because of a genetic mutation. "Sure enough, we kept coming up against something called *Sch9*. Nobody knew what it was at the time, but it was just the most powerful gene. The *ras2* mutation doubled the lifespan [of yeast], but the *Sch9* mutation tripled the lifespan."

When he went looking for what activated *Sch9*, he found a family of genes in a pathway called TOR. Later renamed mTOR, the pathway was turned on and off by amino acids, the building blocks of proteins. The more amino acids a yeast consumed, the more it busied itself processing them and the less time it had for repairs. But when there were no amino acids, the mTOR pathway triggered the release of the instructions encoded in *Sch9*, which caused several restorative chores to be carried out with an almost jaunty enthusiasm. Longo had now found two pathways that made yeast grow old, and in both cases the ultimate culprit was a nutrient: sugar in one, protein in the other.

All of this work presented an obvious next question for Longo: if downregulating the RAS-PKA sugar pathway made a yeast's life twice as nice, and downregulating the mTOR protein pathway made it thrice as nice, what would happen when both pathways were downregulated at once? He created yeast whose RAS-PKA and mTOR pathways were both deactivated, and these double mutants lived five times longer no matter how much he fed them. When he fasted them, they lived ten times longer. They were also "a thousandfold" more resistant to certain toxins. "They're super yeast," he said simply.

Longo and other researchers eventually found more than a hundred genes involved in the aging of yeast, but none were more powerful than those in the RAS-PKA and mTOR pathways. Other colleagues found similar pathways in flies and worms, which prompted Longo to publish a paper arguing that many, if not all, organisms probably aged in similar ways. He predicted that a lot of the genes in lower organisms that could be turned on or off to make them live longer probably also existed in mammals, including humans, and that our genes could likely be turned on or off to help us live longer too.

"This," he later wrote, "was heresy, and the great majority of scientists dismissed it as a crazy idea with no relevance to human aging. . . . It would take another six years for our data on genes activated by sugars to get published, along with the discovery of the pro-aging genes activated by amino acids and proteins."

Over the next decade or so, other labs would confirm his crazy idea. One organism after another, from yeast all the way up to mammals, was shown to have similar pro-aging pathways for protein and sugar. Rather than invent new mechanisms for aging in each species, evolution had conserved the pathways time and again. The pieces were starting to come together.

One of the more interesting pieces was a link between size and longevity: the longest-lived specimens of each species were always small. The super yeast were about one-third the diameter of ordinary yeast, the longest-lived mice were about a quarter as large as their peers, and the longest-lived vinegar flies even had a special name, *chicos*, because they were half the size of normal adult *Drosophila*.

"It's not by mistake that they're all dwarves," Longo said. "It tells us there's a very strong relationship between amino acids, sugars, growth, and aging and anti-aging. If you have a lot of amino acids . . . you grow more quickly and you're able to reproduce more"—a definite survival advantage. But you also age more quickly and die sooner, just as T. Brailsford Robertson hypothesized in the 1920s. Moreover, across all species, the mighty dwarves were not just longer lived but also haler than their well-fed relatives. This was not an easy concept to grasp, as we saw when the odd couple of Carlson and Hoelzel downplayed their longer-lived but smaller mice in favor of shorter-lived but bigger mice. The concept made sense only once you knew the cells of the fasted dwarves, instead of focusing on growth, were constantly protecting and repairing themselves, while the cells of their well-fed and quicker-growing relatives had little time for such measures because they were too busy processing nutrients.

The link between growth and pro-aging pathways became even clearer thanks to Cynthia Kenyon at the University of California at San Francisco. Kenyon was another young researcher who, like Longo, had gone hunting for the cause of aging in a basic organism. Hers was *Caenorhabditis elegans*, a millimeter-long nematode that had the inestimable scientific benefit of being transparent. Kenyon discovered that a hormone called insulin-like growth factor 1 was at the heart of another pro-aging pathway, and its effects were just as dramatic as the protein and sugar pathways Longo had found. When Kenyon knocked out IGF-1 in *C. elegans*, it lived to an unnaturally ripe old age. (IGF-1 is called "insulin-like" because its molecular structure is similar to insulin's.) Kenyon's was an especially exciting discovery because only multicellular organisms have IGF-1, which represents one of the new ways of growing that we and other animals devised on our way to becoming something more exhilarating than yeast. Humans use it to grow properly in childhood, and researchers would ultimately learn that the IGF-1 pathway is controlled by growth hormone (GH), which also controlled the pathway of IGF-1's namesake, insulin, which turned out to be another promoter of aging. Clearly, a complex dance was going on between growth, nutrition, and longevity in multicellular organisms.

The question was, what did it all mean for humans?

*　*　*

In 1957, a young Israeli doctor named Zvi Laron returned home from training at Harvard Medical School and Massachusetts General Hospital and set up Israel's first clinic in pediatric endocrinology, the field concerned with hormones in children. Among his earliest patients was a trio of dwarf siblings, a young sister and two brothers who not only were extremely short for their age but also shared a distinctive physical appearance atypical of dwarves: their foreheads protruded, their nasal bridges were nearly collapsed, their jaws were underdeveloped, their hair was thin, and they were obese. Their grandparents were first cousins, which suggested to Laron that a mutant gene the children inherited might be behind their peculiar dwarfism. He hypothesized that the mutation was keeping them from making growth hormone, but several years later when a test for GH became available, he found he was exactly wrong. The siblings didn't have too little GH—they had enormous quantities of it. Laron revised his hypothesis: either his patients were making GH that was in some way defective, or they were making GH that was just fine but their bodies couldn't figure out how to use it.

Hormones, as I suggested earlier, can be thought of as tiny keys that organs send into the bloodstream in search of the right locks, which are hormone receptors, some of which are attached to the outside of cells. When the right key connects with the right lock, the cell gets a command to do something. The command from insulin, for example, is to open the gate and let glucose in. Trouble arises when a hormone can't deliver its message, either because it can't get to a receptor or because although it has got there, a malfunction prevents the receptor from receiving the hormone's message. In either case, a task won't get done, and for growth hormone, that task is growth.

Around the time Laron was making the acquaintance of his unique dwarf siblings, a scientist at Washington University in St. Louis named William Daughaday discovered a new hormone: the aforementioned insulin-like growth factor 1. Daughaday observed that when GH attached to GH receptor, the specific message it passed to the cell was to make IGF-1. IGF-1, in turn, commanded cells to divide—that is, to grow. In a sense, it was IGF-1 that put the growth in growth hormone.

With Daughaday's help, Laron had the trio of siblings tested for IGF-1 and discovered they were making hardly any of it. The science wasn't advanced enough to say why, but a couple of decades later researchers would learn that people with Laron syndrome, as the condition came to be known, could make GH perfectly well but couldn't use it, just as Laron had speculated. This was because their genetic abnormality left them with almost no GH receptors, so their GH wandered endlessly around their bodies looking for receptors that didn't exist, and the message to make IGF-1 never got delivered.

Larons, as the little people are called, can still grow because other hormones besides GH and IGF-1 contribute to growth, but they top out at about three and a half feet. Over the course of a long career, Zvi Laron would find another thirty or so people in Israel with the disorder and about as many others scattered around Europe and Asia. It was, in short, a very rare disease. But it was about to become very big in the field of aging.

* * *

In 1988, a generation after Laron identified the first Larons, an endocrinologist at the University of Florida named Arlan Rosenbloom decided to go to Ecuador and inject six kids with growth hormone. The children all suffered from GH deficiency, and Rosenbloom had been treating them twice a year at his Gainesville clinic. But their flights to Florida were expensive, and the injections weren't cheap either, so Rosenbloom opted to go to his patients. It was one of the longer house calls in history.

When the head of the children's hospital in the Ecuadorian capital of Quito got word of Rosenbloom's arrival, he sent him a steady rivulet of patients with hormonal disorders, including two sisters aged eight and six but no taller than one-year-olds. They had protruding foreheads, the bridges of their noses were sunken, and tests showed they had plenty of GH. Just four years earlier, Laron had published a paper explaining that patients with Laron syndrome, despite their shortness, had plenty of GH, so Rosenbloom knew he was looking at two more Larons. But while it was satisfying to tell the family what ailed their children, and while it was interesting to note two more of these rare cases, there was no treatment, and that was that. Or so Rosenbloom thought.

What he didn't know was that his diagnosis had piqued the interest of a young doctor named Jaime Guevara-Aguirre, who had just founded the Institute of Endocrinology, Metabolism, and Reproduction in Quito to study and treat conditions long neglected in his country. The seed money for the institute had come with an unusual condition. Guevara-Aguirre's father was a wealthy road builder who had ordered his two eldest sons off to college to study engineering and his two youngest to study medicine.

"We weren't asked," Guevara-Aguirre later said. "We were told to come back when we had the degree."

Jaime came back with his medical diploma and told his father he meant to start a world-class research institute in endocrinology. To his surprise, the road builder said he would buy him a building and outfit it with equipment, but he had a proviso.

"He asked me for the name of the world's best medical journal. When I told him the *New England Journal of Medicine*, he said I had ten years to publish a paper there or close the place. I was so nervous I couldn't sleep for fifteen days."

When Guevara-Aguirre learned Rosenbloom had identified two cases of this incredibly rare disease, he realized with an excited flash that he had seen several other Larons as a boy. In fact, there were enough of these little people in the southern Ecuadorian province where he grew up that they had been given a nickname: *pigmeitos*, "little pygmies," which they understandably disliked. Guevara-Aguirre set out to track down as many Larons as he could, and by the time Rosenbloom came back to Ecuador six months later, he had turned up seven, which amounted to ten percent of the world's known Laron population. He also turned up stories of many more who were said to be scattered across Ecuador's mountainous southern hinterland. He tracked down several and learned of still others, and it gradually became clear he was making it his life's work to traverse some of the least accessible parts of the country on some of its most unforgiving roads to find, study, and serve as doctor to what would eventually prove to be more than one hundred Larons.

As it happens, Guevara-Aguirre is just the sort of person—gentle of voice, kindly of smile, a little soft around the edges—whom people enjoy having knock on their door, offer a warm handshake, introduce himself as one of the world's experts in their exceedingly rare condition, and volunteer his services, should they be of interest, as their new personal doctor. It perhaps didn't hurt that Guevara-Aguirre had his own genetic distinction, his hair having decided to gray in stripes—black on top, white on the flanks, black mutton chops, white mandibular whiskers, black soul patch.

Guevara-Aguirre and others learned the Larons of Ecuador were all part of one big extended family, and the same would prove true of all Larons everywhere, or at least all who have been tested. Every Laron was begotten by a primogenitor in medieval Spain who carried a single genetic mutation, a nick on chromosome 5p of the gene *GHR*, the growth hormone receptor gene. Almost certainly the original Laron was a Sephardic Jew, which accounts for the relatively large number of Israeli and Jewish Larons today. Some of the early carriers of the mutation probably converted to Christianity under the gentle coaxing of the Spanish Inquisition, and in the sixteenth century emigrated to South America, perhaps because their former Judaism still weighed heavily on their prospects in Europe. Most of the people with the mutant gene weren't then and aren't now dwarves. To develop, Laron syndrome needs two copies of mutated *GHR*, one from each parent, and even when both parents are carriers, only one of their four or fourteen children might turn out to be a Laron. To intermarry within your extended family increases the odds of mating with another mutant, and the Laron families of Ecuador, living in remote mountains with few opportunities to leave, tended to marry from within their own villages or ones nearby, which after half a millennium was as good as marrying within their extended family.

In 1990, Guevara-Aguirre and Rosenbloom wrote the most extensive paper to date characterizing the Laron phenotype, "The Little Women of Loja." (The first Larons they found were almost all female; many males have since been identified.) The paper revealed several novelties, for instance that Ecuadorian Larons, unlike Larons elsewhere, showed no tendency to mental retardation and in fact were usually academically successful. Fortuitously for the future of endocrinology in Ecuador, the paper was published in what a road builder's son might call the best medical journal in the world. Guevara-Aguirre had beaten his father's ten-year deadline for publishing in the *New England Journal of Medicine* by a cool seven years.

Over the next decade, as Guevara-Aguirre tracked down more and more Larons, two things became clear: they were almost always overweight, often obese, and yet they almost never got diseases associated with overweight and obesity. In fact, it took Guevara-Aguirre so long to find a Laron with diabetes or cancer that for a while he wondered if they could even get those diseases. Although a few cases of each eventually turned up among Larons in Ecuador and elsewhere, in his first twenty-odd years ministering to more than a quarter of the world's 350 known Larons, Guevara-Aguirre watched only one die of cancer and none of diabetes. The relatives of his Larons—people who live in the same households as the little people, eat the same foods, work the same jobs, share the same pastimes, pump the same blood through their veins—die of cancer and diabetes at ordinary Ecuadorian rates: 17 percent and 5 percent respectively. The Larons' genetic defect, it seemed to Guevara-Aguirre, was not such a defect after all, or at least not only a defect. His patients were little X-Men, mutants whose genetic abnormality had endowed them with a superpower: they were all but impervious to some of the most wicked diseases nature could throw at a human body.

*   *   *

On a fortuitous day in 2006, a colleague of Valter Longo's said to him, "You know that pro-aging protein pathway you've been studying in yeast? Well, there's a guy in Ecuador who's been studying it in humans."

Longo, who had moved across town and joined the faculty of the University of Southern California, had never heard of Laron syndrome, and when he looked into it, it seemed too good to be true. He and other researchers had recently figured out that in multicellular organisms, GH and IGF-1 were something like master switches for the protein and sugar pro-aging pathways, the mTOR and RAS-PKA pathways he had spent so much of his career on. When researchers created mutant mice with their IGF-1 receptors knocked out, those pathways were downregulated, their bodies spent more time repairing cellular damage, and they lived about a quarter longer.

The evidence that life could be extended and health improved by shutting down IGF-1, GH, mTOR, and RAS-PKA was as good as it could get, but it was gettable only for non-humans. Neither Longo nor any other researcher would ever get a chance to knock out IGF-1 in people, and even could they have done so, they would have had to wait decades to see whether their mutant humans lived longer and were protected from various diseases. Longo assumed he would never know for certain whether the IGF-1 pathway had quite the same effect in people as it did in other mammals, but suddenly he was being presented with human equivalents of IGF-1–knockout mice, and Jaime Guevara-Aguirre had two decades of data on them. He felt as if he had won the lottery.

He had been feeling like a lottery winner a lot lately. A few years earlier, his paper on yeast longevity was finally published in *Science*, one of the world's most respected research journals. Evidently he and other researchers had amassed so much evidence about pro-aging pathways and the nutrients that controlled them, they could no longer be ignored. He called Guevara-Aguirre and at the first chance was on a plane to Quito.

"One thing that was clear right away from these subjects," Longo said after meeting several Larons, "was they did not calorie-restrict at all. The fasting and calorie restriction is not what they do."

They ate in bulk, their plates piled high with fatty meats, cheeses, and fried foods, and when they could get their hands on the processed and sugary foods Americans ate, they didn't stint on those either. Photos of an ordinary Laron meal could be mistaken for most people's Thanksgiving. Some years later, Longo brought several Larons to Los Angeles for study and each morning fed them a continental breakfast of bagels and coffee.

"They did this for a couple of days," he recalled, "and then they came to me and said, 'We thank you very much for this very nice breakfast, but can we have a *real* breakfast? Can we go to McDonald's?'"

There was no great scientific mystery about why the Larons, notwith-standing being obese at twice the rate of other Ecuadorians, were nearly immune to diabetes. The shutting down of their nutrient-signaling path-ways made them very sensitive to insulin, so sugar was efficiently ushered out of their blood and into their cells. Laron syndrome, in a sense, was anti-diabetes.

There was, however, a mystery about why the Larons' obesity didn't hurt them in other ways. Why didn't they get more cancer or gallblad-der disease, more high blood pressure or strokes? An increase in cellu-lar repairs surely explained some of it, but Longo and Guevara-Aguirre thought more was going on. They suspected, for a start, that the Larons' particular brand of obesity didn't impair their liver function. In most obe-sity, fat predominates in the midriff, where it latches on to and suffocates abdominal organs, but Longo and Guevara-Aguirre discovered Laron fat was distributed more evenly around the body and stayed near the sur-face rather than enveloping the organs below. When they scanned Laron livers, they proved indistinguishable from those of more traditionally healthy people. Longo found the same thing in mice. When he blocked their GH receptors and let them eat freely, they grew up stunted and obese but with fat spread evenly and subcutaneously, their livers healthy and unsmothered.

As for cancer, the Larons were protected in part by their lack of IGF-1. In non-Larons, IGF-1 may be a blessing for childhood growth, but after puberty the blessing is more mixed because IGF-1 shares the same core mission as cancer—to make cells grow and divide—which is why can-cer often hijacks the IGF-1 pathway to do its injurious work. Take away IGF-1, and cancer cells have to find other ways to divide. Cancer can find them, but they're not as convenient, and if the Larons are any indication, they're not nearly as fatal.

"Let me give you the perfect human," Guevara-Aguirre told Longo one day as they rattled down a battered road in his battered truck to meet some of his little friends. "It's a Laron patient who has been given IGF-1 in childhood until he reaches full height, and then it's taken away and he never sees it again."

Another version of the perfect human would be a normal child who is allowed to grow in the usual way until maturity, after which her IGF-1 is inhibited. That kind of human, Longo thought, was one he might be able to work toward.

As it happened, a researcher at Ohio University named John Kopchick was already working on her, although he didn't know it at first. Kopchick was a student of another rare disease, acromegaly, which might be thought of as anti-Laron syndrome. Acromegaly is caused when the pituitary gland turns hyperactive, usually in middle age, and pumps too much GH into the bloodstream. Too much GH leads to too much IGF-1, which leaves sufferers of the disease with painfully prominent brows and cheekbones, oversized lips, and giant hands. Researchers haven't found a way to convince a hyperactive pituitary gland to make less GH, but Kopchick realized he could help victims of acromegaly if he could block the excess GH in their blood from binding with GH receptors, exactly as happens in Laron syndrome. With the receptors blocked, IGF-1 would stay low, which should stop the abnormal growth. Kopchick developed a drug, pegvisomant, that did just that, and it has proven a godsend for victims of acromegaly.

Pegvisomant had an unanticipated and altogether pleasing side effect. When Kopchick gave it to the control mice in his trials—healthy mice, unafflicted by acromegaly—they got even healthier, with less diabetes and fewer cancers of the breast and prostate. Intrigued, Kopchick knocked out GH receptors in mice and found, as Longo had, that they became overweight dwarves with minimal IGF-1 and far less cancer. This was gratifying but by now not particularly newsworthy. One day, however, one of Kopchick's lab technicians asked him what should be done with all the elderly mice. Kopchick runs a big shop and wasn't aware he had elderly mice that needed attending. The lab tech explained that some of the mice with the knocked-out GH receptors were turning four years old. They were supposed to have died at two and a half. They went on to become, at four years and change, the longest-lived mice in any laboratory in the world. One mouse nearly made it five years—in effect, a 160-year-old mouse.

Longo and Guevara-Aguirre got in touch with Kopchick to compare notes, and soon Longo and Kopchick were working to develop a drug similar to pegvisomant but for healthy adults: a medication that would block GH receptor after puberty in the hope of conferring a Laron-like protection against cancer, diabetes, and other ills. Currently pegvisomant exists only as a short-lived injection, sold under the trade name Somavert for $200 a day. To be widely accepted, Longo and Kopchick's drug would need to be long-lived, swallowable, and ideally more attractively priced, although for a shot at several extra years and immunity to some of the most ferocious diseases, there would be takers at any price. Whether they'll develop such an elixir is anyone's guess.

*   *   *

The Larons may be nearly immune to certain disorders, but they live no longer than the rest of us because discrimination has made them dispro-portionately suicidal and alcoholic and because they die more often in accidents—drivers are not accustomed to looking for little people cross-ing the road. Guevara-Aguirre wants to change all that, at least for young Larons. He wants to create his perfect human by giving synthetic IGF-1 to Laron children until they reach physical maturity, after which they would live free of IGF-1. He believes we have a moral duty to help a group of people who have subjected themselves to decades of poking, scanning, and invasive questioning in the name of a science that might one day help all of us live longer and healthier.

The hurdles are the price of synthetic IGF-1, some $20,000 a year, and the rapacity of pharmaceutical companies, whose moguls are loath to donate their product, even though only a few score Laron kids would need it annually. Guevara-Aguirre isn't surprised by the wintry hearts of Big Pharma, but their lack of enlightened self-interest still takes him aback. Why, he asks, wouldn't a pharmaceutical company want to create a non-Laron Laron? Imagine what a drug maker might learn from someone who grows normally for eighteen years, then enters protected Laron mode for the rest of her eighty, ninety, or—who knows?—hundred and thirty years.

The argument isn't lost on Longo, who understands better than any-one what the Larons have given us: proof that the age-inducing effects of IGF-1, which scientists had shown in other animals, translate fluently to humans. Laron biology offers a strong suggestion that if we can keep our IGF-1 low, we'll increase our odds of living to a healthy seniority. Longo had turned to lower organisms to find mechanisms that might help us live better. Now, thanks to the Larons, he was ready to move back to humans, and he would start by taking on one of the most ruthless diseases of all, cancer. Laron biochemistry could fight it, and Longo had an idea or two about how to put a little Laron in all of us. One of those ideas was fasting.

*   *   *

In 1988, a cadre of young rats who were guests of Chicago's Mount Sinai Hospital fasted every other day for a week, perhaps not entirely willingly, after which they were injected, most certainly unwillingly, "intraperitoneally with 15 million Mat 13762 ascites tumor cells." That is to say their abdomens were shot full of breast cancer. Another group of rats who ate normally for a week were injected likewise, and both groups ate normally after that. Nine days after the injections, four-fifths of the normally fed rats were dead, but only one-third of the fasters were. The researchers concluded that fasting every other day could dramatically slow the growth of breast cancer, at least in adolescent rats, but they didn't know why.

Thanks to the work of Longo and others, we now know fasting downregulated the rats' IGF-1 and other pro-growth pathways, which made it harder for the tumor cells to grow, divide, and kill their hosts. We also know the rats' cancer preferred to grow on glucose and struggled when it couldn't get it. During a fast, healthy cells switch from glucose to other fuel, mostly ketone bodies, but the mutations that turn a healthy cell cancerous also turn it slightly stupid and make it slow to adapt to change. Fasting is one hell of a change for a cell whose mantra is "Burn glucose, divide. Burn glucose, divide. Burn glucose, divide." Cancer does not thrive on ketone bodies.

Building on this and other experiments, Longo ran some tests of his own to see what sort of fasting might give cancer the most grief. Fasting every other day did pretty well, but fasting in short bursts of consecutive days did even better. In a few mice, such fasts even eradicated their cancer. Most of the time, however, the fasts just kept the disease at bay by shoring up the body's natural defenses until eventually the cancer outflanked them and continued its rampage. Still, the delay was a big gain. The extra months of life Longo's mice got from fasting might be the equivalent of extra years for a human.

But where fasting really came into its glory was when Longo combined it with other treatments like chemotherapy and radiation. He had hypothesized that since fasting protected cells from all sorts of brutality—cold shocks, heat shocks, oxidation, submersion in acids or bases—it would also guard healthy cells from the onslaught of chemo and radiation, which in turn should reduce side effects in patients. In 2008, he gave the question a quick run-out in yeast. Yeast don't get cancer, but cancer-like yeast cells can be created, and he brewed up several million of these, dumped them into flasks with healthy yeast, starved the lot of them for a few days, and then bathed them in cyclophosphamide, a common chemotherapy drug. Within two days, the cancer-like cells were all dead while the healthy ones were alive and perkily dividing. He couldn't have asked for better.

Moving on to fasted mice, he tested first how they fared with chemotherapy alone, in the absence of cancer. He fed one group of mice normally, fasted another for forty-eight hours, and then gave both a monstrous dose of chemotherapy—proportionally three times the maximum for humans. Ten days later, 43 percent of the fed group were dead, and those who survived were a sorry lot: lethargic, weak of stomach, patchy of hair, clearly not long for this world. The fasted group, on the other hand, looked an entirely different race: only 6 percent of them had died, and just a few of the survivors were visibly toxicated. When Longo repeated the experiment with an even stronger blast of chemotherapy and a slightly longer fast of two and a half days, the control group made for grim watching, all of them gasping their last within five days. Every one of the fasters, meanwhile, not only survived but showed no hint of toxicity and indeed positively frolicked around their cages. Clearly fasting could protect healthy cells from chemotoxicity, at least in mice.

So far, so good, but none of those mice had cancer. Longo needed to make sure fasting wouldn't protect the cancer cells from chemo as it had the healthy cells, so he repeated the last experiment, only this time injecting his mice with neuroblastoma before the chemotherapy. Neuroblastoma is one of the most homicidal of childhood cancers. Only one in five humans survives the advanced stage Longo induced in his mice. If fasting protected cancer cells from chemo, his fasters should have died sooner than his controls, but that didn't happen—the reverse did. Within a week, half the fed mice died from either the cancer or the chemo, but nearly all of the fasters were still alive.

When Longo explored what was going on at the molecular level, he saw that the mice's healthy cells, when fasted, entered an almost dormant state in which they turned away from the toxic chemicals. The cancer cells, however, kept gobbling up inputs, including the toxins. He ran the same experiment on human cells in test tubes and got similar results. The promise of his discoveries was radiant. He had found an entirely new method of fighting cancer.

"When I began my cancer studies," Longo said, "every researcher was looking for a magic bullet that would seek out and destroy only cancer cells. But I got the idea from fasting that we don't need a magic bullet. We can achieve the same thing through a magic shield that protects healthy cells. When I realized that's what fasting was, I thought, 'This is perfect. Now we have a way to distinguish all normal cells from all cancer cells.'"

In Longo's metaphor, fasting is a command to cellular soldiers to kneel behind their shields, but it's a command only healthy cells can understand because the mutations of cancer cells turn them deaf to it. The sole order cancer understands is "Grow at all costs," so its cells continue their march, ever intent on gathering the resources to swell their ranks. Chemotherapy (or immunotherapy or radiation) mows them down while the fasted healthy cells, kneeling behind their shields, are only dinged and nicked.

With not a little excitement, Longo took his research to oncologists and asked if they would help with a clinical trial. Few shared his eagerness. "Would I be enthusiastic about enrolling my patients in a trial where they're asked not to eat for two and a half days?" said Leonard Saltz, a prominent oncologist at Memorial Sloan Kettering Cancer Center in New York. "No."

The oncologists told Longo their patients already lost enough weight during chemotherapy and they didn't want them losing more by fasting. Longo explained that fasted mice who underwent chemotherapy regained their fasted-off weight very quickly, probably in part because they were less nauseated and not put off by food, but the doctors were unmoved. Their patients were people, not mice, and anyway fasting was just too unknown. Untutored in fasting's long history, they weren't interested in the remedial education Longo was offering.

While Longo was struggling to convince doctors, cancer patients who had learned of his work in mice called and emailed to ask whether they should fast during their chemo. Longo had to tell them there was no data in humans and he couldn't recommend fasting until there was. Some of them replied that was all well and good, but they might be looking up at a coffin lid by the time he got his data. They were willing to take the chance. This discomfited Longo, but he knew a research opportunity when he saw one and said if they were going to do it anyway, would they fill out some questionnaires and submit to some tests? Many said yes. Their oncologists were another matter. Some wouldn't even take calls from Longo's lab.

In the end, Longo got data from ten self-experimenters who fasted for two or more days before chemotherapy. Each had already undergone the misery of chemo unfasted, and they all said that after fasting they didn't have the same weakness, fatigue, or gastrointestinal torment they had previously suffered. Most still had some side effects, but not nearly as bad, although since there was no control group, it's possible they merely enjoyed a placebo effect. Whether fasting helped the chemotherapy kill more of their cancer was anyone's guess, but tumors shrank in all six of the patients for whom measurements could be obtained. At a minimum, fasting didn't seem to have interfered with their chemotherapy.

Eventually Longo cajoled just enough oncologists to let their patients participate in a pilot trial on the safety of fasting during chemotherapy. A couple dozen patients made a partial fast on 200 calories a day for either twenty-four, forty-eight, or seventy-two hours before their chemo treatments. The results, which Longo reported in 2016, were all he had hoped for. Not only were his subjects unharmed by fasting; the longer they fasted, the less nausea, fatigue, and gastrointestinal upset they had. A look at their blood suggested why. In the longer fasters, the chemotherapy killed fewer white blood cells and platelets, which suggested the bone marrow where the cells and platelets were made hadn't been badly damaged. The chemo also did less harm to their DNA. It wasn't clear if fasting protected the DNA or if the DNA had been damaged but, thanks to fasting, was quickly repaired. A later study by other researchers hinted at speedy repair. In that experiment, two groups of mice who either fasted or ate before chemotherapy showed DNA damage in their small intestines ninety minutes after treatment, but after another ninety minutes, the DNA of the fasted mice was already mostly fixed. Not so in the fed mice. The upshot of these findings was immensely important. If fasting could indeed guard against or quickly repair the ravages of chemotherapy, oncologists should be able to give higher doses of chemo (or radiation or immunotherapy) to fasting patients to kill more of their cancer without killing more of them.

But though the results of Longo's trial were sparkling, he was downhearted. He had labored mightily not just to recruit doctors and patients but to get them to comply. Several patients had eaten more than their allotted 200 daily calories, others had dropped out, and a study that should have taken two years had taken five. Ultimately he decided fasting couldn't be widely adopted and that it would be a mistake to ask the public to do it. Fasting was just too counterintuitive, especially for people already ill. The future, he believed, lay in a protocol that could mimic fasting while avoiding the actual fast.

Two options presented themselves. One was the standard route for modern research: develop a drug, in this case one to mimic fasting, which patients would surely be more willing to accept and would no doubt be pecuniarily satisfying to its creators. There was even a logical drug to start with. Researchers had recently learned that when they gave skin cancer to mice and inhibited their IGF-1 through a certain mutation, the mice fared exceptionally well. Two months into one experiment, cancer had killed all of the control mice, but 60 percent of the mutant mice were still alive. In another experiment, when the mutant mice were given the chemotherapeutic drug doxorubicin, they all remained free of cardiotoxicity—heart damage—while only 40 percent of the control mice did. The mutation in question caused the upregulation of a binding protein of IGF-1 known as IGFBP-1, which fasting also upregulates.

"If you canceled everything else that fasting does," Longo said, "what it does to just IGFBP-1 would be a very powerful drug." But there was a hitch. "To develop this action as a drug, it would take five hundred million dollars and fifteen years to just get to the point where you can test it and see if it works against cancer. Seven pharmaceutical companies are doing exactly that."

Ultimately, however, Longo didn't think it was such a good idea. Not only would it be time-consuming and pricey, but such a drug would undoubtedly have its own side effects and, most damningly, would target just one of the pathways by which cancer spread, whereas fasting shut down multiple cancer pathways at once. So Longo went to the National Cancer Institute and pitched a different option to mimic fasting: a targeted, calorie-restricted diet. The institute wrote him a fat check, and he and his team went to work.

They decided that of all the biochemical changes that fasting triggered in mammals, four were essential for fighting cancer: steep declines in both glucose and IGF-1 and sharp increases in both ketones and IGFBP-1. If their diet were to truly mimic fasting, it would need to do at least those four things. Longo's group spent five years testing diets ingredient by ingredient and came up with one that was very low in proteins, sugars, and total calories, very high in healthy fats and nutrients, somewhat satisfying to the murine appetite, and able to keep mice in a protected, fasting-like state. Mice who ate the fasting-mimicking diet (FMD) for four consecutive days every two weeks became magnificently healthy. Their IGF-1 dropped an impressive 75 percent on the days they ate the diet and stayed low even when they returned to normal eating. Although overall they ate the same number of calories each month as the control mice (they ate more on non-FMD days to make up for the diet days), they were slimmer and had less abdominal fat than the controls. Apparently the FMD put them into a fat-burning mode that lingered even after they resumed normal eating. As a result of these and other improvements, they developed only half as many tumors as the controls, and they got them later—on average at twenty-six months, compared to the usual onset of twenty months. For humans, that's like pushing back the first cancer diagnosis from sixty to seventy years. In all, the FMD mice lived 11 percent longer, although their maximum possible lifespan wasn't extended. To put that in human terms, the FMD didn't enable them to live 135 years—death still came to even the most genetically gifted before 120—but now it came for the average mouse at 90 instead of 80.

One of Longo's most startling findings came in diabetic mice— mice whose beta cells (the insulin-making cells of the pancreas) he had destroyed. When these mice ate the FMD regularly, their bodies regenerated their ruined beta cells through the same sort of process a fetus uses to grow new cells. Once more they could make normal amounts of insulin. Their diabetes was entirely reversed, their pancreases essentially reborn.

Next Longo put mice with breast or skin cancer on four days of either the FMD or a normal diet before giving them chemotherapy. The tumor-infiltrating lymphocytes of the FMD mice became nimbler at invading and hacking away inside tumors, and their regulatory T cells, which cancer dupes into protecting its tumors, were weakened. In another trial, this one of melanoma, the tumors of normally fed mice grew to an average of 2000 cubic millimeters, the size of a robust pea, but in mice who underwent two cycles of FMD and no other treatment, the tumors grew only to 1300 cubic millimeters—the same size as tumors in normally fed mice who received two cycles of immunotherapy. That's a point worth underscoring: the FMD performed as well as conventional cancer treatment. But the best results of all were in mice who did two cycles of FMD *and* received chemotherapy. Their tumors were even smaller, growing to just 700 cubic millimeters. Tests with other cancers and chemo drugs yielded pretty much the same results.

Longo's team created two versions of the diet for humans—one for cancer patients and one for everyone else—each consisting of five days of vegan soups and snacks. In the non-cancer version, dieters ate about

1,000 calories the first day (roughly half what the average active woman is advised to eat) and 750 calories each of the following four days. It wasn't enough food to sate a person, but it kept Longo's subjects from storming their pantries. The cancer FMD had only 300 calories a day. In Longo's first randomized, controlled trial of the non-cancer FMD, seventy-one volunteers used it once a month for three months and saw gains similar to those in mice: improvements in body-mass index, blood pressure, fasting glucose, IGF-1, total cholesterol, and the inflammatory marker C-reactive protein. The unhealthiest volunteers improved the most. People with high triglycerides enjoyed an average drop of 26 points, people with high LDL cholesterol got a 15-point decline, and the fattest volunteers lost nearly nine pounds even though they, like the FMD mice, made up the lost calories of their FMD days by eating more on other days.

Longo founded a company named L-Nutra to manufacture and sell his FMDs, which, at more than $200 per five-day kit, don't come cheap. On the other hand, if they save someone from diabetes, fatty liver disease, or chemotherapy-induced vomiting, they're a steal at twice the price. (Longo says he donates all profits from his shares in L-Nutra to research.) To date, hundreds of thousands of people in the United States have used his FMDs under the supervision of more than ten thousand caregivers. Studies of their effects are in progress.

*   *   *

A fasting-mimicking diet, whether for cancer or general health, is an unqualified boon to those who will not or cannot fast. It's also a stupendous scientific achievement, and the partisans boosting Longo for a Nobel Prize have my vote. But to my mind, Longo abandoned actual fasting prematurely, and his claim that his FMDs are "as effective as fasting" is regrettable overstatement. Fasting changes thousands of metabolic processes in the body, many still unknown, and even Longo has tracked only a portion of them. While it's possible a body digesting hundreds of FMD calories a day could go about its myriad repairs every bit as well as a body digesting nothing, it would be surprising if it were so. More to the point, it hasn't been proven.

Someday I expect we'll learn that a combination of FMD and other therapies (chemo-, immuno-, or radio-) can send this or that cancer into remission for an average of ten or twenty years. But if it were my cancer, I'd want to know if actual fasting would banish the disease for thirty years—or forever. This isn't far-fetched speculation. In 2019, when researchers compared how well FMDs, fasting, and caloric restriction restrained the pro-cancerous IGF-1, they found a dose-dependent relationship: the fewer calories ingested, the more IGF-1 was inhibited.

I also have my doubts about Longo's claim that most people won't fast. Many of course won't, but the tens of thousands who visit the world's fasting clinics every year are proof many will, and other scientists have had success fasting even gravely ill patients. In a cancer trial at Leiden University in the Netherlands, patients who fasted on nothing but water for twenty-four hours before and after* each of three rounds of chemotherapy reported few problems sticking with the protocol, and the results were promising. The fasters had more red blood cells and platelets than non-fasters, and the DNA of their white blood cells was either protected from chemotherapeutic damage or quickly repaired. No doubt one reason Longo had such trouble was that he was working through oncologists who didn't particularly support their patients' fasts. Supported fasters fare better. In a trial in Berlin, women with breast or ovarian cancer were put on a Buchinger-style fast that ran from thirty-six hours before each chemo treatment to twenty-four hours after and were also given counseling and instruction on what to expect when fasting. Only five women found the fasting onerous enough to quit, while thirty-four others saw it through. Thirty-one of those said they were so pleased with the reduced side effects that they would willingly do a modified fast again during chemotherapy.

It doesn't take a scientist to see that what the field needs now are head-to-head studies comparing how chemotherapy (or radiation or

---

* In such trials, the fast is continued beyond the administration of chemotherapy to keep healthy cells kneeling behind their shields until the chemical toxins have been eliminated.

immunotherapy) fares against cancer in patients on either an FMD, a modified fast, a water-only fast, or a normal diet. Such trials would be simple to execute but would come dear, which is the rub. No giant corporation stands to make money from fasting, so none cares to underwrite the trials, which is why most of the research funds are going to FMDs without a fasting arm. Capitalism, not for the first time, has queered the science.

CHAPTER 13

A GENTLE DEPRIVATION, 2

On the third morning of my fast at the Buchinger Wilhelmi Clinic, a nurse whom I had christened Nurse Brokenhearted because her eyes expressed a sadness beyond knowing and her shoulders sagged beneath a somber weight—a jilting, I decided—said, "Today eez zee eeneema, yah?"

"Yah," I said, matching her frown. "My first enema ever."

She gave me a woebegone look, and I went off to an hour of yoga in which I torqued into all sorts of positions that I hoped would contribute to the unpuckering of a certain sphincter. Back in my room, Nurse Brokenhearted appeared almost as soon as I rang the call button, as if she had been eagerly awaiting the moment. Perhaps even giving an enema was better than moping over a jilting.

The enema was intended to flush from my intestines whatever the Glauber's salt hadn't—a few remnants from my last meal, I supposed—as well as any new secretions, sloughed-off cells, and such parts of my broths and honeys that my body had declined to absorb. Otto Buchinger had said an enema wasn't strictly necessary during a fast because the body would push out this gunge on its own, but absent an enema there would be "'critical' situations before and during the bowel movement," which might include nausea, abdominal pain, diarrhea, and vomiting. This was all news to me, who had fasted without enemas and had no such problems, but since I had signed on for the full Buchinger, I submitted.

Beforehand I attempted to learn what an enema was like and was frustrated that doctors, nurses, and recipients, both in the flesh and online, waltzed prudishly around the details in a little box step of elision and euphemism that did nothing to calm the worry-prone mind. I have rectified the problem below, but if the particulars of intestinal irrigation do not enchant you, skip the next two paragraphs. Never let it be said I don't look out for my readers.

Nurse Brokenhearted bade me lie on my side on a towel at the edge of the bed while she filled a medical bag with a liter of water and explained that the tube emerging from the bag was lubricated with petroleum jelly, for which we were both grateful. The bag filled, she had me pull down my pants and slid the tube into my rectum. The sensation is foreign to nobody who has ever had to work a toilet-papered finger an undignified distance into his anus, the only difference being the tube went a bit farther. Then it just stopped, although whether it actually stopped or reached a place where I lacked nerves to feel it, I don't know. She squeezed the bag, and the water began to flow into me, which I experienced only as an awkward pressure in my bowels lasting a few seconds. Then I felt nothing at all. After a minute of gentle squeezing, she pulled the tube out, advised me to remain lying for three minutes to let the water do its work, and shuffled dejectedly out the door. She was in the room all of five minutes.

Other guests at the clinic had told me I might struggle during the three minutes' wait not to soil the bed, but the time passed peacefully. When finally I went to the toilet, a small plug popped out, followed by a brief gush of liquid, a pattern that repeated itself several times over a few minutes. The only discomfort was a slight feeling of nausea at the back of my jaw. Evidently, with my innards acting diarrheal, some vestigial warning system was telling me this wasn't the best time for an éclair. When I judged the liquidation complete, I arose triumphant, only to be instantly glad the toilet was still beneath me. A vast gush forced me to plop right back down, and for another several seconds I was a garden hose turned on high. It was hard to believe Nurse Brokenhearted had pumped that much water into me. When it finally ended, the toilet bowl looked as if small creatures had had a mud fight with soil of the darkest shade. The reek easily surpassed the abilities of the bathroom's ventilation fan, and I had to open the balcony door for a quarter hour to defumigate. The sharp chill was welcome.

I have no idea whether I subsequently felt better than I would have without the enema, but I went about the rest of the day with a light step, perhaps in gratitude at having the enema behind me, as it were.

Two days later when it was time for my next enema, the nurses of Villa Larix, my dormitory, were all hustle and drive because Nurse Brokenhearted hadn't shown up that morning and they had to share out her patients. I decided the lover who had jilted her had seen the error of his ways, returned to sweep her off her feet, and they were now having torrid elopement sex in Marrakesh. An exuberant nurse bustled into my room with an enema bag and bustled into me with such unsentimental efficiency that I started and arched my back almost theatrically. With the exception of an awkward moment at a Pride parade in my youth, never had anyone been so keen to get up my ass. Her double load of patients beckoning, she exited both me and the room as quickly as she had entered.

For my third and final enema, two days later, Nurse Brokenhearted was still AWOL—satisfyingly entwined on a beach in Zanzibar by now, I hoped—and another ebullient, patient-strapped nurse arrived. She paused just before entry and said in a chipper voice, commanding as much as asking, "Ready?!" Unfortunately, as became instantaneously clear, she hadn't taken enough time to let the tap get hot. In a part of me never before breached by anything not already warmed by digestion to 98.6 degrees, the stream was extraordinarily enlivening—not painful precisely but also not the kind of thing you'd book a return ticket for. On the toilet, the sensation of cold water flowing the other direction was also new and disorienting. However, either because of the cold or because I was becoming an adept at enemas, I had none of the mild nausea of my first two irrigations. I strode off confidently to a cooking class only to realize the confidence was recklessness, and was supremely grateful for the well-placed bathroom outside the demonstration kitchen. As I landed with an appreciative crash on the commode, I thought I probably wouldn't rate enemas among the top five things I would miss about Germany.

* * *

After the Second World War, Otto Buchinger again had an overflow of patients whom he stashed around Bad Pyrmont, and the surfeit motivated his daughter and son-in-law, Maria Buchinger and Helmut Wilhelmi, to found a new clinic in 1953 a few hundred miles to the south in Überlingen. Eventually Otto joined them. The Buchinger Clinic in Bad Pyrmont, which Otto handed over to his son, is run by his great-grandchildren now but has been eclipsed in capacity and fame by the Buchinger Wilhelmi Clinic in Überlingen. One reason for the success of Überlingen was the social touch of Maria, which is felt everywhere at the clinic today. Maria thought community at mealtimes, during classes, and on hikes enhanced fasting, and she had a knack for knowing her guests' interests and artfully mixing them together. Her habitual cry was "Darling, you really must meet . . ." More than one of her dinner pairings ended in marriage.

In 1973, seven years after Otto's death, Maria opened a second Buchinger Wilhelmi Clinic in Marbella, Spain. It was a brash endeavor. Spain had no history of therapeutic fasting, and the tourism that would eventually overwhelm the Costa del Sol and on which the clinic would depend was for the moment little more than a developer's febrile dream. But after a few lean years, a Spanish actress named Carmen Sevilla began talking up the charm and sagacity of the *dueña* of the clinic and proclaiming that fasting had positively revivified her. Other celebrities arrived, and the clinic became known as the place the rich and famous went to starve. They were not always easy.

"Famous people are capricious," Maria told *People* magazine in 1986. "They sit in their room and smoke, and we tell them it's their last cigarette or they're out."

The most capricious of all was the heiress Christina Onassis, whose arrival was preceded by twenty-four suitcases, one filled with bottles of Coca-Cola, later surrendered on threat of exile. Onassis took a suite with half a dozen retainers, snuck out of the clinic after the gates closed at 2 a.m. to frolic in Marbella's discos, and kept a private jet at the airport for weekend getaways. At the end of her stay, Maria invited her not to return. Onassis complied for several years, but in 1984, on the eve of her fourth marriage and desperate to lose some of her more than two hundred pounds before taking her latest vow of eternal devotion, she begged clemency. Maria relented, and Onassis arrived with just one nanny. She kept a low profile for three weeks, lost thirty pounds, and enjoyed her life's most successful marriage, all three years of it.

Other celebrities were less troublesome. Sean Connery spent a placid week in Marbella, lost fourteen pounds, and pronounced himself glad to have done it, "but once was enough." For a time, the Spanish royal family took their reservations in ensemble and, like everyone else, were required to leave their bodyguards at the gates and queue for their broth. The rich who were put out by rubbing shoulders with the proletariat could soothe their wounded pride in a 900-square-foot top-floor suite that lets today for €12,000 a week. (Plebeians can get in the door for under €2,000 a week, same as at Überlingen.)

While Marbella blossomed under Maria, Überlingen continued to burgeon, and to date the two clinics have hosted better than four hundred thousand people, more than a quarter million of them fasting, the remainder on a low-calorie diet. The payroll of five hundred includes about twenty doctors, sixty nurses, and whole platoons of massage therapists, dietitians, psychologists, life coaches, and yoga instructors. No fasting clinic anywhere in the world comes close to its scope. America's largest, the TrueNorth Health Center in California, has treated only fifty thousand patients, twenty thousand fasting, since its founding in 1984.

It was remarkable to me that Buchinger and his descendants had built this small empire, a satrapy of fasting, at a time when fasting clinics in America were being chivvied out of existence. Largely because of the success of Buchinger Wilhelmi, Germany today is dappled with other fasting centers, most of humble scale but few in danger of insolvency and none accused of quackery. Meanwhile in the United States you can count the thriving fasting clinics on one hand and still have enough fingers left to give an enema. (In Spain, fasting also keeps to a modest footprint—Maria's enthusiasm did not overspread the peninsula.) Buchinger Wilhelmi succeeded, as I've said, by making fasting so very pleasant, and for many visitors, part of the pleasure was the sense of community that Maria had engendered. But my feelings about our little commune were more mixed.

The trouble was the density of parvenu dukes and duchesses, the type whose stories always seemed to revolve around the getting and spending of their lucre. Sometimes I thought I could hear the rustling of bills as they strode the grounds of the clinic, but it may just have been the autumn leaves they crushed under their heels. Their sybaritism was rivaled only by their solipsism. I would often plunk down at a table in the delightful saloon where broths were served before a majestic prospect of the lake (the dining room, where we took our meals on eating days, could overlook the garage without injury, but on fasting days, the panoramic saloon was a balm) and find my fellow fasters discoursing about bottles of wine that cost more than my mortgage, or the best moorages in the Seychelles, or why one really must get a Porsche for the country home but a Mini Cooper for town (so much easier to park), or why one's child, having grown up with horses, needed to take one to college. One luncheon I arrived to hear Charles, the financial adviser from chapter 10, exclaiming to friends about a twelve-bloody-percent stamp tax on homes over £1.5 million.

"And on second homes, it's fifteen bloody percent." He pushed away his bowl of carrot-fennel broth with a disbelieving shake of the head. "It's just criminal."

My heart ached for him, but my soul did not soar in quite the way Maria envisioned.

Before I came to the clinic, I had a notion it would be peopled by as many pipefitters as periodontists. My misconception was rooted in the fact that German health insurance typically pays for fasting, which led me to assume the working class would be well represented. What I didn't know was the insurance payments are somewhat chintzy, and while Buchinger Wilhelmi's base rate of €250 a night may have been cheap compared to other healthcare facilities—a third the cost of a rehab center, an order of magnitude cheaper than a hospital—it was still more than most German insurers, including the German state, wanted to pay. The pipefitters frequented cheaper outfits whose full cost was covered by insurance.

But the unwashed weren't entirely unrepresented. In fact, the most frequent faster at Buchinger Wilhelmi was a man of the people who had first come in 1972 at the age of forty and had returned for three weeks every six months—ninety-two stays in all at the time of my visit. "Do you know how I paid for all these stays?" he once said to Françoise Wilhelmi de Toledo. "Because I deposited a fortune at your place. I never regretted it, but it is very much." And by way of answer he pulled from his pocket a little key. Before retiring, he had been a metalworker, and his trade had been the fabrication of keys that turned the heat up and down on radiators.

"This," he said, brandishing the piece, "is how I could afford to come to you almost one hundred times."

He believed investing in a long, healthy life had been a wiser expenditure of his salary and vacation time than going on cruises that would have left him fatter and more drained than before. And he was indeed the picture of health, his only complaint a loss of hearing from shelling during the Second World War. So rarely did he get sick that he had long ago dismissed his general practitioner and now relied on the clinic for primary care. The clinicians had given him his own robe, lettered C H A M P I O N across the back in the style of a boxer's wrap.

It would have done my heart good to meet a few more hardscrabble types like him, although I'd have settled for patricians of palpable generosity. Those, however, were thin on the grounds. Only twice in two weeks did I hear anyone speak of giving a titch of their wealth or time to others. It parched the soul, theirs and mine.

*   *   *

My body, however, flourished. In fact, I was enjoying another small miracle. Despite the most appalling nights of restless limbs, once I arose and shuffled blearily off to the reunion of the robed at the nurses' station, my exhaustion vanished, and for the rest of the day I was rarely fatigued. The hypersomnia that had been creeping back since arriving in Spain evaporated, and an unexpected sprightliness propelled me through a full schedule of classes, hikes, interviews, and long stretches of splendidly productive writing. We writers often look back at spurts of alleged luminosity and find our prose self-indulgent and flaccid, but not this time. It was my best writing in months. Otto had said "there is nothing more powerful to stimulate the creative spirit than fasting," and over the years many writers had left the clinic with completed manuscripts. One composer came regularly to write concertos.

My mood also soared, notwithstanding the autumnal gloom that usually sent me into the funk that psychiatrists call, in their dehumanizing jargon, seasonal affective disorder. As part of the detox studies in which I was participating, I had been asked on arrival to rate how cheerful and good-spirited, how calm and relaxed, how active and vigorous I had been in the two weeks before my fast. I gave each of those traits a sad little 2 out of 5: "less than half of the time." But when I left the clinic two weeks later, every 2 had magically become a 4—"the great majority of the time"— notwithstanding gray skies and short days. In fact, every self-assessed metric of my mental and physical well-being, save sleep, ticked felicitously upward during my fast. The transformation was more thorough than I had dared hope for, and if I could have bottled the vital force coursing through me, future generations would know me by my statue on every town square. Not since the birth of Elliott seventeen years earlier had I felt so moved by human biology. I was, it seemed, cured again—for now anyway.

*   *   *

Françoise Wilhelmi de Toledo first fasted at the age of seventeen, when she was the less thoroughly denominated Françoise de Toledo. The year was 1970, the liberationist spirit of 1968 was still thick in the European air, and every month a new idea—*ecology, feminism, meditation*—intruded into her conservative Swiss upbringing. She chanced upon fasting in an organic grocery store that with noble disregard for its bottom line sold a French edition of one of Herbert Shelton's books about not eating. She read it with an avidity that grew by the page. Shelton made fasting sound a panacea, a Leatherman tool to mend the broken body, the enervated family, even the enfeebled nation. Wilhelmi de Toledo was a nervous, exhausted adolescent who had been bulimic ever since her father, disapproving of her twelve-year-old pudginess, offered her ten francs for each kilo she lost. She began to fast the moment she put Shelton down.

"It was like I could suddenly breathe again," she recalled. "It was so extraordinary. I had really this ecstasy, like a trip. I am what the fasting doctors called a good responder."

Liberated from food, she was liberated from her eating disorder. Each morning she awoke feeling fresher than the last. Her skin cleared up, she felt more in touch with nature, and for the first time in her life she was comfortable with everyone. "Why can't I always feel this way?" she wondered. Friends remarked favorably on the change, but after six or seven days they said she was daft not to eat for so long, and on the eleventh day, quite thinned, she knew she had to stop but had no clue how to refeed properly. She asked acquaintances, went to see a doctor, but no one had the slightest idea. In the end, she binged—disastrously, falling into a fever and developing a temporary but frightening angina. Eventually her health returned to its pre-fast, bone-tired state, but the memory of the euphoria stayed with her.

Sometime later at the organic farm where she worked, she came across a flyer about a fasting clinic in Austria and wasted no time packing her bags. For sixteen days she fasted on water and then partially fasted ten more on a little milk and bread. Again she had an almost ecstatic experience in which everything felt right. The doctor who supervised her wasn't unskilled, but the limitations of his craft can be seen in the meal with which he routinely broke fasts: trout cooked in butter, an assault on the intestines no fasting doctor would dream of serving today. To her immense disappointment, Wilhelmi de Toledo returned once more to her weary, anxious baseline, her motor constantly running but always on fumes.

A short time later a dentist noticed a bulge in her neck that proved to be Hodgkin's disease—cancer—and she submitted to a surgeon for what she understood would be an investigation of the tumor. She awoke from the operation with a scar running from sternum to pelvis. The priestly authority of doctors was still awesome in the early 1970s, especially in conservative Switzerland, where patients had about as much say over their treatments as parishioners over their mass. The surgeon, who was talented, had rooted around her abdomen and removed all manner of lymph nodes and for good measure her spleen. Although he may have saved her life, his excision of the spleen, whose role in the immune system is critical, was excessive. Years later an avuncular doctor would tell her, "Madame, your spleen was sacrificed on the altar of Medicine."

After radiation and recovery, Wilhelmi de Toledo went to medical school, in part to understand her illness and how to live without a spleen, both of which her doctors comprehended poorly. Among much else of a dubious nature, they told her she could go back to her previous way of life—eat whatever she wanted, do as she pleased—which made no sense to her. Surely something in her lifestyle had contributed to her illness. Eventually she found a more sensible medicine, although not from her professors, who were equally benighted, but from another doctor. Catherine Kousmine would become one of the great influences of her life, and in some respects it is as much Kousmine's spirit, channeled through Wilhelmi de Toledo, as it is Otto's or Maria's that pervades Buchinger Wilhelmi today.

Kousmine was a Russian émigré whose family fled the revolution of 1917 and settled on Lake Geneva, where the capitalist breezes blew more favorably on her industrialist father. She became one of a very few women of her era to earn a medical degree, which she took at the top of her University of Lausanne class because, she said, women always had to perform better to be taken seriously. Her career was shaped early by the loss of a twelve-year-old patient to a savage form of lymphoma called reticulosarcoma. The disease ate away the back of the girl's nose and took one of her eyes, and she died agonizingly of cachexia, a general wasting away. One day the fading girl told Kousmine, "I am very lucky. My illness allowed me to meet you." All doctors have a case that haunts them the length of their career, and this was Kousmine's.

Moved to look into the research on cancer, she was alarmed to find cases were rising steeply yet no one knew why. Worse, medical schools and the doctors they produced seemed interested only in battling cancer once it was contracted, not in preventing it in the first place. Most experts didn't even think it could be prevented. They thought through bad genes or bad luck, cancer either had your number or didn't. But if this were true,

Kousmine reasoned, why was there more cancer this year than last, more over the past decade than the decade before? Surely it was unscientific to say that in the first half of the twentieth century Fate suddenly decided to deal us a crueler hand. Something novel must be harming us, probably something we were doing to ourselves. Her unconventional ideas were met by her conventional colleagues with a disdain Herbert Shelton would have recognized.

Kousmine decided to do her own research, and for a laboratory she substituted the kitchen of her flat in a suburb of Lausanne. From the Curie Institute in Paris she bought a strain of mice bred so that 90 percent developed cancer by the age of four months. The mice were typically fed pellets that mimicked healthy human food, but the pellets were expensive, so Kousmine used them only every other day. The other days, the mice ate actual food: old carrots, castoff bread from bakeries, milk, a little brewer's yeast. Then a marvelous and unforeseen thing happened. The cancer rates in her mice fell by half. At first Kousmine resisted the conclusion that the "healthy" pellets were in fact cancer-producing, but after further experiments, she concluded that the pellets, which resembled highly processed human foods, did in fact cause cancer while minimally processed foods somehow protected against the disease. She assumed the problem lay in the refining of the pellets, which stripped away valuable nutrients. It was a formidable discovery in so rudimentary a setup, and both her finding and her speculation about the cause have since been corroborated by studies in animals and humans.

Kousmine began paying attention to what her patients ate and observed that those who got cancer and other grave ills seemed to eat more meat, which she also concluded was harmful, as well as more refined foods. To her eyes, the most damaging of the latter were white sugar, white flour, and, especially, highly processed oils, whose use was growing rapidly. (The global explosion in heavily refined sugars and flours was still decades away.) An acquaintance who worked in a vegetable-oil mill told her that during the Second World War manufacturers had learned to keep prices down through a new process that squeezed more oil out of the same quantity of seeds, nuts, and vegetables. The process involved heating the foods to extremely high temperatures before pressing them, and the heat destroyed almost all of their nutrients, including many that nutritionists today extol, like omega-3 fatty acids, antioxidants, and vitamin E. Kousmine called hot-pressed oils "dead oils," and she advised her patients to use only cold-pressed oils and build the rest of their diets around whole grains, vegetables, and dairy, all organic. She was decades ahead of her time and would later be vindicated on most counts, although not dairy. In its essentials, the lightly processed Kousmine diet is the one on which Buchinger Wilhelmi refeeds its fasters today.

In 1949, Kousmine tested her ideas on her first cancer patient, a man in his early forties who had the same disease, reticulosarcoma, that killed her twelve-year-old patient. His had spread throughout his body, and his oncologist had told him he would be dead in two years. Kousmine put him on her diet, and within four months the cancer went into remission. When he later drifted back to his old eating habits, the cancer came back. He returned to the diet, once more the disease remitted, but again he strayed and again the cancer struck. For nine years he kept up this precarious back-and-forth until another doctor told him he had to choose between a clean life or an indulgent death. He chose to live, renounced his old habits for good, and survived into his nineties. Kousmine published accounts of his and similar cases and for her trouble was ridiculed a quack by doctors and researchers who said nutrition and cancer had little to do with each other. It's a dogma with all the scientific grounding of phrenology, yet it persists today.

Wilhelmi de Toledo was captivated by Kousmine. She ate Kousmine's diet, her long-standing enervation disappeared, and she resolved to be a doctor in the Kousmine mold. But when she suggested on one of her student rotations that a cancer patient follow the diet, a superior rebuked her.

"Let the man eat what he wants," the doctor said. "It's his last pleasure."

Even without the reprimand, Wilhelmi de Toledo was coming to realize it was impractical to ask patients in a conventional medical setting to overhaul their eating habits. They always had a dozen questions, and she never had more than a few minutes to answer. She needed a setting more sympathetic to her aims. She would find it on the hillside above Lake Constance.

*   *   *

The reincarnated lama who led our meditation session one morning was fortyish and bald, a little pasty in the way Canadians often are, and possessed of a tone an orator might have called North American Bland. As he guided eight of us in becoming aware of the moment, he managed to project both kindness and a barely suppressed irritation, as if his fast were going poorly. He seemed, in short, an altogether ordinary Joe, and yet he purported to be a reborn Tibetan master last seen in earthly form six decades ago. Often he would pause in the middle of a sentence to think of a word, and he had a knack for choosing one that didn't quite fit, which struck me as odd in someone who had spent more than one lifetime immersed in the teachings he was imparting. Maybe he was still getting used to English this time around. During the long moments of meditative silence, my mind strayed irresistibly to the usual questions: Why do Westerners always reincarnate from Tibetan lamas and Egyptian princesses rather than Tibetan scullery maids and Egyptian slaves? Did the Tibetan and Egyptian lumpenproletariat reincarnate only as weevils and leafhoppers, or were they in fact all around us in human configuration, just less interested in touting their ignoble predecessors? My lama suggested we focus our wandering minds by returning to a simple mantra, like a gentle rain falling on a lake. My rain kept saying, "You *can't* be serious."

The session was part of the clinic's understated and nondenominational program to enrich our spirits, a program with its origins in Otto's writings on the "point of inner repose" that his patients often discovered while fasting: "Analytic thinking is hampered at first; intuition, by contrast, deepens and eases. . . . Later we find thoughts easier, more spiritually productive. . . . We sometimes also experience a release of neurotic fixations. The true core comes to light—it is a coming home to ourselves." That homecoming, Otto allowed, didn't always unfold so idyllically, and many of his fasters struggled through depressive plunges, manic surges, and extreme hypersensitivity. But he believed the faster who opened him-self to change could eventually find equanimity—the very sort of mental transformation that religious fasters had long gone in search of, the kind I suspect Mr. Pidge meant when he said fasting could stir up emotions and psychological events.

Most researchers skirt this terrain, partly because emotion and other qualities of the mind resist quantification and partly because when people like Otto speak in spiritual rather than psychological terms, the words leave a residue of irrationality. For just those reasons, I too had long ignored the psychological changes people claimed while fasting, but after my own psyche improved during my fast the previous January, I began to pay them more heed. I had high hopes of investigating further at the clinic, but the lama was a distraction—and perhaps worse. Otto had cautioned, and I concurred, that with the legitimacy of fasting so finely balanced, fast-ing doctors should take care not to bring ill repute to the practice. To my mind, giving a guest-lectureship to a transmigrated Canuck was as good as handing a pry bar to the detractors who would just as soon lever fasting over a cliff.

That said, after meditating with the lama, my recurring migraine all but disappeared and remained quiescent in meditations with more secular teachers. In fact, I found as deep a calm while meditating at the clinic as ever before, and I surprised myself by meditating on my own several times. The composure that gradually descended on me is the nearest I'd ever come to a steady state of serenity, a state no doubt abetted by the physiological changes of fasting: a slower pulse, lower blood pressure, a brain generally less frantic even when not meditating.

Most of my fellow fasters gave the morning meditation sessions a wide berth, but I was mildly shocked to find Charles a regular attendee. After one session that included a bit of Buddhist doctrine on the true nature of happiness, Charles told me with some pride that he was going to start practicing non-attachment. "And I'm going to begin by getting rid of my Hockney," he said.

I was impressed. Earlier he had boasted that his Hockney was one of the jewels of his art collection. I began to think I might have to revise my assessment of the bloke, but he interrupted this premature reverie to say, "And I'm going to use the proceeds to buy a better Hockney I've had my eye on."

Maybe in another five or ten lifetimes he'd have the hang of it.

*   *   *

Françoise Wilhelmi de Toledo came to the clinic on Lake Constance for the modified fasting, which was instantly appealing, but returned for the tranquility of spirit and clarity of mind that arose within her while there. She made the clinic her study hall for medical exams, and on one of these scholarly sabbaticals a chatty fellow Swiss woman sized her up and announced, "I must introduce you to Raimund Wilhelmi, the junior director of the clinic. You have to marry him!"

The introduction was made, the anticipated courtship occurred, and the year she took her medical degree, 1982, she added the name Wilhelmi to hers. Raimund was the son of Helmut and Maria, grandson of Otto, a young businessman like his father, and as of 1985 director of the clinic. Wilhelmi de Toledo became one of the clinic's doctors, and her first task was to unlearn much of what she had learned in medical school. Although she kept the basic science, the diagnostic training, and the methodical curiosity, she abandoned the reflexive reach for a prescription pad and, often, the inclination to treat at all. Time and again she saw fasting reverse illnesses she had been taught were irreversible, illnesses like rheumatoid arthritis, asthma, and fibromyalgia. One young man whose memory stayed with her had multiple sclerosis so severe he could no longer walk by himself or even write his name. Conventional medicine had given up on him, but after three weeks at the clinic he left walking and writing. He wasn't cured, but fasting gave him back pieces of his life that his doctors had told him were gone forever.

Wilhelmi de Toledo was especially moved by women who were unable to conceive until fasting. She knows five of these Hannahs, including herself. After the radiation to her torso, her doctors said she could never have children, and in the early years of her marriage this had proven true enough. But Dr. Kousmine told her to ignore the pessimists and heal her body through diet and regular fasts. After one prolonged fast, she and her husband made a concerted and agreeable effort to reproduce, and she became pregnant almost immediately. A second son followed by the same method. There are no studies to prove or disprove fasting for conception, but Wilhelmi de Toledo is not the only physician to report it. Buchinger and other German doctors noted several instances, and Herbert Shelton told of one young woman who had had twenty-eight spontaneous abortions but became pregnant and gave birth after fasting ten days and eating fruits and vegetables for four months. Wilhelmi de Toledo hypothesizes that since many of the body's stem cells are stimulated by prolonged fasting, the ones involved in conception are probably among them. To infertile couples, she counsels a supervised fast of ten or more days, followed by copious coupling during the woman's next cycle.

Where Wilhelmi de Toledo's career has most diverged from those of earlier fasting doctors, especially the Americans, is in her emphatic embrace of science. "Many of the alternative-medicine doctors, like Dewey in America, were so attacked by other doctors that they turned bitter," she said. "It happened in other places too. When I was a student, I visited the clinic of Albert Mosséri"—one of the deans of the French hygienic school, whose clinic she found ironically unhygienic, filthy even. "The first thing he told me was, 'You are a medical student? Well, you are lost. You are not the right person. If you study medicine, you can never understand what fasting is.' And I had had a lot of experience in fasting! Here at the clinic we always thought it was necessary to have a cooperation even with the people who do not understand what we do, with doctors and scientists. To learn the mechanisms of fasting, we needed their research, which we could never do on our own. And when good medical research emerged, we always tried to go along with it." Buchinger had been similarly inclined, once referring to conventional medicine as "our dear old mother," even if mum often looked at fasting with wrinkled brow. It was all a far cry from Herbert Shelton's damnable *Science*, and with reason: in Germany, conventional doctors and their prosecutorial allies made few assaults on fasting.

But over the course of the twentieth century, Germany produced no more research about fasting than the United States, and when Wilhelmi de Toledo took her post at the clinic forty years ago, its doctors had little more science to guide them than Otto had when he fasted his first patient in 1920. Wilhelmi de Toledo decided, as her mentor Catherine Kousmine had, to start researching on her own, a labor that would eventually make her one of the world's most influential fasting doctors. Her first foray was an analysis in 1994 that found patients who had fasted at the clinic ten or more times weighed two pounds less at their tenth fast than at their first. Two pounds may sound a trifle, but in the modern West the great majority of adults gain a pound or two a year, and since an average of a dozen years had elapsed between the patients' first and tenth fasts, they "should" have weighed fifteen to twenty-five pounds more. Fasting perhaps helped them maintain their weight, although without a control group it was possible other factors played a part.

As scientific interest in fasting grew, Wilhelmi de Toledo co-founded a pair of pan-European associations to share and coordinate fasting research. One starved to death for lack of interest, but the other survives today with hundreds of members. Across three decades, she has co-authored a thick sheaf of observational studies and meta-analyses, and in 2012 she founded a research department at the clinic in Überlingen, one of three in the world dedicated to fasting. (The other two are at the sister clinic in Marbella and at the TrueNorth Health Center in California.) One evening during my stay, Wilhelmi de Toledo, who is petite and elegant and has the calming personality of a therapist and the right scarf for any occasion, said the most critical thing that fasting researchers had learned during her lifetime was not just that the practice rejuvenated people at the molecular level but that it did so with unimaginable precision.

"Fasting," she said, "is an inner cleansing ability with a *selective intelligence* that no surgery can provide. This is why the old doctors referred to fasting as 'surgery without a scalpel.' Old and used material is *selectively* eliminated by fasting. And while we're fasting, stem cells get ready, and they are activated and regenerated after the fast to build new materials."

Her studies have demonstrated several impressive effects of that selective intelligence. In one trial, she reported that a modified fast averaging just 8.5 days eliminated non-alcoholic fatty liver disease in half of her patients. The longer they fasted, the less fatty their livers were. NAFLD now runs riot across the planet, tormenting about 20 percent of adults, 30 percent in sickly America. It's a stronger predictor of type 2 diabetes than waist size or obesity, and conventional doctors have had little luck reversing it, but they have paid Wilhelmi de Toledo's finding no mind. In another study, 84 percent of fasters with serious health problems— disorders like arthritis, type 2 diabetes, cholesterolemia, hypertension, and debilitating fatigue—substantially improved. And in an evaluation of the safety of modified fasting, 99.2 percent of 1,422 patients at the clinic reported no serious side effects. If there is a shortcoming to nearly all of Wilhelmi de Toledo's research, it is a lack of controls, which, however, are expensive to recruit and monitor. Her work has not been showered with funding from the usual underwriters of medical science—the companies that make drugs and devices or the governments and universities that are increasingly beholden to them.

It's an unfortunate coincidence that at the very moment when researchers like Wilhelmi de Toledo have won fasting a degree of respectability, funders are more than ever backing research based on its potential for profit rather than health. Morgan, the medical professor from chapter 10 who once ran a national science foundation, told me one day, "We used to do research. Now we're supposed to generate revenue. And university administrators apply the most intense screws to us to do it. It's no longer enough that we bring in grant revenue to fund our research. They want revenue from startups and spinoffs to fund the whole blasted university." It helps explain Valter Longo's pursuit of a fasting-mimicking diet.

"Valter is following a successful model," Wilhelmi de Toledo said tactfully, "which is to find something that will be reimbursed by the insurance industry and to make it so that hospitals and doctors are obliged to offer it as a possible prescription. The trouble is, it will then make other treatments, which are not covered, less available. We see it all the time, and the outcome is not always good. Take statins, a horrible product, probably necessary only for one percent of people with high cholesterol, but it's covered by insurance, so it's prescribed to craziness."

If there was a gleam of hope, she saw it in the partial democratization of medicine the internet has brought about. For the first time in her life, millions of people were excited about fasting, and some of their doctors, unenthused though they might be, had been forced to look at the science and acknowledge fasting's worth. It was a slender reed to jam the cogs of the mighty capitalist engine, but it was all she had.

*   *   *

Of the many tales of wonderful cures that rippled through the clinic during my stay, none impressed me more than those of fibromyalgia, the disease in which signals from the brain and spinal cord go haywire and turn muscles, bones, and joints into so many points of agony. For most sufferers, sleep becomes elusive, fatigue mounts, and under the strain mood and memory slip. Year by torturous year the disease progresses, a creeping bellflower of the frame, and nearly every medical organization, from the Mayo Clinic to the British National Health Service, says it can only be managed, not cured. Their doctors ought to visit the Buchinger Wilhelmi Clinic.

When I met Adrienne, a vibrant Swiss of seventy-eight years, she had been fasting at the clinic regularly for seven years. She had developed polyarthritis at sixty-seven, fibromyalgia at sixty-eight, and for three years had lived in an ever-worsening hell of pain and dwindling mobility. In the end, she was unable to fully extend her arms or legs and could do little more than lie shriveled and coiled in the corner of a sofa. She was in a deep depression when a friend told her to go to Überlingen, where there was a clinic that cured all kinds of diseases that other doctors were powerless to treat. Stooped and broken, Adrienne hobbled into Buchinger Wilhelmi and a month later walked out upright carrying her own suitcases. She even hiked during her stay. All that was left of her two diseases was, in her estimate, twenty percent of her previous pain. The next year she returned, fasted another twenty-one days, and the remaining pain disappeared.

To keep her diseases away, she overhauled her life, starting with her diet. She had had a busy career as a contract negotiator for one of the world's biggest consulting firms, and in all that time, she said, "I never paid attention to what was on my plate. I was too busy working, meeting with people. There were business lunches, business dinners. You can live all these patterns for years, and then one day it catches you. Maybe it's cancer, maybe it's heart attack, but it catches you." She eliminated most of the meat from her menu, although she still had a weakness for veal liver and marrow, and she added vastly more vegetables. She worked less, moved into a Paris flat she had long ago shuttered and never gotten around to reopening, and gave the boot to a husband who burdened her as much as her previous diet.

"It was a small revolution for me," she said. "Despite the years of hell, I'm glad I got my diseases. They gave me my life back. They did, and fasting."

Roughly once a year she made a long fast and despite her age had no plans to retire.

The other fibromyalgia transformations were no less resplendent, although Adrienne's was the only one to provoke marital dissolution. One of the hiking guides on staff, a spry woman of sixty-odd years, had been so crippled by her fibromyalgia that she needed a Tanneresque fast of six weeks to send it into remission. To watch her on the trail, you would never have guessed her former disability.

If an experimental compound had cured this incurable disease in mice, let alone humans, half a dozen clinical trials would have followed to document its efficacy. But I could find only two small experiments on fasting for fibromyalgia, one in Germany, one in Japan, both showing marked improvements with fasts as short as a week. Among rheumatologists, fasting to cure fibromyalgia remains entirely unknown.

*   *   *

Five days into my fast, I walked the three-quarters of a mile into the lovely historic center of Überlingen and happened upon a supermarket, which I entered on a whim to see what Germans liked to eat. (Answer: brightly colored packages, same as us.) For didactic bonus, I discovered my sense of smell hadn't sharpened. The odors of the fresh-baked pastry case didn't overfill me as they would have if I had been fasting on water instead of broth, and the produce carried hardly any scent either, whereas on a water fast I can sniff an orange in Tampa from my porch in Boulder. On my way back to the clinic, I walked along a clamorous feeder road and found I also wasn't overly troubled by sounds or fumes even though during my water fasts in Barcelona the din and diesel exhaust that sometimes invaded our flat from the plaza below were simply insupportable. Since one of the joys of water fasting is a reawakening of the senses, I judged the dullness of mine now a minor drawback of the broth fast. There was, however, one sensory compensation. My libido, which would have died with a whimper by the third day of a water fast, didn't entirely expire in Überlingen until day six or seven, although as I had left Jennifer in Spain, the consolation was less considerable than it might have been.

I took all these signs to mean a modified fast probably wasn't overhauling my innards as deeply as a water fast, and the keto strips I peed on each morning gave numerical weight to the assumption. On a water fast, my urine usually contained about 80 mg/dL of the ketone acetoacetate, which is right about what most men average, but at Buchinger I marked a steady 40. A study by Wilhelmi de Toledo showed I was not alone: men at the clinic typically produced between 50 and 60 mg/dL, while women averaged 40 to 50.

I found further corroboration for my hypothesis in the taste buds of my fellow fasters. On a water fast, as I've said, taste buds reset dramatically, and simple foods like vegetables and fruits, previously unexciting, taste delicious again, which in turn makes it easier to eat healthily. But at Buchinger the salted broths and honey-sweetened teas were enough to keep some people's taste buds from resetting, and they complained that the vegetables on which they refed were tasteless. They would, I feared, soon be drawn back to the sugary, fatty, and salty foods that had driven them to the clinic in the first place.

If I was right that our insides weren't being renovated quite as profoundly as they would have been on a water fast, it stood to reason that deeply ill fasters might heal more quickly or thoroughly when fasting on water instead of broth. Adrienne, for example—whose first broth fast reversed her fibromyalgia eighty percent—might, on water, have reached one hundred percent and been spared another year of pain. That isn't to say everyone needs a water fast. I spoke to people who shook their asthma, eczema, or colitis on a single broth fast, and many others enjoyed a deep reset of their taste buds. Charles, after just six days on broth, said he had never experienced such flavor as when he broke his fast on a plain yogurt. And the happiest breakfaster I've ever encountered was another broth faster. He passed me on his way out of the clinic, rollaboard in hand, then stopped, walked back to the bench where I was sitting, and said he was so overjoyed he just had to share his happiness with someone. He was Greek, and he explained in a rush of broken English that he was departing after two full months in Überlingen. He was still a large man but apparently had been far larger. A healthy glow radiated from him now. He hadn't fasted the entire time, but, as he put it, "I never stop working," which I took to mean he was always trying to improve his health even in the intermittent refeeding periods.

"And then," he said, "a miracle happens. Suddenly I like chocolate no longer. Chocolate was for me a problem. Very big problem. I go yesterday to town to buy chocolate for my family, and you know what? I do not like it. I do not want it. Chocolate holds me no more. I never experience this before. Always I love chocolate. It is not everything different, but it is an important small thing."

He paused, frowned, and added, "But now I go back to Greece." No doubt he was imagining all the dangers awaiting him, which clearly included more than just chocolate. But the frown vanished as quickly as it had come—nothing could repress his euphoria over his new self and his newly acclimated taste buds. It was beautiful to see, as was he, and for the rest of the morning my spirit took flight in just the way Maria Buchinger had hoped it would.

* * *

There was one more question to explore before I took my leave of Lake Constance, and that was how the clinicians thought I should eat after returning home. Otto had been of the same opinion as his mentor, Siegfried Möller, whom he quoted, "Whoever fasts only so that afterward he can stuff himself all the more with food and drink, and whoever during the fast revels in thoughts of doing so, hasn't understood the purpose and meaning of fasting. He will never find true health."

The old doctors would have been dismayed at how often my fellow fasters reveled in just such thoughts, how regularly the talk in the saloon turned to the fantastic homecoming menus they were composing. One or two fasters even went to cafés downtown just to watch other people eat, and three Lebanese guys went them one better by stopping at a bar each night for a cognac—the brandy fast.

Much like American fasting doctors, Otto thought the two most important reforms to make after a fast were to give up meat, which could obliterate any cure achieved by fasting, and to eat in moderation. "That man digs his grave with his teeth is a truth so general," he wrote, "that awakened people everywhere have always considered noble moderation a most special virtue. . . . Moderation protects, fasting cures."

His successors at the clinic were of the same mind about moderation but somewhat less so about diet, as I learned at a lecture on refeeding. The lecturer, a bright nurse, implored us to remember that just because we would soon be eating again didn't mean we would be done with fasting. In fact, refeeding was arguably the most important part of our fast. Our fasting bodies, she said, had torn down many complex structures that we would soon be rebuilding in a great hum of construction, the quality of which would depend on the materials we provided. If ever there was a time to eat well, it was now. The shade of Otto surely nodded his approval as she urged us to eat plants, always organic, the less refined the better. To refeed on meat, refined sugars, fried foods, or alcohol would, among much else of a disagreeable cast, incite harmful gut bacteria to flourish and undo most of the good we had done fasting.

It was excellent advice rooted in current research and long clinical experience, but she spoiled it by saying after two weeks we could gradually work back in all the old sins: the meat, the refined and sugary foods, the fatty snacks, the alcohol. I know of no reputable science to say good health flows from such a menu, and I thought she'd have done her listeners a better turn by saying those substances could still hurt us and we should eliminate the ones we could and reduce the rest. She might have added that with our taste buds partly or fully reset, our bodies reinvigorated, and our confidence brimming, we would never have an easier time giving up harmful but previously beloved substances. Her lecture helped me understand the rotundity of many repeat fasters, including Morgan, the physician-professor, who once said to me, "I catch my profile in the mirror—my room here's got plenty of the damned things—and I'm just horrified by my convexity. How did I arrive at this sorry state?" He was genuinely confused about why, after his previous four fasts, he always reinflated.

I suspected the nurse blessed our return to delinquency because she didn't want to tell the customers things they might not care to hear, and her employers didn't disabuse me of the idea. "We don't want to give bad feelings or make them feel guilty," Wilhelmi de Toledo said. And her son Leo Wilhelmi, who has run the clinic since 2019, added that the clinicians today were consciously gentler than his great-grandfather had been. "In Otto's day," he said, "there were rules to follow. Now we have guidelines to consider. Back then you had to rid yourself of the bad things that brought you here." Now, you improved small pieces of your life as it suited you or not. Leo believed that to expect people to change their whole lives in a few weeks was as fanciful as expecting someone to speak fluent French after a three-week language camp. The clinic, he said, gave people little blocks to build on, and if they came back they could add more blocks. A staggering 70 percent of fasters came back, so on one level the formula was clearly successful.

Still, I thought some of those who returned, like Morgan, returned in worse health than they need have. I got a glimpse of how this played out on my last hike with Charles shortly before he departed. He pronounced himself "entirely chuffed" that in six days of fasting he had shed nearly seven kilos—fifteen pounds—which brought him to within a couple of pounds of his ninety-kilo target. And he was practically giddy that his abdominal circumference had shrunk from 42½ to 41 inches and his blood pressure had dropped from 150/100 to 125/80. But when I asked if anyone had told him how to maintain those gains, he said, "No, not really." He hadn't gone to the lightly attended, entirely optional lecture on refeeding, and his doctor told him at his exit appointment that after refeeding on plants, he should, in his paraphrase, "just eat sensibly" and keep reducing his waist. He had no idea what eating sensibly meant and was already salivating over the end of his refeeding period, which coincided to the hour with a Champions League game between Liverpool and Napoli for which he had tickets. He planned to gorge on gloppy stadium food and swill beer by the tub, and the menu for the rest of his year was hardly less noxious. This was perhaps cosmic revenge for the shocking sums he told me he was investing in one of England's largest purveyors of larded-up pot pies, the sort of "food" that sent Britons to an early grave by the thousand, but my heart sank for him all the same. He had made great strides toward health during his fast, and he looked the part. The profound bags under his eyes had shrunk, his skin had snugged and lost its jaundiced hue, and his baby belly, which might have housed twins a week ago, couldn't have held more than a single infant now. He still walked stiff-backed and stiff-legged, and he must have been a sight when he jogged, but he was discovering health, and I hated he would soon give it all back. I thought ruefully of a line of Otto's: "The grocery, the tavern, and the 'bourgeois kitchen' are year after year the tireless providers of the clinics and sanatoriums."

Some months after we parted, Charles sent me an email. He was fresh from the Super Bowl (midfield seats) and said he had just booked another fast at Buchinger Wilhelmi for the coming fall. It was proof of concept for the clinic's business model, and I was happy for both him and the clinic. But I would have been even happier if I had thought he would return a little slimmer and healthier instead of, as I feared, re-bloated and bewildered in the manner of Morgan.

*   *   *

On my last day, I conferred with one of the clinic's nutritionists about what I might eat to keep my hypersomnia and migraines away. Things went cock-eyed from the start. The nutritionist was a generous soul who intended only the best for me, but after reviewing my current diet she uttered the oldest canard to pollute the vegan ear: I needed to eat more protein. The moment someone counsels a vegan to eat more protein is the moment you know she knows nothing about plants, because it is virtually impossible to consume even a modest diversity of plants and not to get enough protein.* I was still reattaching my jaw when she topped that shocker by urging me to combine my foods carefully at each meal (by eating rice, say, whenever I ate beans) in order to get the right mix of amino acids to build complete proteins—another hoary myth, debunked more than forty years ago.

Far more concerning, however, was her suggestion that I adopt a keto-genic diet or something approximating it. Her thinking was that since my hypersomnia and migraines had improved dramatically while fasting, I should stay in ketosis as long as I could—a fallacious logic common among fasters but startling in a nutritionist. I've yet to see the trial showing a diet extremely high in fat is healthy for the long term, while we have liter-ally thousands of studies showing high-fat diets increase the risk of heart attack, stroke, diabetes, cancer, dementia, and many other odious condi-tions. It's true that in the short term a ketogenic diet can improve some biomarkers, notably blood pressure and weight, although much of the lost weight is water, and some of it is muscle. But even short- and mid-term studies have found a keto diet can systemically inflame the body, narrow arteries, lay waste to healthy intestinal bacteria, cause deficiencies in up to seventeen vitamins and minerals, and send markers that predict cancer, gallbladder disease, stroke, diabetes, and dementia in the wrong direction. This internal disorder manifests, again per multiple studies, in headaches,

* The best science suggests most adults of healthy weight need no more than about 30 grams (an ounce) of protein a day, although nutritional authorities typically counsel around 50 grams because a minority of people absorb protein poorly. A handout the nutritionist gave me, citing the recommendations of the German Nutrition Society, said exactly that, and the American Nutrition Association says much the same. Either she hadn't read her own handout, or she wasn't aware of just how hard a vegan would have to work *not* to get 50 grams a day. If, for example, I took my 2,000 daily calories in nothing but oats, I would get 90 grams of protein; if nothing but tomatoes, 110 grams; if only black beans or broccoli, 160 or 180 grams respectively.

constipation, diarrhea, atrial fibrillation, leaky gut, and, most alarmingly, early death. In one trial, after just a week on a ketogenic diet, volunteers' attention spans and reaction times declined, and after only five days in another trial, volunteers had trouble remembering things and performing a complex task. Those, to repeat, are just the short- and mid-term findings.

When I told the nutritionist I wasn't aware of research suggesting we should stay on a ketogenic diet for the long haul, she allowed she knew of none either and said simply, "Well, there are people who eat a ketogenic diet for a long time."

"Before dropping dead of a coronary," I thought.

Other practitioners at the clinic put a more moderate spin on keto. Wilhelmi de Toledo, for instance, favored eating "in a ketogenic direction," with more healthy fats, à la Dr. Kousmine. But several of my fellow fasters told me their doctors in Überlingen had advised them to go enthusiastically ketogenic for as long as they could. I doubted the doctors meant a Hopkins-style diet of 80 percent fat, but my acquaintances certainly took the directive to mean the more fat, the better. Meanwhile, other fasters told me *their* doctors had said just the opposite: eat a low-fat, nearly vegetarian diet. I groaned inwardly at two sets of doctors at the same institution prescribing diets so utterly at odds. It was like finding rival sects of astronomers in a single university, one teaching Copernican celestial movement, the other Ptolemaic. Either the earth went around the sun or vice versa, but both couldn't be true.

*   *   *

I had comprised 140 pounds on check-in, and by the time I broke my fast on the ninth day, only 127 of me were left. "I want to hug you," Jennifer said on a video chat near the end, "but I think I'd break you." She had warned me years earlier that if I ever weighed less than she, she would have to divorce me. Only her pity at my depletion stopped her telling me now how close I had brought us to disunion.

I broke my fast on a small bowl of pureed apple, as I had done many times before. The first spoonful had always been a riot of flavor, but while this one was excellent, the daily honey had kept my tongue familiar with sweet things and ruled out superlatives now. The lush texture, on the other hand, was a true novelty after nine days on broth and transported me to a perhaps unbecoming rapture. For dessert I was given two cashews, but though they're my favorite nut, they were disappointingly bland. A few hours later, however, I bit into an apple that proved spectacular from the first crunch. Clearly, breaking the modified fast was a qualified bliss, like a sexual encounter with a lot of fumbling.

While packing to leave, I experienced more sensory oddity as I was overcome by a feeling of hollowness. At first it seemed to strike from nowhere, but on closer examination I discovered it originated in a realization that my everyday life lacked the tranquil composure I had enjoyed during my fast. Soon I found myself grieving the years I had spent unsettled and dis-eased, and I passed a weepy couple of hours deep in one of Mr. Pidge's psychological events. It verged on the maudlin, but the feeling wasn't false, and I didn't regret it later. Once it lifted, I was seized by an unusually clear and undreamy determination to make myself whole, to bring some of my fasting composure to my normal life. I would go back home, meditate regularly, take more spirit-filling walks in the middle of the day, and make time for the things I had for years been saying I would. It sounds like the tritest of New Year's resolutions, but somehow I knew the reform would stick this time, at least for quite a while. And so, I'm happy to report, it has mostly turned out in the years since. I think the reason is that although I had long known I was passing too much of my life unmindfully, I had never so thoroughly *felt* the pain of it, nor had I enjoyed the health to make good on whatever resolve I had. Fasting not only gave me my health back but helped me feel the loss in a new way— a bit, I suspect, as psychedelic drugs help some people make psychological breakthroughs when years of therapy and medication have not. Fasting was my psilocybin. When I walked out the doors of the clinic next morning, I felt as well in body and spirit as I'd felt in years, and I very much hoped I'd be back.

* * *

A few weeks later in Barcelona, Jennifer shaved off an expanse of my dor-
sal hair for the clinic's detox study, and after some months I got emails
with the results. The hundred of us who had given blood and urine, having fasted an average of ten days, enjoyed a vertiginous decline in the poisons inside us. The arsenic in our urine, for example, measured 28.7 µg/L
(micrograms per liter) before our fasts and 7.2 after. (Most of us soak up
arsenic from agricultural pesticides in food and from petroleum residues
in the atmosphere.) My own arsenic dropped from 5.92 to 1.13 µg/L. I
figured it had started so low either from eating organic and lower on the
food chain—plants accumulate less arsenic than animals—or from fasting
shortly before coming to the clinic. We also enjoyed modest declines in our
stock of lead and nickel, although not mercury, which remained the same.
Nearly all of my metals were too low to be detected, with the exception of
nickel, and I resolved then and there to stop eating five-cent pieces.

The study's results were both expected and exciting. Fasting doctors
had long supposed that fasting detoxified the body, but they had little
proof. One of the few trials to test the question was of sixteen Taiwanese
who had been poisoned by PCB-contaminated vegetable oil. (PCBs, poly-
chlorinated biphenyls, are used in industrial coolants.) Two to three years
after their poisoning, they still had headaches, pain in their joints and back,
numbness, skin pustules, hacking coughs, and excessive sputum. But after
a partial fast on juices of just seven to ten days, most of their symptoms
either receded or disappeared entirely. Wilhelmi de Toledo's study added
heft to the detox hypothesis, although as with her other research, a control
group would have made the finding heftier. It was possible, after all, that
we had been detoxified just from hiking in the clean Überlingen air and
basking in the presence of reincarnated Canadians.

The results of the hair study were more complicated. Most of the
heavy metals in our hair stayed the same or, in the case of lead, decreased
after our fasts, which suggested we remained detoxified weeks after
leaving the clinic. But most of the organic pesticides, like glyphosate,
increased. The cause was not known. Our fasts may have started a process of slowly expelling the pesticides, which we were still shedding
weeks later through our follicles. It was also possible we were rapidly

reacquiring pesticides as we refed, and these were showing up in our hair. More research was needed.

For the first few weeks after I returned to Barcelona, my migraines and hypersomnia stayed away, and every day was a rhapsody of feeling normal again. But little by little the familiar migrainous clenching on the left side of my face crept back, and then the fatigue did too. Once more I grew almost too weary to exercise, to write a taut sentence, to mate. When Jennifer and I video chatted with Elliott at college—ordinarily the highlight of my week—I had trouble holding my focus more than twenty minutes. Two months after Buchinger Wilhelmi, my fast was looking like an Alamo, not the San Jacinto I had sought.

I was not, however, without hope. Exasperating as the hypersomnia and migraines were, they were less severe than before, and most days I could still work several hours, be a semi-engaged husband, and stroll through the old city in the afternoon sun. Every once in a while at the heel of an evening there was even a little left over to read or people-watch on the balcony. Life was like jogging through sand, but at least it was jogging. Previously I had crawled. I hoped repeated short fasts and dietary diligence might chip away at my afflictions bit by bit, and to my immense delight they did. After three or four uphill months, the hypersomnia and migraines gradually faded, and everything returned to how it had been after my first liberating fast a year earlier. It felt another miracle.

Over the next several months, each time life took a demanding turn, I braced for the hypersomnia to pounce again, but none of the great changes of my 2020—the COVID lockdown, returning home mid-pandemic, or, trickiest of all, relearning how to cohabit with a teenager—undid my gains. It was gloriously, implausibly wonderful. I figured the wonderment would fade after a few months, but two years on, it's still there. More days than not, I still feel one of the luckiest people alive.

CHAPTER 14

WHAT THE SOVIETS KNEW

In 1880, the year Henry Tanner made his forty-day fast in New York, a thirty-eight-year-old from Haddonfield, New Jersey, began his own endurance trial under round-the-clock observation. Alas for poor Henry Clark, his performance unfolded in the Camden County Insane Asylum, just across the Delaware River from Philadelphia. Clark was said to suffer from a "dual consciousness," and during periods of "acute mania, brought on by religious excitement," he prophesied he would ascend to heaven an apostle. Occasionally he grew violent enough to need restraining, but at other times he was lucid, eager to please, and fully aware of his insanity. The psychiatry of the age amounted to little more than wait and see, but when a year and a half of waiting brought no improvement to Clark, he announced to the matron of the asylum, a Mrs. Stiles, that he would fast in search of a cure.

"I hardly credited what the man said at first, having been accustomed to hear all sorts of ideas from patients," Mrs. Stiles told a reporter. "But on the day following, Clark refused to come to the table."

Clark had gotten the idea from his brother, who also went insane and resorted to fasting, apparently receiving some benefit. But he took his fast too far and died on the fifty-first day. Clark told Mrs. Stiles "he did not intend to carry his experiment to such an extreme, but that the moment he felt it would be proper for him to break the fast he would do so."

We don't know whether Clark and his brother came to their fasts independently of Henry Tanner or if they perhaps read some of his musings on psychology. Tanner had said, for example, that he thought his mind had changed in some way during his Minneapolis and New York fasts and "that his delightful mental experiences," in the paraphrase of one reporter, "were adequate compensation for the physical tortures he suffered."

After Clark stopped eating, Mrs. Stiles and the asylum physician, a Dr. Brannin, implored him to return to table, and when that failed tried to tempt him with dainty nibbles. But day after day Clark allowed no more than a small cup or two of water to pass his lips. After twenty days, he looked a little haggard and was feeble of step but said his head felt better. Five days later, he brightened notably, and observers adjudged his mind uncommonly clear. He declared his experiment a thoroughgoing success, but still he fasted. At thirty days, Mrs. Stiles and Dr. Brannin redoubled their efforts to get him to eat, but he continued in foodless good cheer until the thirty-fifth day, when he took a turn for the worse and grew weak. Next day he was so spent he took to bed, where he remained for some days more. Matron and doctor feared he would go the way of his brother, but on the afternoon of the forty-first day, a frail Clark begged an attendant to tell Mrs. Stiles he should like a cup of coffee, and after drinking it he broke his fast on a cup of milk.

Clark refed cautiously—none of Tanner's bingeing for him. He seemed to think that if abstaining from food had cured him of his disease, maybe there was something about his diet that had made him ill in the first place. For the first week he took nothing but a cup of milk a day, and for the next three weeks his only addition was strawberries. Much pressed by Mrs. Stiles and Dr. Brannin, he subsequently added oatmeal. "Not once," a reporter marveled, "has he tasted fish, flesh, fowl or vegetables."

Asked whether she thought the fast made any change in Clark's condition, Mrs. Stiles said simply, "Well, he will probably be discharged as cured at the next meeting of the Board of Freeholders."

It was a most extraordinary tale. In a time with no cure for insanity and virtually no palliatives—no pills, no electroshocks, no talk therapy— an insane man seemed to have cured himself simply by not eating. Several prominent newspapers reported Clark's recovery, but neither doctors nor scientists were stirred to investigate, and only one learned medical journal appears to have picked up the affair—and only if you strain the definitions of "learned" and "medical." That organ was the *Phrenological Journal*, the literary arm of the pseudoscientific creed that held a person's character and intellect could be divined by measuring the lumps on his head. The editors of that fishwrap, muddled though their brains otherwise were, seemed to have understood the possibilities in Clark's story, for they titled it "Fasting as a Remedy for Insanity." But even they gave the case the shortest of squibs, and there it died.

* * *

After ridding myself of my own mental disorders through fasting, I began looking for stories of other sufferers who claimed (or whose doctors claimed for them) a similar cure. The past two centuries turned out to be lightly stippled with such narratives, including several as credible as Henry Clark's. Some of the earliest reports came from Germany. At the start of the nineteenth century, one doctor of some renown, Christoph Wilhelm Hufeland, who directed the medical college at the University of Berlin, reported curing two-thirds of his cases of madness by aggravating the abdominal nervous system, as he called it. Long before the gut-brain connection was established, Hufeland believed the stomach and intestines could influence the mind, and although he mostly aggravated them with toxins like calomel and hellebore (the latter a plant of the buttercup family that deer and rabbits are wise enough to leave alone), he also used fasting. I wasn't able to find the specifics of Hufeland's fasts, but one of his colleagues, the psychiatrist Anton Müller, wrote of two mentally disturbed patients who were cured with a near-fasting diet. One of the two patients had become mentally unbalanced after suffering epileptic attacks and languishing three years in a madhouse. But when his diet was reduced to two daily meals, each consisting of two ounces of meat and two ounces of bread, he recovered his sanity in days. Apparently he maintained his recovery for some time only to relapse when he went back to his habitual diet. The other patient was an insane adolescent who returned to sanity after being put on a similar low diet and didn't regress when returned to his usual viands.

Our acquaintance Dr. Benjamin Rush, the father of American psychiatry and a contemporary of Hufeland and Müller, was "disposed to think favorably" of low diets for the mentally ill, although he believed, fancifully, that they worked partly by diminishing the patient's blood and partly by "exciting the disease of hunger in the stomach to such a degree as to enable it to predominate over the disease of the brain." In other words, a near fast was such an ordeal, it snapped the insane back to reason.

Tales of fasting for mental illness are somewhat sparse across most of the nineteenth century, but after Henry Clark's fast in 1882 a handful of intriguing cases emerged. One was the brilliant recovery of Estella Kuenzel, a twenty-two-year-old milliner who in the summer of 1899 became so depressed she lost the will to live. She deteriorated in Philadelphia's insane asylum for three months until a friend named Henry Ritter prevailed on her family to remove her to a house under his care. Ritter was a chemist with no medical training, but he had read Edward Hooker Dewey's odes to fasting and thought a break from food might help Kuenzel, a fact he neglected to tell her parents. He didn't intend a long deprivation, but Kuenzel improved so much in her first week that neither she nor he was inclined to interrupt her healing. Ultimately she fasted forty-four days.

"I did not in the least feel tired or weak," she subsequently wrote, "but happier and brighter each day of the fast, as I could feel the effects of a new life throughout my whole body. My mind also became clearer and dizziness became a thing of the past." Life, she italicized, was once again *"joy supreme to me."* The same might be said for Henry Ritter, who married his rejuvenated friend.

Ritter went on to help dozens of others fast for as long as fifty days, and he received a mild and surprisingly thoughtful press. A writer for the Philadelphia *Public Ledger* said Kuenzel's case was one that "a judicious editor ponders in no little perplexity" because on the one hand the result spoke for itself but on the other hand "there is the danger of having a lot of ignorant or impulsive people risking their lives . . . forgetting the adage that a little knowledge is a dangerous thing, especially in therapeutics."

This was exactly right, but not many doctors took so nuanced a view. Even to medical minds expansive enough to acknowledge that fasting had likely healed Kuenzel, her experience was thought one of a kind. "I am a firm believer that in selected cases the fasting method would be efficacious," one doctor said, clearly emphasizing *selected*, "but I do not believe in its general application"—unless, he added, some respected authority first undertook a "most thorough investigation." But no investigation, most thorough or otherwise, followed.

After fasting blossomed in the early twentieth century, various practitioners reported curing mental illness through fasting. In the 1920 edition of *Macfadden's Encyclopedia of Physical Culture*, one of Bernarr Macfadden's ghostwriters said neurasthenia (an ill-defined mental disturbance coupled with fatigue) was routinely remedied by fasting patients for a week, refeeding them on a minimal diet for a week, fasting them another week, and so on until a cure was effected. "The results," the writer contended, "are little less than miraculous. The exhausted nervous system seems to gain new life and power as the elimination progresses."

Herbert Shelton later wrote that he fasted the mentally ill to good effect and that "when the insane person refuses food, this is an instinctive measure designed to assist the body in its reconstructive work.... All who have had extended experience with fasting have seen cases of insanity recover health while on the fast and many others make great improvement while fasting."

One of Shelton's contemporaries, a New York chiropractor named Robert Gross, reported the compelling case of Ms. Lynn S., a twenty-one-year-old schizophrenic who had been hospitalized, electroshocked, and drugged without finding the slightest relief. When Ms. S. checked in to Gross's Hyde Park clinic, "her behavior was illogical, bizarre, erratic, and she was ambivalent toward those trying to help." Her mental state during her fast oscillated between psychotic and normal, but after thirty-five days of fasting, her psychosis was gone. Later she fasted for eighteen, six, and fourteen days and went on to marry and have three children, "although," Gross temporized, "some intellectual and emotional limitation remain."

Virtually no researchers could be bothered to investigate such provocative anecdotes, although the University of Chicago's odd couple,

Anton Carlson and Frederick Hoelzel, touched on the topic. In the 1950s, Carlson said he was impressed that his own fasts of five to ten days alleviated his mental funks, and Hoelzel reported that his mental improvement after a fast of twenty-six days lasted about six months. The pair also said, without much specificity, that some of their human subjects enjoyed mental gains after fasting, but it apparently never occurred to them that if fasting helped people of sound mind, it might also help the unsound.

For the longest time, the only Americans to undertake a trial of fasting for mental health were a team of Missouri researchers who made a complete farce of it. In the mid-1960s, they plucked twenty-one obese schizophrenics from the St. Louis State Hospital and subjected them for ten days to what they described as a "total fast," which, however, included soft drinks of up to 180 calories a day, black coffee, multivitamins, and supplements of potassium and calcium. It was a trial less of fasting than of severe dieting on sugar, caffeine, and supplements. The patients seem not to have been consulted about their fate. Three quit after the first day, seven more dropped out over the next four days, and one who had been a firestarter before her committal set three fires on the ward before she was fingered and excused from the trial. The remaining ten patients continued sipping soda and coffee without problem, but tests showed no improvement in their mental status. The investigators concluded not that a short spell on sugar and caffeine failed to help schizophrenics but that fasting did. Fasting for mental health was at a dead end in America.

Five thousand miles to the east, however, it was blooming behind the Iron Curtain. In fact, Soviet doctors were achieving recoveries so breathtaking, their counterparts in the West would scarcely have believed them had they learned of them. To this day, they remain all but unknown outside the Russian Federation.

* * *

Born in 1905, Dr. Yuri Nikolayev grew up with the idea that fasting was restorative. His father Sergei was a writer, editor, and translator, and one of his translations was of Upton Sinclair's *The Fasting Cure*. The elder

Nikolayev and Sinclair enjoyed an illuminating correspondence, and Sinclair paid homage to his friend in his novel *Oil!* with a brief sketch of a Bolshevik student named Nikolaieff. The elder Nikolayev had probably known of fasting even before translating Sinclair, for in Russia the practice advanced much as it had in other countries, with tentative explorations by doctors in the late eighteenth century, a gradual awakening across the nineteenth century, and finally vigorous claims for its therapeutic use in the early twentieth century. The Nikolayev family fasted when sick, ate a mostly vegetarian diet, and were part of a circle of friends who did likewise. One member of that circle was Count Leo Tolstoy, who appreciated fasting as a fortifier of both body and soul. "Fasting is an indispensable condition of a good life," Tolstoy wrote. "A man may wish to be good, dream of goodness, without fasting; but in reality it is just as impossible to be good without fasting as it is to walk without getting up on one's feet." Young Yuri played on Tolstoy's knee.

Yuri hadn't intended to be a psychiatrist. He went to university to study mechanical engineering before deciding he'd rather tinker with minds than machines. To change faculties, he had to find a medical student to take his place in the engineering school, and I've sometimes wondered whether the field of engineering owes as big a debt to Nikolayev as the field of psychiatry does to that nameless engineer.

For two decades after graduating, Nikolayev practiced in the brutally conventional manner. Soviet psychiatrists of the 1940s, like their peers elsewhere, treated persistent mental disorders mainly with shocks: electroshocks that produced epileptic-like fits and insulin shocks that yielded first convulsions and then a diabetic coma, from which the patient was awakened with a glucose injection. The shocks were supposed to elicit biochemical changes in the brain that somehow unscrambled the jumbled circuitry behind the patient's derangement. But Nikolayev came to believe the unscrambling could be brought about more gently by the "inner doctor" of fasting.

The timing of his realization was woeful. It was 1948, three years after the Great Patriotic War in which countless Soviets had gone hungry and millions had died of starvation. Everyone had seen the wasted wraiths of

Auschwitz and Mauthausen, and few were prepared to hear that fasting was physiologically distinct from starvation, that it could in fact heal. But Nikolayev had a sympathetic superior at the Moscow psychiatric center where he worked, and he was permitted to fast three patients.

The results were so unpropitious, it's a wonder psychiatric fasting in the Soviet Union didn't die then and there. The first patient was a colonel, a paranoid schizophrenic who thought sinister forces were working to destroy his family. Angry, silent, and indifferent to nearly everything around him, he didn't react when Nikolayev told him his food would be stopped. When Nikolayev asked him to exercise in the hope it would help flush out the toxins behind his illness, the colonel refused. Nikolayev horrified his colleagues by forcing his patient to exert himself, but in the end it was all for naught because the colonel improved not a bit.

The second patient, of whom we know less, was the colonel's opposite. When his food was taken away, he berated his caregivers and angrily demanded its restoration. A week into the fast, he broke away from his handler, ran to a buffet, and tore into a loaf of bread. His illness didn't improve, and neither did the third patient's. The opprobrium of Nikolayev's colleagues was severe.

But Nikolayev was one of those persistent types who populate history books, the kind who, rather than quit after an early rout, ask what went wrong and set about fixing it. He decided the great flaw in his method lay not in fasting but in forcing it on uncooperative patients. At another psychiatric hospital, two understanding mentors encouraged him to try again, and this time he was in luck because he was presented with a young schizophrenic who was practically catatonic and had already refused to eat. Like Shelton, Nikolayev interpreted his patient's refusal as an instinctual attempt to heal, and he ignored his colleagues' calls to put him in an insulin coma. He let the young man continue his fast and gently encouraged him to exercise and take part in the rest of his protocol but never forced him. He counted it a small victory when the man took the briefest of walks or agreed to an enema.

Nikolayev would later write that the happiest day of his life came on the sixth day of the fast, when his patient finally spoke. It was just a few semi-coherent sentences, but that was all the confirmation Nikolayev needed that the fast was altering his mind. Day by day, he spoke a little more, and soon he was getting out of bed on his own and taking fuller part in Nikolayev's prescribed activities. After a month of fasting, he was fully recovered.

"A miracle seemed to have occurred!" Nikolayev wrote many years later. "But no, it was not a miracle, not a miracle. What occurred was the logical result of a well-thought-out method of treatment." As other suitable candidates appeared on his ward, Nikolayev fasted them too. Most were also schizophrenics, and the results were just as encouraging.

In 1952, four years into this tentative beginning, therapeutic fasting caught a break in the Soviet Union. The good fortune was the fruit not of Nikolayev's work but that of a childhood friend, one who had also grown up fasting and become a doctor and was now fasting his patients, albeit for somatic (that is, physical) rather than psychiatric conditions. Dr. Nikolai Narbekov had ventured into unconventionality as early as 1934, when, serving in the Pacific Fleet, he fasted sailors with gastrointestinal disorders for one to three days. But not until 1947, while stationed in Crimea, did Narbekov propose fasting as a first-line treatment for a range of diseases. His colleagues, openly hostile, marshaled against him the same arguments long used in the West: fasting weakened the body, wasn't scientific, was cruel.

Narbekov persisted and in 1952 won the support of the Soviet minister of health, Efim Ivanovich Smirnov. Smirnov had served as chief medical officer of the Red Army during the late war and took an interest in fasting because soldiers often had to fight on inadequate rations. Smirnov gave Narbekov twenty-five beds in a Moscow center for thermal bathing, and his patients, having failed other treatments, reportedly fasted their way to relief from asthma, pneumonia, heart problems, phlebitis (inflammation of the walls of the veins), sciatica, cholecystitis (inflammation of the gallbladder), and sundry disorders of the skin. But the program was short lived. When Smirnov left the ministry in 1953, the ward was eliminated, and Narbekov descended into a depressed alcoholism from which he never recovered. He died in 1956.

Fortune didn't neglect Soviet fasting for long, although she did bestow her favor in a curious shape. In 1955, Lev Bulganin, the son of Premier Nikolai Bulganin, showed up in the office of Yuri Nikolayev's wife, Valentina Nikolayev, who was also a psychiatrist. Lev Bulganin was hell on wheels, a spoiled and reckless aristocrat (or what passed for an aristocrat in the supposedly classless Soviet Union) whose alcoholism had survived more than one attempt at rehabilitation. He, or perhaps his father, was in search of another fix. As it happened, Valentina Nikolayev's husband had noticed that his mental patients often lost their addictions to alcohol, drugs, and tobacco during their fasts, and she referred this tinderbox Bulganin to him. It was at once the most dangerous and promising assignment of Yuri's career, one that could win him either a Siberian confinement or the favor of the most powerful man in country.

Nikolayev was relieved of his quotidian duties and sent to the premier's heavily guarded dacha to oversee the young Bulganin's fast. Mostly he made sure his charge didn't sneak off to town for a bender, but he also became a kind of elder confidant to the lonely prince, and after three weeks Bulganin dried up and lost his taste for booze. We don't know how long he maintained his sobriety, but it was long enough for his grateful father to give Nikolayev a small ward dedicated to fasting in a large psychiatric hospital in Moscow.

The contrast with midcentury America could not have been starker. In the USSR, a conventionally trained doctor with the sanction of the highest office in the land was to carry out fasting in one of the country's biggest hospitals. Meanwhile in the United States every practitioner of fasting, irregular to a one, was being harried and hounded, often out of practice and into prison. Fasting was as poised to flourish in the Soviet Union as it was to collapse in America, and over the next four decades that is just what happened.

*   *   *

Nikolayev would ultimately fast perhaps ten thousand patients. He was said to be a kindly caregiver, "unconstrained by clinical coldness" and blessed with "a warm curiosity for the soul of man, an enormous tolerance, and constant attentiveness to his patients." The stories of three of those patients suggest what his regimen could, and could not, achieve.

One young man we can call Ivan was brought to Nikolayev during a suicidal spell. Ivan had been a lively, sociable child with an infectious eagerness, but one day a teacher dressed him down for botching a lesson, and when he blushed extravagantly, a classmate cried, "What red ears and nose you have!" From then on, Ivan feared he would blush at the least provocation and that his red nose would be mocked. His curiosity and joy evaporated, he became a teenage recluse, and he thought his nose was red even when it wasn't. At university, he interpreted every look in his direction and every peal of laughter down the hallway as contempt for his nose, and he fled to a factory where the workers' faces were covered in soot. It was a kind of heaven for him, but after some years his boss told him his exceptional skills merited a transfer to a less grimy job, and he fled again.

He consulted a dermatologist, a neurologist, a psychotherapist, and a homeopath, but none saw a problem with his nose, and a couple even ridiculed him. As his despair mounted, he decided to prove he was ill by bringing an axe down on his fingers. This earned him a visit to a psychiatric hospital, but he left after five months worse than the day he entered. He tried to kill himself, first with poison, later by opening his veins, and relatives finally sent him to Nikolayev's hospital.

"I'm not crazy," Ivan told Nikolayev's staff. "I don't have delusions or hallucinations. I just have an abnormal development of the capillary network in my nose, but the doctors don't pay attention to my complaints."

Nikolayev's team paid attention. They told Ivan a fast might help him, and they didn't mind that he assumed they meant fasting would fix his capillaries. He agreed to their program, and four days in, he said the feeling of swelling in his nose that had bothered him for years was all but gone. Three days later he complained of headache, weakness, and dizziness, but those complaints quickly vanished and he said that on reflection he didn't think having a red nose was such a tragedy after all. Day by day his thoughts grew healthier, and when he broke his fast at three weeks, he had almost no abnormal views. Two weeks later he said, "Why this ridiculous idea took so much time and such prominence in my life I don't understand."

He was discharged in fine health and at his one-year follow-up was still in good form. At his two-year follow-up he was married, employed in a gas plant, and reading medicine and biology on the side. At three years, he was successfully balancing the demands of medical school with those of work and family.

*   *   *

The second patient, a schizophrenic from Central Asia whom I'll call Azim, developed a sudden fear as a young man of contracting a sexually transmitted disease. Either he had a creative notion of how such diseases are transmitted or he soon lost his grip on reality, for he became obsessed with washing his hands. He was still sane enough to know that twenty scrubbings a day were abnormal, and sought help, but the drugs his doctor prescribed did little for him. He checked in to a psychiatric hospital and received a horrific thirty insulin shocks before being discharged in a sorry state: weak, hands trembling, and with a new phobia of the number 1 because Department 1 had been the hospital's most fearsome. Later he became phobic of the numbers 4 and 9, and after another hospitalization he added to his fears the number 10, the letter C, the church, and the cross. By then, Azim's life was a misery of hygiene. He touched nothing he didn't have to, insisted his mother feed him with a spoon, and became terrified on reading a Jack London novel that the leprosy of one of its characters could be transmitted to him through the pages. He passed each night from 10 p.m. to 1 a.m. in a relentless ritual of scrubbing.

Ten deteriorating years into this neurosis, Azim arrived at Nikolayev's ward and agreed to fast. He had a rocky time of it. His hunger was intense, and after a week his schizophrenic symptoms reached new heights. He washed endlessly, all the while fearing that water drops splashing off the sink would convey germs to his skin. His hunger, whose origin must have been psychological rather than physical, finally passed after ten days, but his schizophrenia persisted. When nurses came to his room, he covered his head with blankets to guard against their germs, and if he saw an orderly mopping a floor, he beat a retreat lest cancer, leprosy, or trachoma splatter off the mop and onto him.

Most patients who recovered under Nikolayev began to do so during their fast, with the peak of their recovery coming two to three months into refeeding. But twenty days of fasting brought almost no change to Azim. Nor did the start of refeeding, which he did on juices. But the first day he took solid food, he went to bed without washing. "On the third day," he recalled, "I touched door handles myself, and again went to bed without washing. On the fourth day I stopped the doctor in the corridor and said with delight I was perfectly healthy. I ran my hands along the floor and over his face. I knew it was unhygienic, but I overcame my feeling of squeamishness—I wanted to prove I had gotten rid of my fears."

By the time Azim was discharged, he was fully recovered. Nikolayev sent him home with the same instructions he gave all his patients: follow a vegetarian diet similar to that used by fasting doctors in America and Germany, and make short, repeated maintenance fasts. For a time all went well, but one day Azim crushed a spider and became disgusted by its oozing innards, and from that moment he grew afraid once more of contracting disease. He tumbled back into his obsessive washing and eventually returned to Moscow for another fast. This time fasting freed him of his affliction much more quickly—a common occurrence among Nikolayev's repeat fasters, as if the body, having once fasted, knew what to do.

Azim wanted to know why he had relapsed, and Nikolayev thought he had an answer. Fasting was a powerful therapy, but he believed the vegetarian diet was at least as critical, although he couldn't say why. What he could say was that his patients who went back to meat, fried and salty foods, alcohol, tobacco, coffee, or even overly strong tea often relapsed. The maintenance fasts of three to five days, up to ten total days a month, were also essential. Azim, in his joy at being restored to normality, had neglected this regimen.

Nikolayev sometimes told a cautionary tale about the relative merits of fasting and diet. Its protagonist was a sixty-eight-year-old who came to him with a grim potpourri of maladies: cerebral atherosclerosis, cerebrospinal syndrome, chronic coronary insufficiency, postinfarction cardiosclerosis, atrial fibrillation, emphysema, and pneumosclerosis. Nikolayev had been astounded to learn the man was a devotee of fasting who for forty years had regularly gone without food for three to eight days. But he had also consumed enormous quantities of meat and alcohol and had fasted in hope of balancing his indulgent lifestyle. No amount of fasting, Nikolayev believed, could level a scale so weighted with gluttony.

Azim had not been nearly that decadent. He had simply neglected the vegetarian diet and maintenance fasts, but such was the depth of his illness that even a modest straying from discipline was enough to do him in. He left the fasting ward a second time vowing reform.

*   *   *

The third patient was a schizophrenic named Valery who came to Nikolayev at the age of twenty-two, having fallen into a hypochondriacal hell similar to that of red-nosed Ivan. In a high school anatomy class, Valery learned about the disorder of the pituitary gland called acromegaly, which we learned of in chapter 12, the one that causes hands, feet, and certain facial features to grow to exaggerated prominence. Valery had a slightly protruding jaw that he decided was acromegalic, and he became convinced that classmates, family, doctors, and even strangers on the street loathed his hideousness but pretended not to notice it. He didn't think he was mentally ill. He just had an obvious physical disorder that everyone affected not to acknowledge.

"Well, if you consider yourself sick," Nikolayev said, "and you agree to therapeutic fasting, we will treat you and hope it will help you."

Valery agreed, and his delusion vanished during his fast. After his discharge, he returned to university and became an art historian at a museum in Moscow. For eleven years, he lived a full and seemingly happy life, but when his father died prematurely, previous stresses became magnified, and something in him snapped. His schizophrenia reemerged, this time manifesting as paranoia rather than hypochondria. He blamed his mother for his father's death, thought a coworker was trying to get him arrested, and abused another colleague for taking credit for one of his discoveries. Three years into this descent, Valery sliced open his wrists but was found before he bled out and brought back to Nikolayev.

Unlike with Azim, Nikolayev found little fault in Valery's diet or habits. He had, it seemed, simply been overwhelmed by years of untended psychological troubles that surfaced after his father's death. Valery fasted thirty days, and once more his illness completely receded. He left the hospital in good form, patched things over with his mother, returned to the museum, and passed thirty more years without relapse. It was, so far as we know, a happy conclusion, but Nikolayev drew a more guarded inference. Fasting, he said, couldn't cure schizophrenia. At best, it sent it into remission, and some remissions were more fragile than others. The best chance for long-term success was to adopt not just a vegetarian diet and periodic maintenance fasts but also some kind of psychological therapy. Life's buffetings were perilous to the battered souls who left his ward, and nothing short of constant vigilance and psychological upkeep could preserve their sanity.

*   *   *

Every case had its own trajectory, but Nikolayev noticed certain patterns. During the first week without food, the symptoms of the disease often intensified, as happened with the obsessive washer Azim. But they usually began to dissipate after about ten days, at which point patients became calmer, almost sedated. Before thirty days were up, the last of their deliriums, hallucinations, and other troubles usually disappeared, their tongues became clear, and their foul fasting breath vanished. Often their skin acquired a healthy glow and they developed a "wolf's appetite." Refeeding—first on juices, then fruit and yogurt, next cooked vegetables and boiled grains, and finally other plants and milk—made patients calmer still, although many were understandably elated with their newfound health.

By 1970, Nikolayev had fasted about fifteen hundred mental patients, three-quarters of whom were schizophrenic and nearly all of whom had failed other treatments. Despite so hopeless a pool, he reported restoring nearly 70 percent of them to full functioning. At their six-year follow-up, half of the cured were still cured, and another 15 percent maintained part of their remission. (In the Soviet Union, mental patients were followed for up to ten years after their hospital discharge, with visits from doctors at both home and work.) Nikolayev believed two factors best predicted long-term success: how closely his patients followed the vegetarian diet and how long they had been sick before their fast. For the most common types of schizophrenia, 80 to 90 percent of his patients enjoyed complete, long-term remissions if the disease was caught very early and they stuck to the diet. For those who had been sick up to two years before treatment, the remission rate dropped to 70 percent; for those sick five years, 50 percent. He also found that some schizophrenias were more resistant to treatment than others. For example, fewer than 40 percent of paranoid schizophrenics enjoyed substantial improvement over the long term, although oddly enough they usually did quite well during the fast itself. Even 40 percent, however, was a great improvement on other therapies.

These kinds of numbers earned Nikolayev official support, and by the early 1970s his fasting unit grew to eighty beds and a staff of ten physicians, which, however, was still a tiny part of the vast Moscow Psychiatric Institute, with its three thousand beds and five hundred physicians. In 1973, he published a book, *Fasting for Health*, to bring his quarter century of knowledge to the public. It sold two hundred thousand copies and was translated into Japanese, Bulgarian, and Greek but not English or any other widely spoken language of the West. That same year, the Soviet government granted a request he had long sought: an expansion of his fasting program to somatic disorders.

From the beginning, Nikolayev had observed that when his psychiatric patients fasted, they often lost their physical illnesses, and he was of course familiar with the somatic work of his late friend Nikolai Narbekov. But conventional Soviet doctors who treated somatic disorders were no more eager to subject their patients to fasting than conventional American doctors were, and the small unit of twenty beds that Nikolayev was granted for somatic diseases struggled to find favor and was disbanded after just four years. Fortunately, successor units sprang up elsewhere, and in the

1980s thousands of Soviets fasted in Moscow and Leningrad for a range of conditions that read like the index to *Gray's Anatomy*: arthritis, asthma, benign prostatic hyperplasia, bronchitis, cerebral atherosclerosis, cholecystitis, colitis, coronary artery disease, diabetes, eczema, gastritis, glomerulonephritis, gout, hives, migraine, pancreatitis, psoriasis, Raynaud's disease, stomach ulcers, and umpteen more conditions. For many of these disorders, doctors reported rates of success approximating those in Nikolayev's mental patients: roughly two-thirds of their patients got substantial relief.

The doctors compiled masses of data and wrote scores, maybe hundreds, of clinical reports testifying to fasting's efficacy. In one retrospective study of 700 asthmatics, 65 percent of patients demonstrated good to excellent near-term results after a three-week fast, 25 percent showed satisfactory results, and half maintained complete remissions for the long term. Pulmonologists in Leningrad discovered that when the spasms of asthmatics stopped during a fast (typically after about twelve days), their mastocytes underwent a remarkable change. Mastocytes are bronchial cells that in asthmatics become overly rich in allergy-fighting histamines, but as the airways of the fasting asthmatics opened, their mastocytes emptied of histamines, which partly explained the relief they enjoyed. In another paper, doctors reported that 75 percent of patients with sarcoidosis of the lungs (a growth of inflammatory cells that causes scarring and labored breathing) improved after an average fast of two weeks. Most of the patients maintained their improvement through a one-year follow-up. Although the studies were almost always uncontrolled, unblinded, and not peer-reviewed, they probably represent the largest set of clinical observations about fasting ever gathered. Today most of them are moldering in archives, and the few that have found their way to the internet haven't been translated from the Russian. Whatever insights they hold remain nearly as hidden from the West as if the Iron Curtain had never fallen.

Within the USSR, though, the studies helped Nikolayev win another victory he had long pursued: the establishment, in 1984, of a freestanding clinic and research center dedicated solely to fasting. No longer would fasting be confined to the small wards he and colleagues had carved out of larger hospitals against the opposition of other doctors.

Nikolayev hoped the Scientific Center for Medical Fasting in Leningrad would be the first of many around the Soviet Union, but in fact it was one of fasting's last hurrahs.

The turning point had actually come a few years earlier, in 1981, when a pair of Nikolayev's colleagues at the Moscow Psychiatric Institute led a two-week fasting walk through two hundred miles of Ural foothills. Nikolayev had long argued that fasting was not only a cure for the ill but a safeguard for the healthy, and the walk was meant to suggest that vigorous health could be maintained without food. The trekkers demonstrated that much but also kicked up quite a controversy. According to one report, one of the USSR's leading nutritionists was an opponent of fasting, and at his instigation the director of the Moscow Psychiatric Institute censured Nikolayev for fasting healthy people who had no need of the therapy. Nikolayev, then in his late seventies, was no longer in charge of the fasting unit in Moscow, but the criticism took, and within a couple of years he was forced to retire and the unit was shuttered.

For a time the country's other fasting clinics, including the center in Leningrad, continued to fast patients, but two forces combined to do them in. One was perestroika. After Mikhail Gorbachev opened the Soviet Union to Western-style "reforms" in the mid-1980s, many state assets were sold to modern-day robber barons, and what remained of the state health-care system came under intense pressure to cut costs. Doctors were pushed to provide more "efficient" care, which meant minimizing the time they spent with patients, which in turn left scant room for fasting. The other destructive force, medication, antedated perestroika. When neuroleptic drugs were invented in the 1950s, Soviet psychiatrists took to prescribing them as fondly as psychiatrists anywhere. Neuroleptics helped many patients only in the near term, failed to help others at all, and had severe side effects, but they were easy to administer, cheaper than hospitalization, and far more humane than shocks. As better drugs emerged, the partiality to pills only grew, and when this preference met perestroika's pressure for a quick fix, the laborious practice of psychiatric fasting was in deep trouble. A similar story could be told of fasting for somatic illnesses. Shortly after the Soviet Union fell apart in 1991, the Russian government abandoned both the study and practice of therapeutic fasting as expensive and unnecessary. After forty-three years, fasting's exceptional run under the Kremlin was nearly at an end.

*　　*　　*

But Nikolayev wasn't quite done yet. Despite fasting's decline, the minister of health in the Russian Republic of Buryatia was a fasting enthusiast who thought Nikolayev's method just the thing to rejuvenate his people and the fading resort town of Goryachinsk. In 1994, Nikolayev traveled to Goryachinsk, which rises from the comely shore of Siberia's Lake Baikal, and fell in love with the tranquil setting. He agreed to help establish a fasting center and train its first doctors. With the warm support of the republican government, the little center thrived and has since fasted perhaps twenty thousand people. Most come today to lose weight, but a substantial minority fast for angina, diabetes, asthma, high blood pressure, or eczema. Sadly, in recent years the support of the republic has been inconstant, the program has contracted, and in 2019 some of the center's buildings were put up for sale. The remaining days of the only sizable fasting outpost in Russia may be few.

Nikolayev was spared witnessing the downturn, having died in 1998 at the age of ninety-two, able to do yoga on his head until near the end.

*　　*　　*

There was a brief moment in the 1970s when scientists in the West might have been moved to explore Nikolayev's method. The opening arose from the curiosity of an American psychiatrist named Allan Cott, who somehow heard of Nikolayev's work and traveled to Russia to observe it. Cott was amazed by several "miraculous" cures he witnessed, including one of a nuclear scientist whose senile psychosis was so severe that, as Cott wrote, "he could not recall his own name. But after an extended fast his memory was completely restored and he regained full possession of his intellectual powers."

Cott went home and fasted thirty-five schizophrenics over three years at New York's Gracie Square Hospital. All of them had been diseased for at least five years and had failed numerous other treatments, but after an average fast of twenty-five days, most got well. In 1974, Cott reported two of his first patients were still healthy after four years and ten of his more recent patients remained well after two years. He agreed with Nikolayev that a vegetarian diet and monthly maintenance fasts were essential for long-term recovery and said three of his patients who neglected the protocol relapsed but returned to health after a second fast and more rigorous maintenance. It was promising stuff, but the promise was never fulfilled.

"Unfortunately," Cott wrote Nikolayev, "I was not able to establish therapeutic fasting at Gracie Square Hospital. The new director feared he would get into trouble with the state department of health if he allowed me 'a new, drug-free, experimental treatment.' How strange! Fasting is called 'the new experimental treatment,' despite abundant evidence of its safety and efficacy and the fact that we have thousands of years of experience using it. And yet the same doctors who say this prescribe 2000 mg of chlorpromazine or other potent psychotropic drugs with acute side effects."

Cott's work did not go entirely unremarked. A few obscure journals and a scattering of newspapers ran articles, the most important of which appeared on the front page of the *Los Angeles Times*. But this modest publicity sparked only a couple of other North American psychiatrists to dabble in fasting, and scientists paid no attention at all. So far as I could tell, in only one country beyond Russia were studies of psychiatric fasting ever conducted. (I'm discounting the farcical Missouri trial.) A group of Japanese doctors in the 1960s and 1970s fasted patients for ten days and reported remission rates as high as 86 percent for depression and 82 percent for other mental illnesses. But as in Russia, fasting in Japan was no competition for pills, and the uncontrolled trials were never expanded on with more thorough experiments. For more than a generation, fasting for psychiatric health has been a dead letter everywhere.

* * *

A happier ending could be fermenting. In the 1980s and 1990s, as scientific interest in fasting suddenly sprouted, a small number of researchers began looking into what fasting does to the brain and discovered—to the surprise of nobody familiar with the practice—that it becomes healthier when fasted. Partly this is because fasting does for the brain what it does for the rest of the body: downregulating the pro-aging gene-regulatory pathways, decreasing insulin and inflammatory cytokines, repairing DNA, and increasing autophagy. But fasting also induces changes specific to the brain that scientists are just starting to understand. One of the most important seems to be the boost fasting gives to brain-derived neurotrophic factor (BDNF), a protein that helps us grow new neurons, maintain the neurons we've already got, and form new synapses between them. BDNF, which was discovered only in 1982, is essential for learning and memory, and it's no coincidence that people with some of the most dreaded neurodegenerative diseases—Alzheimer's, Huntington's, Parkinson's, multiple sclerosis—tend to be desperately short of it. Scientists have discovered that when we fast, one of the ketones we release, beta-hydroxybutyrate (BHB), stimulates the brain to make BDNF, which in turn stimulates the creation of new neurons, synapses, and mitochondria. These last are the proverbial powerhouses of the cell, and healthier powerhouses make for healthier brains.

In lab animals, these and other fasting-induced changes have been shown to sharpen the mind. When scientists fasted vinegar flies, they became more skilled at creating long-term memories. (You test a fly's memory by giving it a tasty reward or an irksome deterrent cued to a particular circumstance and later repeat the cue to see if the fly remembers how to get the carrot or avoid the stick.) When researchers fasted mice every other day for several months, the mice learned new tasks better than their free-eating peers, and when mice were fasted every other day for nearly a year, they got through mazes more quickly and responded more prudently to threats. Old rats who ate every other day for three months learned to swim a water maze faster and remembered it better. In humans, comparable trials have only just begun, but in one ongoing experiment, when people at risk of cognitive impairment did a modified fast of two days a week for several weeks, their verbal fluency and executive function seemed to improve.

Fasting has also been shown to protect animal brains from a wide range of degenerative diseases. In mice with a mutation that leads to Alzheimer's, every-other-day fasters had better short-term memory and learning as they aged, even though their brains still developed the plaques and tangles that characterize the disease. In mice who were fasted every other day for three months and then afflicted with a Parkinson's-like syndrome, their neurons were far more resistant to degeneration, and they had fewer motor problems. In a similar experiment in rhesus monkeys, a combination of caloric restriction and daily fasting (in the form of a very narrowed feeding window) failed to save them from Parkinson's, but compared to normally fed monkeys, they had fewer motor impairments, a greater quantity of the pleasure-producing neurotransmitter dopamine, and more of the neurotrophic factor GDNF, which promotes the survival of neurons. In yet another experiment, mice with a mutation for Huntington's disease who were fasted every other day showed less neural degeneration, less motor dysfunction, and less muscle wasting than normally fed mice. They also lived longer.

Fasting has also recently been shown to protect against strokes and their aftermath. When scientists gave fasted mice an ischemic stroke by blocking one of their cerebral arteries, they suffered far less damage to their brains than normally fed mice, with fewer dead neurons and neurological deficits. The researchers speculated that fasting made their neurons more skilled at guarding against and repairing stroke damage in roughly the same way fasting protected Valter Longo's healthy cells from chemotherapy—in effect by telling them to kneel behind their shields and then prioritizing reconstruction.

What goes for stroke goes for concussion. When researchers surgically concussed adult rats and then fasted them just twenty-four hours, they had less neural damage, less cognitive decline, and better-functioning neural mitochondria than normally fed rats. The NFL should take note. So should other researchers. One group of scientists who reviewed these and related studies concluded that since we have no effective treatments to heal the concussed or stroked brain, it would be "prudent" to test fasting in humans after brain trauma.

To my thinking, it would be far more than prudent. It would be the only decent thing to do. But since no pharmaceutical company can make money off fasting, and since decency to patients is so infrequently the determining motive for funding research, I wouldn't bet the back forty on trials anytime soon.

* * *

None of the above experiments bears immediately on mental health, but I cite them because they show fasting protects the brain in myriad ways, which, in the near absence of research on psychiatric fasting, is about all we've got. Among the very few studies to look directly at fasting for mental health is one in mice, half of whom were fed normally while the other half were fasted daily and fed a calorically restricted diet. All of the mice were tested periodically in an elevated-plus maze, which isn't a maze at all but rather a platform in the shape of a plus sign elevated two feet off the ground. Two of the platform's arms are lined with guardrails, the other two are open to the drop, and anxious mice will spend more time in the safety of the railed arms while calm ones will venture onto the unrailed planks. Young mice are pretty fearless, and the ones in the experiment spent plenty of time in the open arms whether they ate freely or were on the fasting regimen. As mice age, they become more anxious, and when the free-eaters in the trial grew old, they spent much more time cowering behind the guardrails. The fasters, however, spent only a bit more time there. Apparently their fasting and diet made them less anxious.

A similar effect was demonstrated in aged rhesus monkeys. After years of either fasting and caloric restriction or normal eating, they were subjected to "aversive contexts" like being put in restraints or placed alone in a new cage in an unfamiliar place. The normal eaters freaked under the duress, but the fasted monkeys remained fairly calm. To make sure the fasters' brains hadn't simply been dulled by their dietary regimen, the researchers ran other tests and found the fasters were just as active, attentive, and attuned to their surroundings as the normal eaters. MRIs showed that parts of the monkeys' brains that were involved in emotional regulation—the prefrontal cortex, hippocampus, amygdala, and hypothalamus—were larger and denser in the fasters than in the normal eaters, possibly because the fasters had been making less of the stress hormone cortisol, which can shrink the brain.

Scientists expect similar effects will someday be demonstrated in humans, but we know already that fasting increases several mood-lifting molecules in which the mentally ill are often deficient, including neuro-trophic factors like BDNF, hormones like endorphins, and neurotrans-mitters like serotonin (whose increased circulation Prozac stimulates) and endocannabinoids (your body's own cannabis). But discoveries that translate into therapy probably lie well in the future, in part because the field isn't crawling with discoverers. More scientists are needed to carry the work forward.

Doctors needn't wait for more bench science. For three-quarters of a century we've known how to safely fast—and heal—psychiatric patients. What's needed now are more Nikolayevs. For want of an American doc-tor of his perception and persistence, I endured half a lifetime of grief, and the same goes today for countless others in my mentally ill clan. I wrote this chapter in the hope that a few doctors, of whatever nationality, would decide their careers were better spent picking up where Nikolayev left off rather than prescribing pills to yet another generation. We have the knowl-edge. All that's wanting is the courage to use it.

CHAPTER 15

A WINE COUNTRY ABSTENTION, 1

No patient, I will hazard, has ever arrived at the TrueNorth Health Center in Santa Rosa, California, and mistaken it for a New World outpost of the thoughtfully designed and meticulously tended Buchinger Wilhelmi Clinic. America's oldest fasting clinic, indeed the country's only one of any girth, is housed in a converted apartment compound built in an era when the motto of suburban developers everywhere was "Just how crummy can we get away with?" Its two stories—sided above, bricked below in the manner of an Allentown split-level—are fronted by a too-shallow eave whose ersatz colonial columns are meant to transmit an air of history but waft only cheapness. It's a building you could walk by a hundred times without seeing.

TrueNorth is domiciled thus because its founder, Dr. Alan Goldhamer, keeps the rates low in hope people will stay long enough to get well, which in turn bolsters the studies he conducts to prove fasting's worth. At the time Jennifer and I visited, the tariff hadn't been raised in thirteen years. For $199 a night, the single guest got not only a room and educational programs but, if she wasn't fasting, three all-you-can-eat meals and a twenty-four-hour salad bar. The price was so low for spendy Northern California that business travelers occasionally lodged there in preference to nearby hotels, which could not compete.

It was all very noble, but in our two weeks in residence in the summer of 2021 I felt wistful for Überlingen every time my eyes ran across the torn window screen in our bedroom, the wall art bought in volume from Kmart, or the stained and mismatched grout in the shower. At Buchinger Wilhelmi every exquisite door handle and tasteful lampshade said, "You deserve to be looked after," but at TrueNorth the guests had with cause given the joint the moniker "The Last Resort." Few came unless they had first tried to fix their health elsewhere and failed. The desperate will endure a lot for relief.

Jennifer and I planned a fast of nine and a half days followed by four and half days refeeding. Although the previous year had been one of my healthiest—my hypersomnia and depression dispelled, my migraines all but extinct, my energy boundless—I had, on returning to Colorado from Spain, developed a minor but persistent gastrointestinal disturbance. It announced itself in a cloud of gas and the occasional dash to the commode, and soon I was passing more of my day in the privy than I strictly cared for. For months of nights I dutch-ovened Jennifer with undercover flatulence. The whole-house ventilator ran round the clock.

A stool test revealed I had too many of the wrong bacteria in my intestines, which prompted a gastroenterologist I consulted to declare, "The vegan diet is *not* good for the gut." Perhaps not incidental to that imbecility, he wore cowboy boots, which are an affectation in an office job, and boasted on his website of tormenting calves on the family ranch. It's true an abrupt switch from a low-fiber diet to high-fiber veganism can kick up a lot of gas, but a gradual transition usually avoids the problem, and anyway I had done fine—better than fine—for quite a while as a vegan. I suggested to this Hippocrates that the problem in my viscera more likely originated in some aspect of my return from the Mediterranean to the Rockies, but he kicked the suggestion aside like an unruly calf and told me to try a special diet low in fermentable foods or, failing that, probiotics. I tried both but enjoyed only modest improvement. A subsequent colonoscopy—a gift to self on turning fifty—gave no clue why my bowels weren't improving.

I called Dr. Goldhamer, who said a fast of two weeks, with a third week for refeeding, might help. Unable to spare quite that much time, I did as I had before Buchinger Wilhelmi—jump-starting the visit to

TrueNorth by fasting on my own for a week, then refeeding a week. I felt halfway improved by the time we showed up in Santa Rosa.

Jennifer, for her part, had nothing to cure save a slightly inflamed shoulder from a spill on ice the previous winter. She is one of those frustrating people who never has to contend with troubled sleep, low energy, or mental troughs, and she has been in offensively fine health for half a century, which, however, has left her plenty of time to take care of me.

* * *

Intimacy is compulsory at TrueNorth, where the seventy or so guests are squeezed into a couple dozen two- or three-bedroom apartments, strangers rooming with strangers. Jennifer and I passed half the drive from San Francisco to Santa Rosa speculating about our flatmates, and the suspense was hardly lessened by our encounter with the first of them. As we surveyed the spartan living room of our new quarters, luggage at our side, two young women burst through the front door, scurried past us with neither a glance nor a word in our direction, disappeared down the hall, and slammed the door of their room with a resounding finality. This scene was replayed in various ways over the next day and a half, and I never ceased to marvel at how they had mastered the art of avoiding all eye contact. Eventually one of them nearly toppled Jennifer in a tight hallway, which gave my wife a unique opportunity to introduce herself.

"Oh, uh—" her new acquaintance elocuted. "Oh!"

Several fuddled moments followed before she cast a tentative eye in Jennifer's direction, which seemed to cause a gear to turn. After a few more beats, she remembered the polite thing to do was to offer her name in reply. After that, we got eye contact and pleasant-enough nods but hardly more than four words out of either of them.

Not that they were quiet. Each night they and three or four guests from other suites would wait until precisely 10:01, just over the border of the mandatory 10 p.m. quiet time, before gathering in their bedroom for long sessions of chortling, howling, and other sonorous night music. Every syllable passed through our walls, which were a wonder of engineering in that they somehow held up the ceilings despite being made of tissue paper. I was gratified to learn the women were from Orange County, a locality where I have rarely passed an enjoyable hour and which, in my limited experience, routinely gives the world such exempla of affability and consideration as our roommates.

After four days the cacklers were replaced by a business executive with a thick Noo Yawk accent who was a 350-pound teddy bear with us but who spent half the day on blaring speakerphoned calls reaming subordinates for such grievous sins as dropping a comma from the quarterly report. He swore with the most terrific invention, and he considerately shared his linguistic innovations to the fullest by keeping his door wide open. *His* quiet-hours fetish was war movies at volume. He was, he told us, staying a month. In nearly four decades of fasting patients, TrueNorth hadn't killed one yet, but Jennifer and I held out hope.

The patient in the third bedroom of our flat was another story altogether: a sweet, frail professor of health sciences in her sixties or seventies who, unfortunately for my bigotry, gave Orange County a better name. (Half of TrueNorth's clientele was from California, mostly southern, while a third came from other states and the remainder from abroad.) By her own admission, she was deeply terrified of water fasting. She had been raised in countries where food had been rationed and never recovered from the trauma of missing meals, but she was in such poor health that she wanted to give fasting a try. At the time of our arrival, she had been at the clinic three weeks and was booked for three more but so far hadn't succeeded in fasting more than four days straight before fear overcame her. Most days she drank thick green juices, as did other patients whose physical or mental health precluded fasting. We never learned what her trouble was, but she moved as gingerly as any resident of a nursing home and spent long hours in her room abed.

The rest of our fellow fasters, whom we encountered mostly in the compound's sunny courtyard, were a more downmarket lot than the Buchinger Wilhelmi crowd. They were teachers and secretaries, strategic planners and homemakers, engineers and tech entrepreneurs, a truck driver, a former White House Fellow, a social worker, a carpenter, and a nonagenarian portrait painter. We talked less of Porsches and yachts than of children and pets, hometowns and home renovations, the power of faith (always with the parochial certainty that the listener shared the speaker's), and of course food and health. Jennifer and I met only one certifiable one-percenter during our stay, a woman of middle years from Bel Air who complained that the previous summer she had drunk her way through the social circuit on Martha's Vineyard with such abandon that by Labor Day she felt sick to her stomach. I thought her poor health a physical manifestation of her soul since the party-hard summer to which she referred was 2020, the season of COVID restrictions. She was at TrueNorth before this summer's saturnalia for a preparatory cleanse.

"I'm just doing a week on juices," she said and hastened to add, "No fasting. And I'm *not* becoming a crazy vegan or anything."

We got along gangbusters.

If there was a typical guest, she was sixtyish, female, overweight, and ill. A lucky minority had only their weight to lose, and the luckiest of all, also the fewest, had come, as Jennifer had, simply to maintain their health. The snug courtyard and its inhabitants constituted a homely and comfortable galaxy, and throughout our stay two stars shone brighter than all others. One was Dr. Goldhamer. The other were his cures, which, in the argot of his boarders, were never less than "miracles."

*   *   *

Alan Goldhamer was born in 1959 and raised in Long Beach, just south of Los Angeles. He discovered fasting during a youthful quest to improve his physique with an eye to beating his best friend at basketball. Later, at a health food store where he worked, he happened upon the writings of Herbert Shelton, just as Françoise Wilhelmi de Toledo had a few years earlier in a health food store halfway around the world. Shelton's idea that health results from healthful living was the most sensible thing young Goldhamer had heard on the topic, and at the age of sixteen he decided to make a fifty-year experiment of clean diet, moderate exercise, and good sleep. Forty-seven years into it, he reports excellent health and gives outward evidence of it, his face nearly unlined, his figure trim, his eyes peppy. Unfortunately, his best friend, Doug Lisle, adopted similar measures, maintained his health, and continues to beat him on the court. Lisle is the house psychologist at TrueNorth and the coauthor of Goldhamer's first book, *The Pleasure Trap*. They still play basketball nearly every week.

Goldhamer's choice of career was settled by two events in his youth. One was a conversation with the fasting doctor Gerald Benesh, whose many arrests we learned about briefly in chapter 9. Goldhamer sought out Benesh after asking the healthiest-looking shoppers in the health food store how they stayed so hale. Several said they followed the advice of Dr. Benesh, who was then practicing in San Diego. When Goldhamer drove down the coast and asked Benesh about his work, the elder chiropractor said, "It's the best job in the whole world. The patient does all the work, the body does all the healing, and all the doctor has to do is take credit for the good result."

"*That*," Goldhamer thought, "is the job for me."

The other formative event was Goldhamer's announcement to his family at his next birthday party that he intended to become a chiropractor like Benesh. A hush fell over the table. The Goldhamers were the sort of progressive Jews whose young were encouraged to go to any college they wanted and study any field they liked so long as the letters on the diploma eventually read MD or JD. Goldhamer's uncle was an MD of firm and conventional opinion, and as veins bulged from his neck, he raged that no one in the family was even allowed to *see* a chiropractor, let alone become one.

"Better you should be a Communist spy!" he thundered.

After the party, Goldhamer's father pulled his child aside and said, "Son, I don't know anything about alternative medicine, but anything that makes that man that mad—it can't be bad."

With that benediction, Goldhamer took a degree in 1983 from Western States Chiropractic College (now the University of Western States), one of the oldest chiropractic institutions in the world, and then trained in Sydney under Dr. Alec Burton at the Arcadia Health Centre. Shelton's retirement left Burton the most experienced practitioner of water fasting in the world, and Goldhamer was awed by the supposedly intractable diseases he saw reversed under him. Time and again he found himself thinking, "If this one gets better, I'll believe it. . . . OK, if *this* one gets better, I'll really believe it." Nearly all of them got better.

He returned to California and in 1984 established the Center for Conservative Therapy, the forerunner of TrueNorth, in Sonoma County. The seed money for the clinic was literal seed money, proceeds from a sprout-growing business he had started in high school, which had also put him through college. To open a fasting shop in the beating heart of California wine country was to follow in the contrary footsteps of Shelton with his clinic in the middle of longhorn country. For many years Goldhamer's little operation grew quite slowly, its modest ranch house rarely hosting more than a handful of patients at a time. But fortuitously for both Goldhamer and the future of fasting in America, one of the early patients was T. Colin Campbell, an esteemed professor of nutritional biochemistry at Cornell who was on his way to becoming one of the fathers of the modern whole-food vegan movement.

Campbell is best known today for his seminal book *The China Study*, which has sold more than two million copies since its publication in 2005. In the titular study, Campbell and colleagues discovered that people in poorer parts of China who ate a traditional diet of rice and unprocessed vegetables were largely protected from certain cancers, while people in wealthier areas who adopted a Westernized diet of meat, dairy, eggs, and highly processed foods had soaring cancer rates rivaling those of Western countries. It was one of the biggest epidemiological studies ever performed—possibly the biggest—and was a clarion call for a diet of unprocessed plants. It was also a posthumous vindication of Dr. Catherine Kousmine.

But when Campbell met Goldhamer, much of that lay in the future and Campbell's own health was in a bad way. Early in his career, Campbell had been the first scientist to isolate dioxin, the compound that makes Agent Orange so ghastly, and had poisoned himself in the process. Decades later his blood still contained disturbingly high levels of the stuff, and in the 1980s it gave him a disorder called dystonia, which caused the muscles of his throat to contract involuntarily. He began to lose the ability to speak, and an eminent neurologist at Cornell said that within a year he would be unable to utter a word. An equally prominent neurologist at Columbia showed him how to perform an emergency tracheotomy with a penknife that he was to carry at all times if he wished to save himself from choking to death.

In 1991, Campbell was invited to lecture the American Natural Hygiene Society (today called the National Health Association), the group that Shelton and colleagues founded in 1948. He told his would-be hosts he was no longer much of a speaker, but they said to come anyway and added that their doctors—who, they promised, weren't like any he'd ever met—might have some novel ideas about his dystonia. Campbell stumbled through the speech and then was examined by ten or so hygienists, including Goldhamer and his mentor Alec Burton. Their consensus was that a fast might rid him of his toxic load and help with his dystonia.

Campbell was frankly dubious of therapeutic fasting, but he was impressed with the doctors' knowledge and Goldhamer's keen interest in the science of fasting, and as he had nothing else left to try, he flew to Sonoma and fasted twelve days. He improved only slightly, but he saw other patients get well, and a year later he returned with his wife for a fast of ten days. Her asthma, which had dogged her for years, went away completely, never to return, but again he improved hardly at all.

He nonetheless followed Goldhamer's post-fast prescription, which squared with his own research, to eat a diet of minimally processed plants free of added salt, oil, and sugar—what Goldhamer calls an SOS-free, whole-plant diet, the one I adopted in chapter 7. Six months later, Campbell noticed something changing in the musculature of his throat. Soon his speaking grew easier, and over the next three or four months he regained, by his estimate, ninety-five percent of his lost ability. He believed his two fasts, unproductive though they seemed at the time, had in fact triggered a healing mechanism that his body carried forward as he ate foods that abetted rather than interfered with the healing process.

Goldhamer was as gratified as his patient for the cure, possibly even a little more so, because he had an ulterior motive for making Campbell a believer in fasting. He had long thought that if fasting were ever to gain wider acceptance, it needed to stand on firmer scientific footing, and he had been collecting data from his patients with the aim of publishing the more noteworthy outcomes in peer-reviewed scientific journals. That, however, was a tall order for a chiropractor, but it might not be quite so tall if the byline included the name T. Colin Campbell. Goldhamer asked Campbell if he would help put together a paper on fasting and hypertension, and Campbell agreed.

That fasting lowered blood pressure had been noted in scientific publications as far back as 1915, but no one had ever made a systematic study of a sizable number of patients nor, more crucially, shown how to maintain the lowered blood pressure, which always went back up when the fasters refed. The article that Campbell and Goldhamer put together, which I've alluded to in earlier chapters, was rejected by thirty journals. Apparently the idea that fasting could heal, let alone heal spectacularly, was beyond the comprehension of most scientific editors. In 2001, the obscure but not disreputable *Journal of Manipulative and Physiological Therapeutics* finally published the paper, which showed that of 174 consecutive hypertensive patients who fasted at TrueNorth for an average of 10.6 days, 89 percent became normotensive by fast's end, and the remainder enjoyed substantial drops in pressure. All of the patients who had been on medication for hypertension before their fasts were able to discontinue it, and in those with stage 3 (the most severe) hypertension, the average drop in systolic pressure was 60 mm Hg. Overall, the average drop in systolic/diastolic pressure was 37/13 mm Hg. As I've mentioned, this was and remains the largest drop in blood pressure from any therapy, including drugs, that has ever been reported in a scientific journal. Among the 42 subjects who participated in a follow-up six months later, average blood pressure had risen hardly a jot, and those who did best seemed to be the ones who stuck closest to Goldhamer's unprocessed vegan diet. In 2002, Goldhamer and Campbell published another study, this one of less severe hypertensives, 82 percent of whom achieved a blood pressure of 120/80 or lower with an average fast of two weeks. The mean drop was 20/7.

While Goldhamer was preparing the data for the first paper, he tried repeatedly to get his uncle, the dogmatic MD, to look at the numbers, but the uncle said he wouldn't glance at so much as a digit until the paper had been published in a peer-reviewed journal indexed by a leading scientific service. The *Journal of Manipulative and Physiological Therapeutics* qualified on both counts, but two months before the article's publication, the uncle had a massive heart attack and died. Ever after, Goldhamer's mother said he died out of spite so he wouldn't have to read the paper and admit he was wrong.

Two decades later, Goldhamer and Campbell's cure for hypertension remains all but unknown. A drug company can advertise its latest blood-pressure pill with a budget rivaling that of the Kingdom of Belgium, but the promotional kitty is somewhat smaller for a low-cost clinic whose treatment consists of nothing much. The advocacy groups that might be expected to alert doctors and patients to a cure for hypertension—a disease that nearly half of American adults suffer from—say nothing either. "High blood pressure cannot be cured," the American Heart Association's website asserts. "But it can be managed." It's surely merest coincidence that the AHA takes millions of dollars from drug companies that profit from "managing" hypertension.

*   *   *

An operating engineer is a tradesperson, usually male and often burly, who runs the bulldozers, steamrollers, and pile drivers that build everything from highways to the hospitals where in the 1990s their poor health increasingly landed them. Their decline spurred California's International Union of Operating Engineers to hire Goldhamer at the turn of the millennium to fast some of its most desperate members. The unlikely contract came about because an operating engineer had gotten well at TrueNorth many years earlier. The grateful tradesman told Goldhamer that although he was nobody of consequence just then, he was going to get elected to the board of the union, and when he did, he would get TrueNorth added to its health plan.

"Yeah, right," Goldhamer thought. The IUOE, with four hundred thousand members, was one of California's biggest and most powerful trade organizations, and ascending its hierarchy was no small task. But fifteen years later, his former patient called to say he was on the board and would Goldhamer come make a presentation? Goldhamer gave a pitch to a somewhat wary assemblage of union members, a representative of the builders who hired them, a reviewer for the National Institutes of Health, and a union actuary. He told them that even after the IUOE paid TrueNorth, the union would probably save money because their members would get healthier and need fewer drugs and doctors' visits.

"After we presented our data," Goldhamer recalled, "the contractors' representative objected to the cost. He thought they spent enough on healthcare and didn't want to send people to a resort. I asked if he'd like to come stay at our resort and experience the low back pain, the nausea, the skin rashes, the vomiting, and some of the other interesting symptoms that happen when fasting. He decided maybe it wasn't really a vacation, but they still voted against us."

The NIH reviewer said he thought Goldhamer was right, that getting people healthy would save money in the long run.

"At that point," Goldhamer said, "the actuary objected because union members, if they live long enough to retire, get a monthly pension benefit. He said, 'Dr. Goldhamer, if we do this program and it works, won't it dramatically increase our costs of retirement payouts by making them live longer?' I didn't know what to say, but a guy stood up—I knew he was a crane operator because his neck was twice as big as my thigh—and he said, 'Listen, *little man*. You should remember who you work for. You work for *us*. Why don't you calculate how much money we're gonna save when I come back there and break your neck.' And then they voted to make our program a fully covered medical benefit for any member of the union or their family that had high blood pressure or diabetes."

The first engineer who showed up in Sonoma was an obese diabetic with five prescriptions and a blood pressure of 220/120. The union hadn't told him what he was in for. On surveying the terrain, which had every appearance of a crazy health farm, he said, "I think I'm in the wrong place. I don't belong here."

"Well, you're here because you need to get well," Goldhamer said.

"But I'm not sick," the man replied.

"Of course you're sick. You've got diabetes and hypertension, and you're obese. You're gonna die."

"Oh yeah?" the engineer countered. "Aren't we all gonna die?"

Deciding another tack was needed, Goldhamer ventured, "You're on eight hundred and sixty dollars a month of medications. If we get you off all those drugs, you won't need them anymore. You'll save all that money."

"What do I care? The union pays for my drugs."

"And at this point," Goldhamer later said, "I realize this is not my normal self-selected, highly motivated patient. So I figure I should go with something he does care about. We know that males with diabetes and hypertension often develop 'little problems.' So I said, 'You know, if we get you off all those drugs, I think we can do something about your little problem.'" Here Goldhamer erected his forearm to the rigidly vertical before letting it fall limply at his side. This brought the engineer out of his chair. Putting both hands on the desk between them, he leaned heavily over the doctor, who thought he had made the final error of his career, and demanded, "Why the *hey-ell* didn't you just say so in the first place?"

The man's usual diet, Goldhamer learned, consisted chiefly of Big Macs, up to three times a day, and if the *garçon de café* made the mistake of putting a sliver of lettuce on the tower of patties, he would strip off "that disgusting green crap" and throw it in the trash. Had Goldhamer fasted him directly, such fare would have sat in his gut for days or weeks and given him all kinds of grief, so he sent him straight to the dining room to eat some plants. The engineer proceeded to make such frightful gagging noises that Goldhamer at first worried his clinical team had missed a throat tumor during the intake evaluation.

Sitting down next to his patient, he said, "It seems you're having a little trouble with the food."

"*This*," the man said with a dismissive jerk of his fork, "this is not food. If I have to eat tasteless swill like this, I'd rather just *die*. Matter of fact, why don't you go out to my truck, get my twelve-gauge, and when I'm not looking, just shoot me in the head?"

But he stayed, fasted twenty-six days, lost fifty pounds, and normalized both his blood pressure and blood sugar. The refeeding went better than the prefeeding, and when Goldhamer remarked as much, the engineer said, "Yeah, your damn chef's finally getting the hang of it. This stuff's not bad."

It took twenty minutes for Goldhamer to convince him it was the same food he had eaten when he arrived, only now his taste buds—previously habituated to overly dense foods like meat, cheese, sugar, oil, and salt—had been reset by his fast, so less dense but healthier foods like vegetables and fruits tasted good again.

Some years after the engineer's discharge, Goldhamer ran into him at a crowded event. When he asked how he was, the man wordlessly raised a forearm to upright turgidity and smiled from ear to ear.

The IUOE asked Goldhamer to do a cost-benefit analysis of the first thirty union beneficiaries treated at TrueNorth. He reported that on an average fast of three weeks, the typical patient lost 26 pounds, and their blood pressure dropped 30/11. At follow-ups between two and twelve months later, the patients hadn't backslid—in fact, they were two pounds lighter, and their blood pressure was still down 28/11 from where it had started. The $1,900 a year the union had previously spent on drugs for each of these beneficiaries fell to $1,000, and the $3,900 it had spent annually on their doctors' visits and other medical expenses fell to $2,000. The savings in the first year alone surpassed the cost of treatment at TrueNorth, and the savings multiplied with each year of improved health.

Over the course of a decade, about a hundred engineers fasted at the clinic, but during the Great Recession of 2008 the union axed benefits, and fasting fell under the chop, notwithstanding that it saved more than it cost. By the time the economy recovered, the official who had helped Goldhamer get the contract had retired and there were no enthusiasts of fasting on the board. By then, however, word had gotten out about Goldhamer's cures, and TrueNorth had more clients than it could handle. Today the wait to get in is four months.

*   *   *

If Herbert Shelton arose from the grave, strode through TrueNorth's lus-
terless entry, and observed the work inside, little in Goldhamer's protocol
would surprise him. In addition to fasting on nothing but water, its hallmarks were enforced rest, the SOS-free diet of unprocessed plants, and,
Goldhamer having learned from Shelton's error, medical supervision that
verged on the obsessive. Start with the supervision. Goldhamer held that
any fast longer than eighteen hours should be made only under the watchful eye of an experienced clinician. In this he differed from other fasting
doctors, including his friend Michael Klaper, another dean of the vegan-
health field who practiced eight years at TrueNorth and whom we met in
the prologue. Klaper believes a healthy person—someone with no diagnosed or suspected illness and taking no medications—can safely water
fast unsupervised for five to seven days. But Goldhamer worried about the
rare cases, like the tiny number of people with a genetic defect that keeps
them from completely breaking down fatty acids. Unable to use fat for
fuel, they can slip into a coma when fasting. Another tiny group cannot
safely dispose of the ammonia that is created when proteins are broken
down during a fast, again with dire results.

   At TrueNorth, four MDs, six chiropractors, two naturopaths, and a
swarm of nurses monitored us for signs of these and other troubles. Our
intake exams, at an hour apiece, were the most thorough evaluations
Jennifer or I had ever received from a physician and amounted to more
time than we had spent with our family doctor over the last few years in all
visits combined. Each morning a nurse came to our room to take our vitals,
followed by a rounding doctor who checked our pulses and asked about
our symptoms, and in the evening another doctor repeated the procedure.
If our supervising doctor saw us as he passed through the courtyard during
the day, he often pulled a chair alongside our loungers and chatted about
our progress. We surrendered blood weekly and urine twice weekly, and
when our lab reports came back we got detailed explanations about how
this or that number should behave on a fast and what the plan would be if
the numbers did something else. In half a century of going to doctors, we'd

never been cared for more intimately. A fellow guest had it right when she suggested that Goldhamer adopt the motto "TrueNorth Health, The Safest Place on Earth."

The doctors clearly liked this model of caregiving too, even though they were paid what Goldhamer called "a fraction of what they could earn elsewhere." Elsewhere, however, they'd have to see two dozen patients a day at seven minutes a head. Here they were spending fifteen, thirty, even forty-five minutes with a patient if need be—and for the first time in their careers nearly all of their patients were getting healthier. That we were being thus attended and getting a roof over our heads and meals (during refeeding) for under $200 a night made the dowdy décor far more tolerable.

As if to prove Goldhamer right that fasting should take place only under a competent practitioner, Netflix in 2020 released the documentary series *(Un)Well*, one of whose episodes contrasted fasting at TrueNorth with fasting at the Tanglewood Wellness Center, once of Panama, now of Costa Rica. Tanglewood is run by a man who describes himself as "a Reiki master, a certified permaculture instructor, a poet, the author of a children's book, a body surfer and beginning board surfer." His staff consists not of medical professionals but former guests. At the end of 2010, a thirty-three-year-old Coloradan named Jonathan Kamm fasted thirty-two days at Tanglewood for digestive troubles, and although all seemed to go well during the fast, he began hallucinating a week into refeeding. Over the next week his behavior grew more and more peculiar. One day at breakfast he tried to take off all his clothes, and on several addled occasions he demanded to leave before his refeeding was complete. Astonishingly, Tanglewood finally checked him in to a nearby hotel even though he was, in the opinion of some who saw him, far from mentally stable. The next morning Kamm's broken body was found at the bottom of the hotel stairwell. He died a few days later.

Goldhamer believed the key to heading off disasters long before they came to such a pass was a practiced vigilance about subtle clues that even doctors, if untrained in fasting, might not spot. "When a patient has symptoms," he said, "part of our job is differentiating whether this is a positive acute response generated by the body as it tries to get well or whether it's a problem. Not everything that might look like a healing crisis necessarily is a healing crisis," and not everything that looks like a problem is a problem. The only way to tell, Goldhamer believed, was to constantly monitor vitals, blood, and urine. Evidently the odds of getting it right were somewhat lower with an expat Reiki master than with the trained professionals of TrueNorth.

*　*　*

Goldhamer was happy to give any patient who couldn't fast a few hundred calories a day of green juices, but after thirty-seven years of watching people water fast and juice cleanse for the same conditions, he was certain it was quicker to regain one's health with no input but water. No input but water meant no input but water. Fasters at TrueNorth drank neither tea nor coffee, were tapered off all medications and supplements, and were advised to brush their teeth without toothpaste and forgo deodorant and lotions. The body absorbs small amounts of these substances, and Goldhamer thought the energy to process them could be better used on repairs. He also discounseled showers while fasting, although less to conserve the body's energy than to maintain its integrity. The hot water of a shower, we were told, causes the capillaries of the skin to dilate, which brings an inrush of blood, and gravity ensures that much of it comes from the head. This poses no problem to a fed body, which quickly resupplies the brain, but a fasting body, with its lower blood pressure and diminished blood flow, may have trouble getting replacement blood back up to the head quickly enough to avert swooning. Urgent care visits have been known to follow fasted showers.

Patients who heeded all of these hygienic dicta mesmerized the rest of us with lurid tales of the brown sludge—presumably dead skin and sweat residue—that washed off them in the shower when they broke their fasts. Jennifer and I weren't quite so devoted. We brushed our teeth with the slightest smidge of paste and indulged every few days in an intermittent shower: twenty seconds of lukewarm water to wet ourselves, a minute soaping with the water off, another twenty seconds rinsing. Neither of us conked a head. But even with these nods to sanitation and although we kept our bedroom windows open all night, with the two of us exuding acetone breath and who knows what from our pores, by morning our room smelled as rank as a Tallahassee flophouse on the Fourth of July. It took half the day to air out.

*　*　*

Both Jennifer and I anticipated the hardest part of the Goldhamer protocol to abide by would be the mandate to stay on the grounds while fasting. I had long stood with Otto Buchinger when he wrote, "The doctor of fasting who doesn't resort to nature for help, to the landscape or somewhere that roots are spread . . . *never* will have a *great* success." But Buchinger wasn't water fasting his patients. Goldhamer's charges got weaker sooner, and he didn't want them going for a stroll and collapsing in the neighbors' petunias. He was also concerned that the more a faster exercised, the more energy their body might divert from healing and the more likely it would burn proteins unnecessarily. To lose a little protein during a fast is no problem because there's no evidence of harm to vital tissues like the heart. Moreover, any protein that is burned may be old and damaged, and since it's quickly replaced with healthy new proteins during refeeding, its loss is probably not to be mourned. But Goldhamer feared a water faster whose exercise accelerated the protein burn might be more likely to consume essential proteins like heart muscle.

The proposition is far from certain, and even if it's right, it may take an extravagance of exertion before a patient crosses that dangerous threshold. Yuri Nikolayev encouraged his ten thousand water fasters to exercise at least three hours a day, and he never reported any sign of trouble in their urine, blood, electrocardiograms, encephalograms, or long-term followups. We also have accounts of individuals who have performed Herculean feats of fasted exercise without evident harm, although no formal study has been made. One of these exceptional exercists is a Frenchman named Florian Gomet, who specializes in arduous travel under his own power. In 2018, Gomet hiked the 222-mile Canol Heritage Trail in Canada's

Northwest Territory while fasting. The Canol is so remote and rugged, it lands on nearly every list of the most wickedly challenging hikes in North America. For most hikers, it's a twenty-day slog, but Gomet did it in fourteen on nothing but water, save for on his thirty-fourth birthday when he dressed his drink with salt and pepper. Throughout, his temperature remained normal, his pulse mostly stayed in a narrow band between 40 and 45, his blood sugar was generally ordinary, and his weight dropped the usual pound a day, from 137 at the start to 123.5 at the end. Doctors who evaluated his bloodwork after the hike said they saw no hint of damage, although they probably weren't scrutinizing such specifics as his cardiac proteins.

An evolutionary biologist looking at Gomet and his kind might hypothesize that since humans evolved to fast when food ran out, they perhaps also evolved to travel long distances in search of more food. That's certainly the case with other members of the animal kingdom, some of whom are even designed to lose heart muscle while fasting. When the ruby-throated hummingbird fasts on its annual migration from the Yucatán to the United States across the Gulf of Mexico, it loses 40 percent of its body weight and much of its cardiac muscle, which, however, poses no problem because, weighing so much less, it can get by with a smaller heart. When it refeeds, it regains the cardiac muscle along with the rest of its bulk. A similar, earthbound tale could be told of penguins during their long fasts at their Antarctic nesting grounds.

But for now, lacking firmer evidence, Goldhamer errs on the side of caution and enforces inactivity, although not as insistently as some of his predecessors. David Scott, a chiropractor who for many years ran a fasting clinic outside Cleveland, required his fasters to lie prone much of the day, not even sitting up in bed, let alone undertaking anything so taxing as reading, playing cards, or watching television. A devout man, Scott made an exception only for the movie *The Greatest Story Ever Told*, although whether from piety or because that particular tale made fewer demands on the brain than a round of Go Fish, only he could say. At TrueNorth, we were permitted to engage daily in two educational lectures by the staff, as much reading or TV as we could stand, and an evening session of seated yoga, stretching, or meditation. We were also free to take the air in the courtyard whenever we liked, and most of us passed many a lazy hour basking in the warm Northern California summer while the fountain splashed in the background and a light breeze rustled through the trees.

Neither Jennifer nor I, as it turned out, were troubled by our confinement. We lacked the strength to wander. Whether because I am getting older or because I was starting my fast lighter than ever before, at 131 pounds, the energy I awoke with each morning was usually depleted by mid-afternoon, and even a short walk sounded abhorrent. Jennifer, who hadn't a lot of burthen to shed either, was just as tuckered, and we enjoyed many a bedbound matinee of one of the clinic's scores of educational videos. Certainly nothing else was happening in that bed. Our afternoon ritual may not have been as sublime as a hike in the hills above Lake Constance, but for compensation there were the possibility our bodies were healing more quickly and the certainty our savings were draining more slowly. We were, in our listless way, wholly content.

CHAPTER 16

YOU ARE WHEN YOU EAT

One of the great uncelebrated advances in human biology of the last century was the discovery of just how thoroughly our bodies are governed by circadian rhythms, those metabolic processes that repeat every twenty-four hours with consequences ranging from the trivial to the grand. One circadian rhythm, for example, makes male facial hair grow exuberantly by day but hardly at all at night, which is why if you shave in the morning, you'll have a five o'clock shadow, but if you shave at night, you won't have five-in-the-morning shadow. Another circadian rhythm causes muscle tone to peak late in the day, which makes afternoon a more productive time than morning for some exercise. Still another circadian rhythm prompts certain cells to devour damaged bone at one time of day, while other cells make new bone at a different time. If our rhythms get off track, the bone-making cells won't make enough new bone, the bone-eating cells won't eat enough damaged bone, and our bones will become brittle, which may help explain why older people, whose rhythms are weaker, are more prone to fractures.

We have circadian rhythms for a very sensible reason: the body has too much work to do it all at once, so chores must be staggered. Take the brain, which fires countless neurons all day long to power our thoughts, so circadian rhythms direct it to wait until night, when presumably we'll be asleep, to carry out other tasks like cleaning up the toxic byproducts of the day's chemical reactions, creating new neurons, and making hormones like melatonin and growth hormone. It's easy to understand this kind of staggered scheduling, but other arrangements are a little more surprising.

Our immune system, for instance, has four vital jobs: surveillance, attack, repair, and cleanup. If you or I were to design the system, we'd probably schedule attack, repair, and cleanup to occur in lightning succession after the surveillance crew has perceived a threat like a virus or a cancer cell. But in fact our bodies prefer to do each of these tasks at different times of day, each dictated by a circadian rhythm, because when they're done all at once we're thrown into the wholly uncongenial state known as septic shock.

Circadian rhythms have been observed since antiquity, and not just in rhythms of sleep and wakefulness. You have only to notice a flower opening its petals in the morning and closing them at night to mark the phenomenon. But not until the 1950s did scientists learn that humans have circadian rhythms that operate even in the absence of cycles of light and dark. And only in the 1970s did they learn we have not one but two types of clocks regulating circadian rhythms.

One is the master clock, which resides at the base of the brain in a tiny collection of cells inside the hypothalamus. (The hypothalamus is a command center that directs a great sweep of bodily functions through the autonomic nervous system and the hormone-regulating pituitary gland.) The master clock is more formally the suprachiasmatic nucleus (SCN), so named because it sits above, or *supra*, the optic chiasm, a chiasm being an intersection, itself named for the Greek letter *chi*, which we know as *X*. The chiasm of the SCN is the place where our two optic nerves cross, and that's no accidental siting because it's the light of dawn that keeps the SCN humming to a twenty-four-hour rhythm. More specifically, the abundant blue light of the morning sun resets the SCN each day, which is why blue light from our screens in the evening can trick our SCNs into thinking it's not night and disturb our sleep.

The other type of circadian clock is a peripheral clock, and we have not one but quite a few—trillions actually, because they reside in almost every cell in the form of genes that keep time day after day, year after year. Scientists once thought the master clock ruled the peripheral clocks as a master ruled a slave (in their infelicitous phrase), but the relationship between the two clocks has proved much more complicated. Although the peripheral clocks generally look to the master clock to make sure they're keeping time, they also have the ability to run somewhat independently, much as the clock on your mobile phone checks in periodically with a remote atomic clock but can run serviceably offline for a while. And like the clock on your phone, many peripheral clocks can also be reset to a time completely different from the time kept by the master atomic clock. Only recently did scientists learn the stimulus that resets those peripheral clocks is food.

Researchers made the discovery by feeding mice during the day rather than night (when they normally eat) and observing that the circadian clocks in their livers reset to the new feeding schedule with surprising speed. Even though the SCNs of the mice, taking their cues from light, commanded their livers to run on their normal nocturnal schedule, the genes of their liver cells, cued by food, turned a deaf ear to the SCNs and switched to a diurnal schedule. Scientists have since found that clocks in many other organs can be reset when food arrives out of sync with the SCN's preferred schedule, and this has led to an inescapable conclusion: food is as powerful a superintendent of circadian rhythms as light.

It wasn't hard to surmise why we and other animals had evolved this way. Mouse or man can live an age without sunshine but only so long without food—two or three days in the case of a mouse. When food becomes scarce at the normal time, an organism that can shift its organs to run a little more efficiently as it forages at an odd hour is more likely to survive, mate, and pass on its genes.

In the 1980s, scientists began to explore how these discoveries might benefit humans, and one of the more fascinating developments came from the Argonne National Laboratory, outside Chicago, where a biologist named Charles Ehret devised a regimen he called the Argonne Anti–Jet Lag Diet. Having experimented on protozoa, rats, and his eight children, Ehret recommended that in the four days before flying across several time zones, travelers should alternate between a day of feasting and a day of what he termed "fasting," by which he meant light eating. During the flight, the traveler was to continue nibbling sparsely and then eat a big breakfast at about 7:30 a.m. in the new time zone, no matter that it was still 11:30 p.m. in the time zone he had just left. His reward would be little or no jet lag.

In a study published in the journal *Military Medicine* in 2002, National Guardsmen who followed the diet were 7.5 times less likely than a control group to suffer jet lag after flying from the United States to Korea, and on their return they were 16.2 times less likely to lag. (The difference between the two flights has not been explained, although, as the authors noted, jet lag is more common flying east than west, so perhaps the diet paid more dividends when travel was most demanding.) Ehret postulated that the diet worked because the days of irregular eating gradually unmoored the body's circadian clocks from their usual rhythms, which were then re-anchored in the new time zone by the big breakfast.

The diet was used by the US Army and Navy, the CIA, the Canadian National Swim Team, the Mormon Tabernacle Choir, and an aged Ronald Reagan, who I had previously assumed looked so fresh on arrival in Beijing or Bitburg because he was uncommonly unburdened by the cares of his office. But the regimen had one big drawback, which was that the light eating of the "fasting" days stimulated a gnawing desire for more food. Some people thought enduring days of hunger in order to avoid days of jet lag was the proverbial cutting off the nose to be revenged of the face.

Fortunately, a couple of decades later a team from Harvard and Beth Israel Deaconess Medical Center in Boston concocted a more elegant remedy: the anti–jet lag fast, in which the international traveler simply doesn't eat for twelve to sixteen hours before morning in the new time zone, at which point, as in Ehret's diet, she breaks the fast. Since nearly everyone has at some time gone twelve to sixteen hours without food between dinner and breakfast, the abstention is a minor hardship for most people. The fast has never been tested in a controlled trial, but its mechanism has been well theorized. When food fails to appear at the expected time during the fast, peripheral clocks in multiple organs suspend their circadian cycles, and upon eating again they reset to the new schedule. When a traveler from Los Angeles to London eats breakfast over Dublin shortly after dawn, her peripheral clocks neither know nor care that it's still midnight in California. They know only that the food entering the stomach is declaring a new eating pattern, a fact the blue light of morning over the Irish Sea will reinforce through the SCN. By contrast, in the unfasted traveler on the same flight, when the SCN tells the body it's morning in Mayfair, his peripheral clocks protest that it must be otherwise because his organs are still digesting dinner. It's this disconnection between the SCN and the peripheral clocks that causes jet lag, a disconnection blunted by the fast.

When I learned of the anti–jet lag fast a dozen years ago, I was over-joyed because even short hops to Europe left me with a week of lethargy and brain fog, and my journeys to the Far East were simply incapacitat-ing. As luck would have it, Jennifer was headed soon to a conference in India, and Elliott and I were to be laded with her other encumbrances. We decided to make an experiment of our twenty-four hours in transit from Denver to Delhi. (These were, I'm ashamed to say, the days before our awareness of the climate catastrophe prompted us to whittle our flights to a nib and a nub.) Jennifer and I ate our last food on the Chicago–Frankfurt leg, skipped the airline slop thereafter, and after arriving in Delhi at two in the morning, slept and arose at eight to a glorious banquet of dosas and samosas. To our pleasant surprise, we had more than enough vitality to trade enlivening elbows with patrons of the Delhi Metro, and on subse-quent days we felt not the slightest hint of jet lag. Elliott, who was nine, suffered an altogether different fate. As every traveling parent knows, the young rarely suffer jet lag to the degree of their betters, so we had seen no need to fast him. I also wasn't opposed to having a control group for the experiment—and what a control he proved. On each of the first four or five afternoons in India, he collapsed in an insensate heap, utterly unstirred by his elixir of choice, mango lassi.

On the return home, all three of us fasted. This time the young master was jet lag's master, Jennifer its mistress. They awoke in Colorado full of vim on the morning after the journey. Not so I. In our last days in Mumbai, I had contracted shingles, and on my first days back home I was as sluggish as I would have been had I not fasted at all. Whether I would have escaped fatigue had I been unshingled was a riddle beyond answer. The same air of mystery, of course, hung over our successes against jet lag, which might have been due to a placebo effect. But I was impressed enough with our trial that ever after, when an airline steward has asked me to choose between the rubber stroganoff and shellacked pasta, I've always opted for a cup of water. Sometimes the day after my travel I've been nearly sprightly, sometimes merely not moribund, which, however, is still a vast improvement over my previous sorry state.

*　*　*

While I was conducting these experiments, my fellow scientists were exploring what happened when food decoupled the peripheral clocks from the SCN. What occurred, for example, when the SCN and the peripheral clocks ran on different schedules for longer than it takes to fly across an ocean? Was there a problem if the SCN, cued by light, told the peripheral clocks to do something, but food arrived unexpectedly and the peripheral clocks ignored the SCN? And what of the fact that not all peripheral clocks listened to food? Did it matter that some cells continued to do their work on schedules set by light while others marched to a beat set by meals? This sort of discord might explain why shift workers were so much more prone to diabetes, obesity, cardiovascular disease, cancer, depression, liver disease, and gastrointestinal disorders. Scientists had once assumed that those who labored overnight were bedeviled by their weird relationship to light, but maybe eating lunch at two in the morning also brought trouble. And shift workers, of course, aren't the only ones who eat at odd hours. Many people graze across the day and night, which raised a broader question: are there specific times that humans should and shouldn't eat if they want to live long and healthily?

One researcher who made a deft start at answering these questions was Satchidananda Panda (Satchin to friends and slow-tongued Westerners) of the Salk Institute in suburban San Diego. Panda had some standing in the field, for it was he who made the momentous discovery, in 2002, that blue light entrained the SCN. His starting point on decoupled master and peripheral clocks was the uncontroversial idea that many species evolved to eat by either day or night but not both. Humans, for one, have long eaten in daylight because the full days of equatorial Africa, where our species emerged, afforded plenty of time to find food and prepare meals. Our ancestors had little need to stir about after sundown, when nocturnal predators had every advantage over them. Panda's impelling question was, what would happen if modern humans, rather than eating throughout the day and night, ate in a window more in keeping with the one we evolved to eat in?

In 2012, he published the results of an experiment that may someday prove as important as his blue-light discovery. His team fed a high-fat diet to genetically identical mice, half of whom ate all their food in eight hours during the night, as mice usually do, while the other half ate ad libitum, anytime they wanted, which meant they stretched their feeding across both night and day, much as humans do today. Both groups ate the same amount of food, a chow that had induced obesity and other metabolic disorders in eleven thousand prior rodent studies. Sure enough, after three months, the mice who ate ad lib were stricken with obesity, diabetes, liver disease, and a host of other untoward conditions.

But a most remarkable thing happened to the mice who ate within eight nocturnal hours: they stayed healthy, utterly free of the metabolic diseases their siblings developed. Their weight, blood sugar, and cholesterol were normal, their livers were less fatty than those of the free-eating mice, their motor coordination was better, and their entire bodies were less inflamed. Eating in an eight-hour nighttime window had, in Panda's slightly exaggerated phrase, "completely protected" them. Better still, when Panda later put the sickly ad-lib eaters on the eight-hour feeding schedule, their diseases reversed, even though they were eating the same unhealthy diet. Researchers had long focused on what animals, including humans, should eat to be healthy. But in a couple of simple experiments, Panda had brilliantly shown *when* animals eat might matter as much as what.

What, to be clear, still mattered. When Panda ran the experiment again but with different diets, mice who ate healthier, low-fat chow in the nighttime eight-hour window fared even better than mice who ate high-fat chow in the same window. The eight-hour window, it seemed, could negate much of the harm of a bad diet, but optimal health required good food. Panda also experimented with the length of the window and found his mice were reasonably protected from the ravages of a high-fat diet if they ate across no more than twelve hours a day. Beyond twelve hours, the diet started to make them sick, and by fifteen hours their health was ruinous.

Panda wasn't the only scientist to make such discoveries. In fact, the same week in 2012 that he published his first study, a professor at Hebrew University of Jerusalem named Oren Froy published a paper asking whether time-restricted feeding (TRF), as the practice was known, could protect mice not just from a bad diet, as in Panda's study, but also from a bad eating schedule. Whereas Panda's TRF mice had eaten at night, Froy made his TRF mice eat their high-fat diet in the middle of the day, and he used a much-narrower window than Panda, only four hours. The results were no less dramatic. Froy's mice who ate ad lib grew sicker by the week, but his TRF mice stayed healthy even on the high-fat diet at the weird time. And just as in Panda's experiment, the TRF mice became even healthier when they ate a low-fat diet. In fact, even on their upside-down eating schedule, the low-fat TRF mice were healthier than the low-fat mice who ate ad lib.

Panda, Froy, and others wasted no time trying to determine the mechanisms behind these marvelous results, but other researchers, not caring to wait until the means were parsed, sought to test the grand question that Panda's and Froy's work raised: could eating in a narrower window make humans healthier too?

* * *

The first attempt at an answer had actually been made five years before Panda's and Froy's studies, but the results were so disappointing, most researchers abandoned the effort. A group under Mark Mattson at the National Institute on Aging asked fifteen healthy, middle-aged volunteers to eat all their food for eight weeks either at the customary three mealtimes or in a single window from 5 p.m. to 9 p.m. After an eleven-week washout period in which they could eat however they wished, they crossed over to the other arm of the trial: those who had eaten normally now ate between 5 p.m. and 9 p.m. for eight weeks, while those who had eaten in the evening now ate normally. During both of the eight-week experimental arms, the two groups ate about the same amount of food and stayed roughly the same weight. Unfortunately, the health of the volunteers improved hardly at all during their eight weeks on TRF, and a few of their biomarkers, like cholesterol, actually took a turn for the worse. To many researchers, TRF looked a bust. But after Panda's and Froy's trials, some scientists looked back at the NIA study and realized TRF hadn't failed in humans; TRF *in the evening* had failed in humans. A study that had seemed a dud had actually yielded useful information, and researchers now asked whether an earlier eating window might have more success.

To understand why, we need to dip a toe into the roiling waters of the controversy over breakfast skipping. For decades researchers have quietly wrangled over the merits of passing a foodless forenoon, a practice that in some countries is observed by nearly a quarter of the populace with no obvious harm. But just because the harm isn't obvious doesn't mean it's not there. Multiple large observational studies have shown breakfast skippers are more likely than breakfast eaters to suffer heart disease, atherosclerosis, and even premature death. On the other hand, those who skip breakfast are also disproportionately poor, obese, alcoholic, and given to smoking, which confounds the results. (The poor skip breakfast to save money, the obese to save calories, the alcoholic sleeps or drinks through breakfast, and the smoker's cancer stick suppresses his morning appetite.) But when researchers have controlled for the confoundables, skipping breakfast still appears to lead to illness and early death, although the evidence has fallen short of irrefutable.

My interest in the dustup was keen because eating breakfast had long made me feel soporific, particularly during my hypersomniac days, and I had remedied the problem by becoming a No-Breakfast Plan man in the manner of Edward Hooker Dewey. Countless considerers of my best interest warned that unless I started the day as they did—with, I suppose, a sugary cereal awash in the growth hormone of an animal the size of a sofa—I would drop dead of a coronary or be damned to an early senility. For a long time I took refuge in the minority of studies that found no link between skipping breakfast and ill health, but in recent years new research has emerged that tilts the balance so unmistakably against skipping, I have yielded to the science. If there is anything worse than having to admit you were wrong, it's having to admit it in print.

One of the more convincing studies was published in 2012 by a group of Israelis, including Oren Froy, who set out to study not breakfast skipping but breakfast skimping. Specifically, the Israelis were testing the adage that one should breakfast like a king, lunch like a prince, and dine like a pauper. (The line has been attributed to various eminences, including, in one scholarly paper, the great Jewish polymath Maimonides, who, however, predated it by eight centuries. The maxim was in fact first committed to the page in the 1950s by the nutrition writer Adelle Davis, who was often unreliable, although not on this point.) The researchers randomized seventy-four overweight or obese women with metabolic syndrome to one of two weight-loss regimens. One group ate 700 calories at breakfast, 500 at lunch, and 200 at dinner, while the other group ate the reverse: 200 at breakfast, 500 at lunch, 700 at dinner. The meals weren't precisely the same because the volunteers made them themselves based on sample recipes, but they were all of a piece with the standard Western diet: fatty, meaty, sugary, and low on fruits, vegetables, and whole grains.

At the time, the assumption among experts was that the two groups, eating roughly the same 1,400 calories, would lose about the same amount of weight and make roughly the same gains in health. (Even on a frightful diet, when calories are sharply limited, weight loss and improved health are all but assured in overweight subjects.) But after twelve weeks the group that took breakfast like kings and dinner like paupers lost 11 percent of their weight, while those who dined like kings and breakfasted like paupers lost just 4 percent. The kingly breakfasters also enjoyed slightly better blood pressure, cholesterol, triglycerides, and glucose, and on a composite score known as the insulin-sensitivity index, they were 163 percent more sensitive to insulin than before the diet, while the kingly diners improved only 56 percent.

Why did the king-prince-paupers do so much better than the pauper-prince-kings? One possibility is they moved more. Other studies sometimes found that those who ate larger meals earlier in the day puttered around more often, doing light housework, going for walks, and otherwise acting as if they had energy to burn. A stronger probability, however, is that the king-prince-paupers benefited from eating in sync with their circadian clocks. We know this is likely, because other research suggests there are indeed better and worse times of the day for humans to ingest just about any substance.

This was demonstrated rather startlingly in a 2012 analysis of fifteen thousand attempted suicides in Sri Lanka, where the preferred method is pesticide. The study found that people who poisoned themselves in the evening died only half as often as people who poisoned themselves in the morning, apparently because in the morning their digestive tracts quickly absorbed the pesticide and efficiently shuttled it throughout their bodies. By the time they were found and brought to a hospital, they were usually beyond saving. In evening suicide attempts, by contrast, the poison moved more slowly and the victims could frequently be preserved.

On the same principle, scientists have learned there's an ideal time to give chemotherapy, which is, after all, a glorified poison. Against some cancers, chemo can be up to five times less toxic to the patient and twice as effective against the cancer when delivered at the right hour. The right hour probably varies with the specific chemicals and type of cancer, but for other conditions the timing of medication is more straightforward. In 2010, Spanish researchers reported that patients who took blood pressure pills at bedtime instead of in the morning cut their risk of heart attack and stroke by two-thirds and their risk of death in half.

We now know beyond doubt that our bodies digest, absorb, and store nutrients more efficiently in the morning and early afternoon than in the evening. Our circadian rhythms simply demand it. No matter what we do—no matter when we sleep or eat—each morning around dawn (or what would be dawn if we were living in our ancestral African home), our master clock, the SCN, tells the pineal gland to stop making the sleep hormone melatonin, which cues the body to get ready for the day. In response, our breathing and heartbeat quicken slightly, our blood pressure and temperature rise, and our adrenal glands release cortisol to nudge us into activity. Soon the digestive system stirs to life. The stomach makes enzymes and acids to digest the food it expects to arrive shortly, the pancreas makes the insulin that will move nutrients into cells, and the cells make their own preparations to put the nutrients to work. All of these processes run exceptionally well in the morning but wane over the course of the day.

"We used to think that the digestive system was like a constantly active boiler, where you could add food at any time and it would get metabolized," explained Satchin Panda, a diminutive chap with a soft subcontinental lilt that makes you lean forward to hear and who usually says something that makes you glad you did. "Now we know that this is not the case. Almost every aspect of eating, from craving food or feeling hungry to digestion and elimination, occurs according to strong circadian timing." We can shift the timing of a few of these processes by taking our first calories of the day later or earlier. For example, if we regularly eat breakfast at 11 a.m. instead of 8 a.m., our stomachs will learn to hold off making digestive juices for a few hours. But we can't shift most of our nutrient-related processes, nor can we make them work as efficiently later in the day as in the morning. The breakfast-like-a-king rhythms are etched immutably into our DNA, probably because prehistoric humans who ate early were able to go about the day's labors more zestfully and so were more likely to survive and reproduce, while their cousins who breakfasted like paupers died off.

The best studied of our nutritional rhythms is the one governing insulin, which the master clock in the brain and the peripheral clocks of the pancreas jointly regulate to ensure a ready daytime supply. By evening the supply decreases markedly, as does the sensitivity of our cells to insulin, so by nighttime the body has a harder time moving glucose out of the bloodstream and into cells. If the glucose lingers in the blood long enough, it can damage arterial walls and over years can sow a dark harvest of maladies ranging from atherosclerosis to diabetes, kidney disease, impotence, neuropathy, amputation, and blindness.

If insulin were regulated only by peripheral clocks, it might not matter when we ate because our bodies could shift our insulin production to match our eating habits. By consistently taking our first meal at, say, 11 a.m., our peripheral clocks would be nudged to start releasing insulin around 10 a.m. rather than dawn, and we could efficiently process food well into the night. But the master clock won't be coaxed out of its stubborn rhythm with insulin the way it will with digestive juices. Every morning, blue light cues the SCN to tell the pancreas to start making insulin, and every afternoon the SCN tells the pineal gland to release the melatonin that will shut down the pancreatic insulin factory. Between morning and evening, the core of that factory—the pancreas's clump of insulin-making beta cells—loses a quarter or more of its function.

The clinical effects of this daily insulin swing are dramatic. In one experiment, researchers replaced volunteers' food with a steady IV drip of glucose for twenty-four hours. If you didn't know anything about circadian rhythms, you'd expect the amount of sugar in their blood to have held steady throughout the day and night, but in fact at about 8 p.m. their blood glucose rose markedly as the beta cells in the pancreas cut back on insulin, which left too little of it in the bloodstream to hustle the sugar out of their arteries. This circadian shift in insulin is so great that in another experiment, people whose blood glucose measured a prediabetic 163 mg/dL after a sugary drink at 7 a.m. (prediabetes falls between 140 and 199 mg/dL) tested a fully diabetic 203 after the same drink at 7 p.m. In another trial, when healthy young men in Japan were assigned to eat 2,200 calories spread evenly across either breakfast, lunch, and dinner or just lunch and dinner, the breakfast-skipping group, taking more of their calories later in the day, had significantly higher blood glucose all the way until eight the next morning. It took that long for their pancreases to release enough insulin to clear the night's blood sugar.

Given this circadian swing in insulin, even modest shifts in eating habits can have large impacts. In a trial from 2015 in Spain, where lunch is traditionally the heartiest meal of the day, healthy young women were only half as able to process glucose after eating an 800-calorie lunch at 4:30 p.m. as they were when they ate the same meal at 1 p.m. Not incidentally, generous midday meals may explain what I've come to think of as the Spanish paradox: Spaniards are one of the longest-lived peoples, yet they eat late into the night, which should be bad for them. The reason their nocturnal noshing doesn't overly harm them may be that they keep their late meals small and take most of their sustenance at lunch. In another study of the same principle, overweight homemakers in Italy were put on a low-calorie diet in 2014 and randomized to eat either 55 percent or 70 percent of their daily calories at breakfast and lunch, with the rest at dinner. After three months, the 70 percent group were not only more sensitive to insulin but lost an average of five pounds more fat than the 55 percent group—not a bad return for shifting just 15 percent of their calories earlier in the day. "Eat breakfast yourself, share lunch with a friend, and give dinner away to your enemy," the eighteenth-century Russian general Alexander Suvorov supposedly advised, and he appears to have been bang on.

But if you truly wish to ravage your enemy, modern science says give him a bedtime snack. When researchers at Japan's Osaka City University fed healthy young women a typically sized meal either as dinner at 6 p.m. or as a late-night snack at 11 p.m., the blood sugar of the late snackers shot up so high and remained elevated so long—till nearly lunchtime the next day—some of the women tested as prediabetic. In another study simulating the late mealtimes of shift workers, roughly one-third of the participants became prediabetic in just ten days. And in another Japanese trial, when healthy young men took three equally sized meals either as breakfast, lunch, and dinner at the usual times or as lunch, dinner, and an 11 p.m. snack, the LDL cholesterol and triglycerides of the late-night eaters jumped a respective 21 and 9 points after just two weeks.

You might have noticed a tension between my comment several pages ago that evolution equipped us to shift our peripheral clocks so we could eat at odd times and my comments here that we actually do a pretty lousy job of eating at strange hours. The explanation is that although we have the ability to eat at weird times, it's not ideal. That's because at night our bodies have other important tasks to do, and they can't do them well, and sometimes can't do them at all, if we're still eating. One of those tasks is repair. Consider the renovations that just one part of our digestive tract, the gut, has to make every night. To prepare for the work, the gut slackens its muscles to a near torpor, which slows the passage of food to a creep and frees up resources to repair, among much else, the intestinal lining. The lining, formally known as the epithelium, is a barrier just one cell thick that keeps food and pathogens from leaking into our abdomens. As our food slides across the epithelium, parts of it become worn, so at night the pituitary gland in the brain, cued by the SCN, secretes growth hormone that directs the gut to check the entire lining—all four thousand square feet of it—for damaged cells. Night after night, 10 to 14 percent of that McMansionesque surface area is replaced. It's an astounding amount of work, about like re-carpeting a couple of bedrooms every night, and that's not the only maintenance the gut has to do. One of its many other chores is replacing the lubricating mucus that was used during the day to help food pass across the lining. If the body doesn't make enough mucus because we interrupt it with nighttime eating, the lining will suffer more damage the next day as food drags raspily over it.

All of our other digestive organs are doing similar maintenance on the graveyard shift, and the woes that can befall us when we interrupt them are many. The stomach, for example, not only minimizes its repairs when it has to digest food nocturnally but also produces up to twice as much acid as it does during the day—acid that even in its daytime quantity is caustic enough to dissolve coins. Panda thinks this acidic doubling "may be a defense mechanism of the gut to make sure that if bacteria or other pathogens were to somehow make their way to the stomach at night, the acidity of the stomach could destroy them before they got to the next phase, the intestinal phase, which slows down at night." Because of those slowed intestines, food doesn't move out of the stomach as quickly, which means the acid doesn't either, and when we lie down to sleep, gravity sends the acid seeping in the wrong direction—toward the esophagus. If the acid oozes through the sphincter that seals off the stomach from the esophagus, we get the burning throat of acid reflux. If we persist in eating late, acid reflux evolves into the even less companionable disorder called gastroesophageal reflux disease, GERD.

A still worse consequence of eating late, particularly if our food is bereft of fiber (as it usually is in so-called developed countries), is irritable bowel syndrome. The name sounds innocuous, like the grumpy uncle of your abdomen, so it should perhaps be called the clutch-your-gut-in-agony-and-crap-your-pants syndrome. Its causes are several and still debated, but lingering food in the bowels is a decided contributor, and food that does its lingering at night is almost certainly worse than food that lingers during the day. The same goes for the affliction doctors call increased intestinal permeability—leaky gut to most of us—which befalls us when the gut gets holes in its lining that aren't repaired overnight. When that happens, bacteria, viruses, partially digested food, and toxins leak out and inflame nearby tissues, disturb the balance of our intestinal flora, and make us sick in ways we're only beginning to understand. For years, mainstream physicians and scientists mocked leaky gut as a myth of alternative medicine, and while it's true all kinds of diseases have been blamed on the condition for which there's little or no evidence, studies have at last shown it's no fiction. Leaky gut causes or worsens irritable bowel syndrome, celiac disease, and non-celiac gluten sensitivity and likely contributes to fatigue, skin rashes, joint pain, arthritis, and that mother of all infirmities, systemic inflammation. If that's not reason enough to skip the bedtime snack, I don't know what is.

* * *

I realize I've been mixing the problems of eating late and skipping breakfast. That's because the two behaviors are almost inextricably intermingled, as is the research into them, and *that's* because people who skip breakfast usually eat later at night, which makes them less hungry in the morning, which reinforces their breakfast skipping. Certainly that was the case with me. One interesting thing about the research into eating late and skipping breakfast is that the findings are largely the same for both, and the finding that has gotten more attention than all others combined is that both behaviors tend to make people fatter.

Partly this is because we don't burn as many calories when we process food later in the day as we do in the morning. In fact, to process a meal in the morning can take roughly 25 percent more energy than processing the same meal in the afternoon, and about 50 percent more than the same meal at night. In a crossover trial published in 2015, twenty young men and women in Turin, Italy, ate the same 1,200-calorie meal at either 8 a.m. or 8 p.m. and later did the reverse. When their bodies processed the meal in the morning, they burned about 300 calories, but when they processed the evening meal, they burned only 200, which meant their 1,200-calorie meal "counted" for just 900 calories in the morning but 1,000 in the evening. Over a year, that extra 100 calories a day could add up to ten pounds of fat. (Other studies, however, have put the difference in burned calories at well under 100.)

Why would our bodies, if they're built to eat in the morning, be so much less efficient at processing breakfast than dinner? The answer is they only seem less efficient. In the morning, they're actually doing more work because they're turning our food into fuel reserves to help us through the day. Our muscles, brain, and other organs need a steady supply of glucose, but we can't store glucose as such, so at the morning meal our bodies string glucose molecules together into chains of glycogen and stash them in the liver and skeletal muscle. Over the day, the glycogen is broken back down into glucose as needed. The process of transforming the glucose from our breakfast into glycogen takes a bit of energy, which explains the extra calories used to process morning meals.

By contrast, if we eat at night, our bodies don't convert much of the glucose to glycogen because they expect us to go to sleep soon and foresee no need for stored energy. Moreover, because the pancreas is already half asleep and not making much insulin, there's less insulin in the bloodstream to move the glucose out of our blood and into cells. So the glucose lingers, with all the potential for arterial damage that implies. Insult to injury, our bodies may turn some of the unneeded glucose into fat and pack it away with our other flab. Research shows we can't shift this rhythm by changing our schedule—say by working overnight and sleeping during the day. Our bodies were simply forged by evolution to be stirring about in the daylight, and we apparently ignore this history at our peril.

But that's not the only reason late-night eaters put on more weight. A bigger reason has to do with the body's fat-making and fat-burning modes. To oversimplify a little, the body can usually be in only one mode or the other but not both at once. When we eat, our bodies switch on fat-making mode, and for the next few hours they store fat, either by taking fat molecules directly from our foods and stockpiling them in our cells or, far less commonly, by turning some of the proteins and carbohydrates in our food into fat. (It's a myth, incidentally, that carbs are the prime driver of body fat; fat is—overwhelmingly.) Once the body is certain no more food is coming, it switches from fat-making to fat-burning mode. But because shutting down the food-processing machinery requires a lot of energy, and starting it all up again if food arrives unexpectedly requires even more, the body takes a long time to conclude no more food is on the way. So it waits. About six hours after we ingest our last calories, it finally feels confident enough to start the gradual shift from storing fat to burning it. The more time passes, the more confident it becomes, and the rate of fat burning increases accordingly—"almost exponentially after a full twelve hours of fasting," according to Panda. For most people, twelve hours in fat-burning mode is enough to balance out all the fat they stored during the day and keep them from gaining weight.

But there's another and perhaps even more important reason to prolong fat-burning mode: it coincides with repair mode. Just as it's costly for the body to stop making fat and start burning it, it's also costly to stop the body's ordinary work and start making overnight repairs. So repairs don't get deeply underway either until about six hours after our last calories. And just as with fat burning, the repairs accelerate the deeper we go into the fast. All of which is to say that longer overnight fasts seem to build healthier bodies.

Unfortunately, our overnight fasts have gotten shorter in the last several decades. When surveyed, the average American claims to go twelve and a half hours a night without eating, but a smartphone app created by Panda's team found vast numbers of people all over the world, including Americans, were eating or drinking something caloric across nearly fifteen hours a day virtually every day of their lives. Only 10 percent of adults fasted consistently for twelve or more hours a night. The app also found people were taking their food late—consuming fewer than 25 percent of their calories before noon and more than 35 percent after 6 p.m. There were an awful lot of bedtime snacks. This meant most people, eating and drinking their last calories at 10 or 11 p.m., weren't entering fat-burning mode and repair mode until 4 or 5 a.m. and never reached anything like exponential burn or repair before they took their morning coffee with cream at 7 a.m. (Panda has found that just five calories—one and a half grapes—are enough to keep us in fat-making mode for six more hours.)

On the basis of this and similar evidence, Panda said that when it comes to diet, "eating late at night is by far the worst choice you can make, and it will totally defeat any benefits you've achieved throughout the day." To his mind, late eating is even worse than fasting through breakfast, and a 2013 study from Harvard suggested the same by showing that while the odds of heart disease in older men were about 25 percent higher in breakfast skippers than in breakfast eaters, the odds were doubly bad—about 50 percent higher—in late eaters than in those who didn't eat late.

Does this mean intermittent fasting, which most people do by skipping breakfast, should be avoided? Not at all. The research behind time-restricted feeding, as we're about to see, is robust and encouraging. But as you will have divined by now, there's an optimal time of day to do it. The breakfast-skipping and -skimping studies suggested the eating window should fall in the morning or early afternoon, but before that hypothesis was tested, a group of scientists in San Diego made the rousing discovery that even a less-than-optimal window could yield heady results. In fact, it could better our odds at beating cancer.

*　　*　　*

In 2004, researchers in China and France fed mice either ad lib or in a six-hour daily window and then gave them a bone cancer so savage it usually killed its victims in a few weeks. All of the mice quickly grew tumors, but one week after the growths became palpable, they were only half as big in the mice who ate in the restricted window as they were in the ad-lib mice. Even more impressive, when the experiment was run with mice on a four-hour eating window, the tumors were just one-fifth the size of the tumors in the ad-lib mice. Taken together, the four- and six-hour mice survived about a quarter longer than the ad-lib mice, a tremendous gain for merely tinkering with when, not what, the mice ate.

A team at the University of California, San Diego, under Ruth Patterson took note of these studies as well as the pioneering work of

Panda and Froy and realized that similar data had already been collected in humans. In the 1990s and early 2000s, 2,400 women who had recently recovered from early-stage breast cancer were asked to eat a modestly healthier diet to see if they would stay in remission longer. They didn't, but since most of them couldn't stick with even the small changes asked of them, it wasn't an ideal test. However, they had also been asked to report their eating habits, including how many hours they fasted from their last food at night to their first food in the morning. On average, they claimed a fast of twelve and a half hours, which, given what Panda discovered with his app, was probably an overstatement. Nonetheless, when Patterson separated the subjects into those who said they fasted fewer than thirteen hours a night and those who said they fasted more, she found the shorter fasters were 36 percent more likely than the longer fasters to have a recurrence of breast cancer within seven years. It was a potent finding. Also an ironic one: the original researchers had thought their experiment a failure, when in fact a novel way to thwart cancer had been lurking under their noses. Patterson's discovery was especially encouraging because these were wholly ordinary women—women who, after all, were unable or unwilling to make even small changes to their diet, even with the threat of cancer looming—and yet they were spontaneously fasting for a reasonable length of time every night. If they could do it, surely many other ordinary people could too.

While Patterson was going about her work, a few other scientists began exploring whether time-restricted feeding could help with other aspects of human health. In a trial at Brigham Young University published in 2013, borderline-overweight young men who restricted their eating to between 6 a.m. and 7 p.m. lost a pound a week more than a control group, and in a similar, uncontrolled trial by Panda, overweight volunteers who narrowed their eating window to ten or eleven hours lost weight, slept better, and said they liked time-restricted feeding so much they were going to continue it after the study, which is unusual for a dietary intervention. Italian researchers tested whether the harmful effects of skipping breakfast could be outweighed by a longer fasting period, and the answer seemed to be yes. In their eight-week trial, two groups of Venetian bodybuilders ate either between 1 p.m. and 9 p.m. or between 8 a.m. and 9 p.m., and the breakfast skippers not only remained as strong as the breakfast eaters but lost more fat and had lower IGF-1, testosterone, glucose, and insulin. In an American trial, however, a similar eating window—noon to 8 p.m.— improved overweight and obese volunteers hardly at all. Then again, the volunteers were allowed to drink caffeinated coffee and tea outside the window, which, according to Satchin Panda, can yank the body out of fat-burning and repair mode.

The king-pauper-prince studies suggested it was healthier to eat earlier in the day, and the majority of the human TRF studies suggested it was healthier to eat in a narrow window, but no one had yet tested whether it was healthier to eat early *and* make a long fast each night—that is, to skip dinner rather than breakfast. If researchers were loath to test the proposition, that may have been because dinner is all but sacrosanct in most cultures, the one time of day many of us gather with family and friends for unhurried communion. But a lapsed physicist in Louisiana ignored custom and chased the science, and her discoveries could forever change the way we look at dinner.

*   *   *

There was a time in Courtney Peterson's life when she collected advanced degrees the way some people collect fridge magnets. After a bachelor's at Georgetown in physics and biology, she picked up a master's in math and theoretical physics at Cambridge, then a master's in science communication at Imperial College London, followed by a PhD in physics at Harvard. On her way to the PhD, she realized inner space captivated her more than outer and added a master's in nutritional research from Tulane to her collection.

Peterson was inspired by Panda's 2012 studies, the ones in which TRF not only kept healthy mice healthy on a terrible diet but restored sick mice to health as well. If TRF could do even half as much for humans, she thought, it would be an enormous breakthrough, and she designed two trials to test TRF with an early feeding window. The first asked whether early TRF (eTRF) could keep overweight prediabetics from becoming full-blown diabetics. She wasn't wanting for volunteers. The Pennington Biomedical Research Center, where she conducted the trial, is in Baton Rouge, an obese, diabetic town in one of the most obese, diabetic states in the nation. Nearly one thousand men expressed an interest in the study and were winnowed to the eight who completed it. Peterson assigned four of them to eat three daily meals of equal size in a six-hour window starting between 6:30 and 8:30 a.m. and ending between 12:30 and 2:30 p.m. (Each man's precise window depended on when he awoke.) The other four men ate the same meals in a twelve-hour TRF starting between 6:30 and 8:30 a.m. After five weeks, there was a seven-week washout period in which they ate as they liked before crossing over to the opposite eating schedule for five more weeks.

The great flaw in virtually all dietary trials is that volunteers are left to feed themselves, which means they don't all eat the same food and usually don't accurately report what they do eat. If they get healthier, it's then hard to know whether to credit the variation in their individual menus or the intervention the researchers had set out to test, like a new diet or TRF. It gets even trickier if the volunteers lose weight, because weight loss, no matter what intervention prompts it, can cause people to become healthier. All of the human TRF studies to date suffered from these sorts of control problems, which Peterson endeavored to avoid with a far more rigorous protocol. For both five-week arms of the trial, she paid cooks to prepare all of the volunteers' food, which they had to eat in front of a technician either in person or over video. To eliminate weight change as a variable, they were weighed regularly, and at the first fluctuation in their mass, their meals were adjusted up or down in 100-calorie increments. It was a laborious, expensive undertaking, which is why there were so few subjects, but the results were worth it.

After five weeks on eTRF, the men's cholesterol dropped from 176 to 163, their triglycerides plunged 57 points, and their blood pressure fell from a prehypertensive 125/77 mm Hg to a normal 114/67, which was on par with what the best antihypertensive drugs could achieve. Peterson wasn't certain why eTRF made their blood pressure drop so superbly, but she thought a decrease in insulin in the blood might have relieved some of the pressure on their vessels. Five weeks on eTRF didn't rid the men of their prediabetes—they still had too much sugar in their blood for that—but their cells became nearly 20 percent more sensitive to insulin, which meant their pancreases produced less of it to clear the same amount of sugar as before and were consequently less exhausted. The benefit was surprisingly enduring. Even after the seven-week washout period, which Peterson thought would be long enough to erase the effects of eTRF, three of the four men who did eTRF in the first phase of the trial were still clearing glucose from their meals with less insulin.

She explored the biomechanics further in her second trial, in which she kitted out overweight and obese women and men with continuous glucose monitors before randomizing them, as in the other trial, to either the six-hour eTRF or the twelve-hour TRF. This time they did the intervention only four days and after a washout period crossed over to the other intervention for four days. Peterson found that on eTRF the volunteers had much smaller "glycemic excursions"—sugar spikes to most of us—which surprised her. She had expected exactly the reverse. To eat three meals in a six-hour window is, after all, to send sugar into the blood in a pretty steady stream. She had assumed her volunteers would have trouble clearing the breakfast sugar before the lunch sugar arrived and that the backlog would reach mountainous proportions by dinner. But the six-hour eTRF actually flattened the sugar spikes, whereas on the twelve-hour TRF the volunteers' blood sugar soared to great peaks before plummeting to deep valleys.

Peterson thought eTRF probably smoothed the sugar surges because sugar wasn't the only thing lingering in her volunteers' blood after breakfast and lunch. Insulin was hanging around too. When more glucose arrived at the next meal, the lingering insulin quickly unlocked the gates of their cells and moved it out of the blood. Also, the insulin-making beta cells in their pancreases probably hadn't shut down from the previous meal, so when more insulin was called for, their beta cells needed less time and effort to produce it—another reason their pancreases weren't so tired. Where insulin was concerned, eTRF appeared to work on the principle of the getaway car left idling.

Peterson's second trial was also the first to rigorously test whether people who lost weight on TRF did so because it somehow changed their metabolism or because, not grazing all day, they simply ate fewer calories. She sealed each volunteer inside a respiratory chamber that measured how many calories they burned over twenty-four hours and found no substantial difference between the six-hour eTRF and the twelve-hour TRF. The chamber, however, couldn't detect differences under 80 calories, so it's possible that on eTRF—with meals stacked earlier in the day, when the body spends more energy turning glucose into glycogen—the volunteers burned a few more calories. But if this was so, it didn't change their weight appreciably. Peterson concluded that when volunteers in other trials lost weight on TRF, they probably just ate less.

One reason they did might be that TRF modestly suppressed their appetite. Certainly eTRF could do so. In her five-week trial, the overweight volunteers reported being no hungrier on the six-hour eTRF than on the twelve-hour TRF. And in the evenings on eTRF, when they might have been expected to be ravenous after hours of fasting, they actually reported less desire to eat and a greater sensation of fullness than in the evenings on the twelve-hour TRF. One reason, Peterson discovered, was that on eTRF their bodies made more of the satiety hormone PYY and less of the hunger hormone ghrelin. Ketones, which suppress hunger, may also have played a part. On eTRF, her volunteers burned more fat during their long overnight fasts and had about 25 percent more ketones in their blood in the mornings than on the twelve-hour TRF. These were important findings. Nearly every strategy to help overweight people shed pounds fails because they remain hungry or grow even hungrier on their new diet. If the sole merit of eTRF were that it kept hunger from getting out of hand, it would be worthy of huzzahs.

But eTRF did so much more. Among the discoveries to flutter the scientific heart, Peterson showed that eTRF worked auspiciously on multiple gene-regulatory pathways linked with longevity. One was the SIRT1 pathway, which not only keeps our telomeres (the protective tips at the ends of our DNA) from disintegrating but also reduces inflammation and oxidative stress. In just four days on eTRF, Peterson's volunteers had about

10 percent more SIRT1 protein in the morning, presumably because their lengthy overnight fasts kept their bodies in repair mode longer. A 10 percent bump in a so-called longevity pathway won't, of course, directly translate into 10 percent more life, but it can't hurt.

eTRF also had a winning influence on *LC3A*, a gene vital to autophagy. You'll recall from chapter 11 that in autophagy a cell recycles its damaged parts by first dissolving them in a vat that it fashions for the purpose. The LC3A pathway oversees the manufacture of the vat. The more *LC3A* is expressed, the more autophagy there is, and in all likelihood the healthier and longer-lived the organism will be. After just four days on eTRF, the expression of the LC3A protein in Peterson's volunteers leapt 22 percent in the morning, again presumably because the long overnight fast extended their repair period. There were also hints that the longer a body practices eTRF, the more benefits are to be had. For example, in her four-day trial she found no significant change in genes regulating oxidative stress, but in her five-week trial her volunteers on eTRF produced 14 percent less 8-isoprostane, a marker for oxidative damage.

It was a magnificent set of findings. Peterson had shown that simply changing when but not what her volunteers ate lowered their blood pressure, cholesterol, and triglycerides, improved their insulin sensitivity, smoothed their sugar spikes, gave their overworked pancreases a break, activated longevity genes, and minimized cellular damage. It was all the more groundbreaking because the diet Peterson fed her volunteers—light on vegetables, fruit, and whole grains, heavy on meat, eggs, oil, and sugar—was far from healthy. But by delivering food at the right time, she apparently synced her volunteers' peripheral and master clocks to wonderful effect and overcame some of the problems of the diet.

That's not to say eTRF was a fix-all. She had hoped the regimen would make the stiffened arteries of her volunteers more pliable, but it didn't. She was also disappointed to see only slight drops in inflammatory markers like IGF-1, cortisol, and interleukin 6 and only a slight rise in brain-derived neurotrophic factor, BDNF. Then again, some of the gains she noted may have been understated because even her controls weren't eating the way Americans typically do. By taking three equally sized and evenly spaced meals in a twelve-hour TRF rather than grazing across four-teen hours a day with calories stacked toward evening, they probably got healthier as well.

Peterson's studies were published in 2018 and 2019 in prominent journals, were widely cited by other scientists, yet were all but ignored by the media. A decade earlier this kind of inattention wouldn't have sur-prised me, but it was strange in a moment when intermittent fasting was à la mode. I nursed an uncharitable suspicion that my journalistic kin didn't care to bear the bad news that the family dinner might be shaving years off our lives.

*   *   *

I didn't much care for the news myself. But the studies were so compel-ling that I couldn't stop thinking about the harm my twilight eating was almost certainly doing me. Trouble was, dinner was my favorite meal, din-nertime my favorite hour. I loved everything about the evening ritual: the chopping-block chatter with Jennifer, the house filling with the aroma of sautéing garlic as the sun went down, the chance to catch up on what Elliott was doing and to confirm it didn't require bail or paternity testing. A year or two before I read Peterson's work, other TRF research had con-vinced me to narrow my eating window to eight hours, but my window had always started around 11 a.m. and always included an evening meal. Never in a dozen lifetimes would it have occurred to me to give up dinner. But my desire to put off my rendezvous with the rider of the pale horse is fierce, and I decided to try switching my first meal to 9 a.m. and—in for a haunch, in for the hog—narrowing my window to six hours.

Well, it proved shockingly easy. One reason was that my hunger diminished at both ends of the day, just as it had for Peterson's volunteers. On my former TRF, I had sometimes wrestled with hunger in the last hour or two before my first meal at 11 a.m., but on eTRF what little hunger I felt before my 9 a.m. breakfast was just a pleasant anticipation, like when you sense late in a date that matters will soon end in a gratifying tangle. Even more surprising, in the wide hours between my last bite at 3 p.m. and my first snore in bed, I was almost never hungry. When hunger did poke me a little, it was never sharp enough to tempt me to interrupt the repairs my friends *SIRT1* and *LC3A* were making as we tromped deeper into the evening's fast together.

Not that I had no vaults to clear. When I first sat with Jennifer and Elliott during their dinner, a peevish voice in my head kept nagging, "And why aren't *you* eating?" My gurgling stomach, having made digestive juices at the traditional hour, chimed in to ask why it had gone to all that effort if food wasn't coming and, later, who the hell was going to sluice away all this corrosive juice. But after two or three days my stomach adapted to the new rhythm and was petulant no more, and I was left with only psychological hunger. It wasn't a true hunger because I had already eaten my fill for the day, and felt it. It was more an addictive desire, the kind that has you reaching for the third piece of chocolate cake when the first was plenty. I gently swatted away this yearning of the mind for about a week, after which it hardly ever reappeared, and my old dinner habit, half a century in the making, died with more whimper than bang.

But that wasn't even the best of it. After a couple of weeks on eTRF, I was enchanted to discover that my habitual cravings had departed. For most of the last twenty years, had you entered the Hendricks kitchen at any hour of the day or night, you'd have had a fair shot of finding the man of the house hunched over the remains of a debauch, empty tubs and torn wrappers spread about, crumbs dribbled on the floor, hardly knowing how he had eaten an entire round of gouda, every cracker in the pantry, a pound of hummus, and a mortifying number of cookies. When I switched to eating minimally processed plants, the cravings diminished, but not until I started eTRF did they vanish altogether. In their place were only manageable hankerings. I couldn't have been more surprised or tickled. At a guess, I'd say I was enjoying the glycemic smoothing that Peterson observed, a satisfying absence of sugar spikes and crashes and all the swings of mood and appetite that go with them.

Curiously, it didn't seem to matter whether I ate in three substantial, distinct meals—breakfast at nine, lunch at noon, dinner at two thirty—or browsed steadily across the six hours. Either way, I noticed no difference in hunger, energy, mood, or health. This may have been due, again, to the insulin that was at the ready in my blood to keep glucose moving along. The only exception to this idyllic state was when I fell mindlessly into a morning rush, didn't eat enough food early in the window, and took most of my calories toward the end of the six hours. On those days, my cravings were a little stronger.

But where eTRF most endeared itself to me—in fact, won my heart anew each morning—was in my daily encounter with the scale. For the previous dozen years, as I've mentioned, I had maintained my weight only by fasting periodically for several days. The maintenance grew easier when I switched to minimally processed plants, but the battle between inflation and deflation didn't finally cease until I adopted eTRF. Now when the scale registered slightly high one morning, I had no problem getting myself to eat a little less during the day. I think eTRF somehow made it easier to hear the satiety signals from my stomach. Whatever the case, appetite only rarely overwhelmed intent, and I even had mornings when the figure on the scale came up a little low and the day's happy task, if I chose, was to eat a little more. It felt another small miracle.

After practicing eTRF a couple of years now, I've come to suspect another big reason it has worked so well for me is what I've come to think of as the morning-hunger contradiction. The contradiction is that we're less hungry in the morning than at other times of day (according to both self-report and objective measurement of hunger and satiety hormones), and that's apparently all the more true on eTRF. Yet morning, as we've seen, is precisely when our bodies are primed to eat most efficiently, which suggests we should be at our hungriest then. But on eTRF it seemed to me the modest hunger I felt in the morning was just the right amount. When I ate to satiety early in the day, when I took just as much food as my stomach asked for, I didn't desire outlandish quantities later. It was as if the early eating made my body confident it would subsequently get the food it needed, when it needed it, so never demanded a binge. Whatever was going on, I had no trouble eating what was required and no more. Week to week, month to month, my weight hardly fluctuated: a pound here, two or three there, almost never more.

In the end, I also found ways to maintain most of what I loved about dinnertime. I preserved the nightly chopping-block chatter by dicing vegetables for Jennifer and Elliott's dinner or for mine the next day, and when I sat with them at their meal I was pleased to discover I was a more engaged collocutor because I wasn't distracted by eating. I would have been heartbroken had we never taken a big repast together, but on weekends and school breaks all three of us took dinner at midday, just as millions of families in Europe do. Ultimately it was one of the easiest big changes I've ever made in my life.

* * *

Research into time-restricted feeding in humans is in its infancy, but in other animals it has already been shown to extend both lifespan and healthspan. In a study at the National Institute on Aging, mice on TRF lived 14 percent longer than mice fed ad lib, and the extra months they got were mostly disease-free. TRF has also been proven to enhance the mammalian brain in many of the same ways prolonged fasting does: by strengthening synapses, reducing stress hormones, building stronger immune systems, and protecting against the ravages of Huntington's disease.

Although every trial of TRF in humans has found the practice safe, a few scientists worry about a handful of observational studies from the 1970s and 1980s that suggest daily fasts of more than twelve hours can produce gallstones. In one of those studies, American women who reported fasting fifteen hours a night were twice as likely to develop stones as women who reported fasting only seven hours. Then again, the fifteen-hour fasters had other unhealthy habits that could have given them their stones, like skipping breakfast and eating large amounts of cholesterol, which, however, is no trivial concern since most people in the developed world eat too much cholesterol.

But since no interventional trial of TRF (as opposed to an observational study) has documented a single gallstone in humans or other animals, the great majority of fasting scientists confidently recommend the practice to adults of all ages. (The jury is still out for older children and is a resounding no for infants.) Scientists are less certain about how narrow the eating window should be. Most think somewhere between six and ten hours. Satchin Panda believes "the health benefits that you get from eating within a 12-hour window double at 11 hours, and double again at 10, and so on, until you reach an 8-hour window." Other researchers suspect the improvement continues until six hours, and a few think four. On the strength of such counsel, even the notoriously conservative American Heart Association, long cool to dietary remedies for cardiovascular disease, has recommended TRF as a preventive. It is one more small sign that fasting, after its long ramble in the wilderness, is at last gaining entry to the medical motherland.

CHAPTER 17

A WINE COUNTRY ABSTENTION, 2

In 1994, at the age of thirty-eight, a dentist named Christina Gore was attending a convention when a tent pole worked loose from its stays and smashed into the back of her head. When she came to, she had the worst headache of her life, an excruciation. The blow had torn her dura mater, the tough fibrous covering that shields the brain and spinal cord, and the severely inflamed dura was the source of her headache. As days became weeks, and weeks months, it didn't diminish in the slightest.

Surgeons didn't know how to repair a tear like Gore's without doing more harm, and none of the several drugs her doctors prescribed gave her even modest relief. On a scale of one to ten, the pain was a constant six to eight with occasional stabs of ten that brought her to her knees. She was forced to give up her dental practice, and the only hope her doctors could offer was that sometimes the pain simply went away after two, five, or even ten years. But each milestone passed with her misery unchecked.

Fifteen years after the accident, Gore happened upon the website of the TrueNorth Health Center. She wasn't looking for a cure, just reading a blog that mentioned the clinic and prolonged fasting, and it all sounded so peculiar that she decided to have a look. As she read the website, she noticed many of the disorders that TrueNorth's practitioners claimed to have healed were caused by inflammation, and she picked up the phone. The doctors she spoke to, including Alan Goldhamer, said they didn't know whether fasting would help her, but, yes, it could often work wonders for inflammatory conditions.

Gore flew to California in 2010 and fasted for eighteen days with not a whisper of improvement. On the nineteenth day, she awoke and knew instantly something was wrong but couldn't place quite what. After a minute, she realized that for the first time in sixteen years she had no headache. A few minutes later the pain came flooding back and stayed with her the rest of the day, but that snatch of freedom was all she needed to keep going. Goldhamer was hardly less excited. "It's amenable to treatment!" he shouted. "It's amenable to treatment!"

On each subsequent day of her fast, the pain disappeared for a little longer and was a little less severe when it came surging back. By the time she broke the fast after forty-one days, the pain had fallen to less than one out of ten. She went home for several months, stuck to Goldhamer's unprocessed vegan diet, and after another fast of forty days her pain disappeared entirely and never returned. During that fast, she met Ivonne Vielman, from the prologue, and it was Gore's story of recovery that convinced Vielman to fast long enough to rid herself of follicular lymphoma.

* * *

Sarita Bhola put on weight when she was pregnant with her second child, and sixty-five pounds of it didn't come off—hardly a surprise, she would later say, given the junk food she subsisted on. Now and then she slimmed with crash dieting, but she always yo-yoed the weight back on, and finally her health deteriorated. In 1989, in early middle age, she was diagnosed with chronic fatigue syndrome, the first in a long list of diagnoses that would come to include diabetes, fibromyalgia, congestive heart failure, asthma, adrenal fatigue, sleep apnea, depression, gastroesophageal reflux disease, anemia, urinary incontinence, and ten others. By 1995, she was nearly bedridden and was only able to arise each morning, she believed, because of vitamin B12 injections that she took daily for a quarter century.

Among the dozens of doctors Bhola saw was a blunt naturopath who told her if she didn't make a radical change, she wasn't long for this world, and he referred her to TrueNorth. When she checked in to the clinic in 2014, she brought seventeen prescription drugs and twenty-five supplements, could walk no more than a couple of steps at a time, and considered bathing an almost unendurable workout. She spent a month just weaning off her medications and supplements and eating Goldhamer's whole-plant meals free of salt, oil, and sugar. Then she fasted twenty-one days. By the time she went home, she could walk for thirty minutes and do an hour and a half of yoga. She came back twice more for fasts of one and two weeks, stuck with the new way of eating, and lost eighty-five pounds. Eventually she winnowed her supplements to three and her medications to zero and could exercise for up to two hours a day. Most of her twenty-one illnesses disappeared, and the few that didn't—chiefly chronic fatigue, fibromyalgia, and asthma—improved greatly. She hailed Goldhamer and his staff psychologist Doug Lisle her saviors.

*　　*　　*

Gabrielle Kirby was a young Irishwoman with interstitial cystitis, a harrowing inflammation of the bladder with neither a known cause nor, according to authorities like the Mayo Clinic, a cure. She urinated up to forty times a day, and the pain often grew so savage that instead of sleeping she passed the night standing, sitting, or pacing, always in search of a position marginally less agonizing than the last. Seven years of drugs, diets, and surgery failed to give her relief, and the only other option her doctors could offer was to remove her bladder, but they warned her that in many cases the pain persisted even so.

In 1999, Kirby went to the Center for Conservative Therapy, TrueNorth's earliest incarnation, and had a miserable time of it. Within days of starting her fast, her face flushed scarlet, she ran a rising fever, and she vomited several times a day. Her doctor said she was going through a healing crisis, a consequence of her body repairing itself, but when the vomiting didn't stop, he switched her to juice. The symptoms disappeared,

Kirby fasted again, and once more she became flushed, feverish, and vomitous. Three times she did this jitterbug between fasting and juicing until finally she could tolerate the fast. After seventeen days, her pain disappeared and her trips to the loo diminished. She broke her fast on the twenty-first day, and six months later she still had no pain and remained continent—to all appearances, cured of her incurable disease.

* * *

Gabrielle Fennimore's torment was ulcerative colitis. Her large intestine, inflamed and riddled with sores, assaulted her with twisting pains that she could only incompletely relieve by moving her bowels, which she did eight or ten times a day. Doctors gave her anti-inflammatories and steroids, but each colonoscopy revealed the disease was only getting worse. Her C-reactive protein, an inflammatory marker that in healthy people is below 3 mg/L and in the healthiest below 1 mg/L, was never below 5 and sometimes shot as high as 20. Eventually she developed a perpetual diarrhea and bled from her rectum. When she asked her doctors what she should eat, they said since she had no allergies, food wasn't the cause of her troubles and she could do as she pleased. She tried all sorts of diets anyway—diets without wheat, soy, corn, and beans, diets high in grapeseed oil, coconut oil, and avocado oil—but nothing worked. Life was fast becoming a misery.

Fennimore was a dental hygienist in New Jersey, and one day her boss, a dentist of some perception, introduced her to T. Colin Campbell's *The China Study*. Campbell's explanation of the harmful effects of the standard American diet made instant and convincing sense to her. Her boss also said there was a doctor in Santa Rosa, California, named John McDougall, one of the fathers of the modern vegan-health movement, who ran a ten-day program that taught people how to stop eating the animal products and processed foods that were destroying their health. Fennimore attended McDougall's program, but ten days weren't nearly enough to fix the years of damage to her gut, and her symptoms improved only modestly. The McDougall people said they sent hard cases like her across town to their friend Alan Goldhamer.

Fennimore checked in to TrueNorth but rather than fast ate a very restricted diet of a few select plants and was tapered off her medications. After ten days, her stool was solid for the first time in years. Other foods were very gradually introduced to see which ones triggered her symptoms, and after a month she went back home able to eat fifteen different plants without a flare-up and with the skills to test more plants as she continued to heal. When her C-reactive protein dropped to 1.3, her doctor in New Jersey, who had been dubious of her decision to go to Santa Rosa and had lobbied her to take a powerful immunosuppressant instead, was so stunned that he did something nearly unheard of in American medicine: he called his patient himself.

"What in the world have you been taking?" he asked.

"It's the food!" she cried. It had always been the food.

*   *   *

Not long after Alan Goldhamer founded the Center for Conservative Therapy, his father Harold Goldhamer began having transient ischemic attacks. TIAs, sometimes called ministrokes, often harbinge a worse deterioration to come, and soon Harold began forgetting things, then had trouble thinking clearly, and finally was forced to retire from the job he loved as a math teacher. Conventional medicine offered little hope and no remedy, so he put himself under his son's care, fasted twenty-six days, and became one of the most diligent followers of the SOS-free vegan diet that Alan Goldhamer has ever known. The TIAs stopped. Harold began to remember things and recovered most of his cognitive ability. Later he developed Parkinson's disease, which was not cured by diet or fasting, but his quality of life remained high, and two decades after his first ministrokes, when Goldhamer *fils* and Doug Lisle wrote their book *The Pleasure Trap*, Goldhamer *père*, at nearly eighty, was its editor.

Alan Goldhamer's mother Phyllis Goldhamer also adopted the SOS-free vegan diet and on turning ninety realized she had outlived all fifty-two of her lifelong friends. For decades they had given her grief for giving up all the K foods—kugel, kreplach, knishes—in favor of her son's crazy plants, and she now realized the worst part of outliving them all was there was nobody left to say I told you so to. One day she clapped urgent eyes on her son and said with some heat, "Alan! You need to warn your patients. If they're going to eat this diet: Make. Younger. Friends."

* * *

During my and Jennifer's stay at TrueNorth, remissions less dramatic than those but no less stirring to the heart were thick on the ground. Patients were continually arriving with high blood pressure or diabetes, angina or acid reflux, sleep apnea or insomnia, lupus or gout, and several weeks later departing with normal blood pressure and blood sugar, no chest pain, less reflux, better sleep, and fewer flare-ups of their lupus, gout, and whatever else. In the courtyard, talk of these turnarounds floated atop a broad under-current of dismay that now and then boiled through the surface.

"My doctor *insisted* to me it was incurable."

"Mine said I'd always be on medications."

"Mine said it was genes or bad luck, not the food—the food had *nothing* to do with it."

"Honey," a repeat guest would lean in and say sympathetically, "every one of our doctors told us that."

A couple of our fellow fasters had moved past dismay to cold fury. One older guy had endured fifteen years of angina and shortness of breath, his cardiovascular disease advancing, his doctors giving him more pills every year with the assurance this was the best that medicine could offer. But in just two weeks under Goldhamer's care, he was off all his medications, his angina had reversed, his breathing had eased, his blood pressure was plummeting, and he had learned for the first time that Drs. Dean Ornish and Caldwell Esselstyn had decades ago—*decades*—shown separately in important peer-reviewed journals that cardiovascular disease could be reversed with a diet of plants and a few simple lifestyle changes.

"What the godblasted hell?" was all he could say of his "caregivers."

Every once in a while Goldhamer and his staff achieved a remission even before a patient arrived at TrueNorth. Shortly before our visit, Goldhamer had consulted with a woman long afflicted with bilateral neuropathy—numbness in both legs. She made an appointment to fast, but Goldhamer encouraged her while she was waiting to change her diet. She did, and within a week her neuropathy vanished. She had seen a small battalion of neurologists, orthopedic surgeons, and specialists of other stripe and had had $200,000 of medical workups, and although the doctors couldn't agree on much, when she asked whether her diet was the cause of her illness, every one of them said food had nothing to do with it. She was in a lather of indignation when she called Goldhamer to cancel her fast.

"I spent all this money!" she shouted. "How come those other doctors all said diet wouldn't help—didn't matter at all—and the one person I never even saw resolves it with diet?"

In Goldhamer's experience, frustration with doctors was a common and powerful motivator. His elder brother Mark was a specimen case. Years ago, Mark's wife fasted at the clinic, adopted the SOS-free vegan diet, and overcame her own health problems, but fifteen years later, as Alan told it, "my brother's still eating chicken and getting fatter, he can't play volleyball anymore, and his leg's all swollen up. I'm poking him, but he won't do anything. Finally he calls me and says, 'Alan, I'm in the hospital. I had a heart attack.'

"I said, 'That's great!'

"He goes, 'No, no, no, you don't hear—I had a heart attack.'

"I said, 'I heard you. Best thing that could have happened.'"

A myocardial infarction, Alan had often observed, could be one hell of a prod, provided it was survived. Mark said his surgeon wanted to do a quadruple bypass, so Alan suggested he ask a few questions, like wouldn't the arteries plug up again after the bypass? The surgeon said they would indeed, but a bypass wouldn't clog as soon as stents.

"Well," said Mark, again at his brother's prompting, "what if I made radical diet and lifestyle changes?"

The surgeon practically guffawed.

"Now, Mark," he said, "you are *not* going to make diet and lifestyle changes. Come on."

Miffed, Mark checked himself out of the hospital, got on his brother's diet, lost fifty pounds, went back to playing volleyball, passed a stress test, and kept all of his natal vessels.

A thousand such stories have convinced Alan Goldhamer that conventional medicine is less healthcare than sickcare, a tool for managing the symptoms of disease rather than reversing its causes. Most people, he says, have been so indoctrinated in the model, they don't see how ludicrous sickcare is. "You go to a physician with a disease of dietary excess: the high blood pressure, the type 2 diabetes, the autoimmune disease, and the doctor says to you, 'If you do everything I tell you—if you follow my instructions *exactly*—you're going to be on drugs for the rest of your life. And I also promise you this: you will never, ever get well.'" Anyone who has wrestled for years with a chronic condition under the care of conventional doctors only to find it cured in days by fasting would find his point inarguable.

*   *   *

The medical authorities of California take a different view of healthcare and more than once have tried to shut Goldhamer down. The gravest threat came in 2009, when the California Board of Medical Quality Assurance opined that fasting a patient was so gross a violation of the standard of medical care, it amounted to criminal negligence. The board had earlier sent investigators to TrueNorth disguised as patients to gather "evidence" that Goldhamer, by not feeding his patients, was grievously endangering them. A hearing was scheduled to decide whether to close the clinic.

Goldhamer retained a lawyer in Los Angeles who specialized in medical malpractice, and on reviewing the matter, he pronounced Goldhamer atypical of his clientele because he seemed to have done nothing wrong. Since he was clean, the lawyer said he could make the case go away, although Goldhamer would have to surrender a lot of time and money and, of course, would have to stop fasting people. When Goldhamer explained that fasting was what TrueNorth did, the lawyer said if that was so, the case was unwinnable. The medical board had almost total authority over such affairs, was essentially unappealable, and plainly had it in for him. He told Goldhamer to prepare his professional obituary.

Goldhamer got off the phone and called his friends at the International Union of Operating Engineers, whose members he'd been fasting for eight years. He asked if the powerful union could do anything to help. The official on the other end of the line chuckled and said, "Of course we can help you. It's just a question of what it's going to cost us."

Twenty-four hours later Goldhamer got a call from his lawyer.

"Who do you know?" the barrister sputtered. "I just got a call from the attorney general's office, and you're gonna agree to pay a fine to cover the cost of their investigation, and everything's gonna go away."

And that is just what happened. The lawyer wrote a memo in which he explained fasting wasn't quackery, that even Medicare paid for the fasts of obese patients who needed to lose weight rapidly for urgent surgery. ("But it was only covered if you didn't get well and still had to have your surgery after the fast," Goldhamer said. "If you got well at a place like TrueNorth, the fasting wasn't covered.") The medical board cited the memo and let Goldhamer keep his doors open.

There have been lesser scrapes. A few years after the board fracas, a police officer showed up in TrueNorth's lobby and demanded to interview one of Goldhamer's patients. When Goldhamer asked what the patient had done, the officer said he didn't need to know.

"Well, if you want me to tell you if he's here or not," Goldhamer replied, "I need to know."

Eventually the officer said the department had received a complaint from the patient's relatives, who alleged, in Goldhamer's words, that "he was being held against his will by religious cultists and being starved to death to go to be with Jesus."

Goldhamer said the officer could interview his patient. "But first," he asked, "would you like a nice tall cup of Kool-Aid?"

His psychologist friend Dr. Lisle told him he was not to speak to authorities anymore.

* * *

After Goldhamer and T. Colin Campbell published their articles on blood pressure in the early 2000s, Goldhamer added more stones to the scientific foundation he was laying for fasting by publishing case reports in peer-reviewed journals. It was a well-worn strategy to advance a novel therapy: show through anecdote that a treatment seems to work, and it becomes easier to get funding for the randomized, controlled trials that could put the question beyond doubt. Shrewdly, Goldhamer chose only cases in which the patient had before-and-after scans or tests that could objectively confirm the severity of the disease and its improvement after fasting. The remission of Ivonne Vielman's stage III follicular lymphoma was one such, and he has lately been documenting the reversal of other follicular lymphomas, including, astonishingly, one in stage IV. That reversal was so spectacular that the patient's oncologist, previously antagonistic to fasting, encouraged him to return to TrueNorth and see if another forty-day fast would shrink his lesions even further. The man was doing that during our stay. Goldhamer and his research staff, who numbered half a dozen, hoped the cases would spark a clinical trial to compare fasting for lymphoma at TrueNorth with conventional therapy.

On the whole, Goldhamer's research points to the same remarkable mechanism that Françoise Wilhelmi de Toledo's research points to: fasting eliminates materials selectively, and among the first materials eliminated are those that do us harm. "How do we know this is true?" Goldhamer said. "Let's say you have a tumor and you lose ten percent of your body weight. You would assume that you would lose about ten percent of your tumor weight too, but what happens in follicular lymphoma is you lose a hundred percent of the tumor. So the body is preferentially mobilizing some nutrient stores versus others. And it seems to be able to do that in inverse proportion to the value of those tissues to the body. We see this also with visceral fat, which we think is unhealthy fat. Research we're doing shows the body will mobilize visceral fat at about three times the rate of adipose fat, the other fat in your body, which isn't as harmful. In other words, the body has this intelligence about which toxins to preferentially mobilize. It can do some of this when you're just maintaining a healthy diet and lifestyle, but in water-only fasting it mobilizes these toxins at a much more powerful rate."

Other researchers have begun to take note of Goldhamer's work, and a few have even become his collaborators. At the time of our visit, he was wrapping up a trial with investigators from the Mayo Clinic on fasting for the prevention of stroke. The trial had come about because one of the Mayo researchers, having fasted at TrueNorth for his own health, was impressed by Goldhamer's studies and thought maybe science should focus more on preventing strokes in the first place than dealing with their wreckage afterward. Goldhamer was also working with Luigi Fontana of the University of Sydney, one of the world's foremost researchers of dietary restriction, to examine how fasting affects the gut microbiome and several longevity markers.

A few clinicians have also come to appreciate Goldhamer's efforts. A doctor from the Texas A&M College of Medicine who fared well in Santa Rosa went back to College Station and got the school to approve TrueNorth as a host for third-year students on their functional medicine rotation. I grew up not far from College Station, and if you had asked me which of the country's 155 medical schools would be the first to approve a rotation in fasting, I'd have gone through about 150 before landing on A&M. But Goldhamer didn't seem surprised. He said when he lectured at medical conferences, the air in the hall that used to be filled with hostility was now tinged with curiosity. Young doctors often asked him why they hadn't been taught that fasting and diet could cure various "incurable" diseases, and sometimes even an older doctor wondered aloud why he had spent a whole career failing to heal a single diabetic while Goldhamer was reversing diabetes every month. (Goldhamer claimed 80 percent of his type 2 diabetics who fasted their way to remission maintained the remission if they stuck with the SOS-free vegan diet.)

TrueNorth has a standing offer to train for free, remotely or in person, any doctor to supervise a fast. But the supervision usually takes more time than doctors expect, and it is the rare conventional doctor who has overseen a second fast. If medically supervised fasting is to spread in America,

Goldhamer sees it happening through clinics like his that sit outside the dominant health system. To that end, he annually trains thirty resident chiropractors, naturopaths, and MDs, a few of whom have founded their own tiny fasting clinics, one in Ohio, another in Southern California, another in Puerto Rico. Whether these endeavors will survive longer than the ephemeral clinics of the past is anyone's guess, but thanks to Goldhamer, the climate is more favorable than ever before.

Among establishmentarians, alas, hostility and ignorance remain the wearisome norm. Goldhamer recently finished a simple study showing that when fasters refed on an SOS-free, unprocessed vegan diet, the weight they regained was composed not of fat but of water, fiber, glycogen, and protein. One journal rejected the study with a scathing note that said, in Goldhamer's summation, "that to allow a person to not eat for two weeks was the most egregious violation of human safety standards they'd seen in twenty-five years of publishing." Fasting's path to acceptance remains a stony one.

* * *

To my eyes, the greatest difference between the methods of TrueNorth and Buchinger Wilhelmi was not so much fasting on water versus broth but the extent to which fasters were encouraged to reform their lives. In Überlingen, as I've said, the clinicians preferred the small, gently suggested tweak, but in Santa Rosa we were told flatly that if we were sick, it was usually because of how we lived, above all how we ate and drank, and if we wanted to get well, we had to banish processed and animal foods and eat plants. To do otherwise, to go back home and eat as we'd always eaten, would obliterate many of our heartwarming remissions.

Goldhamer knew the change wasn't easy to make. Most people's taste buds are so conditioned to fatty, salty, sugary, meaty, and cheesy foods that plants no longer taste good, and few people can eat things for long that they find unpalatable. This is the problem at the heart of Goldhamer and Lisle's book *The Pleasure Trap*, in which they argue that the modern epidemic of lifestyle diseases—cardiovascular disease, cancer, obesity, diabetes, dementia, and other afflictions once infrequent but now common—has arisen because for the first time in history we're eating great piles of hyper-rich food, much of it intentionally engineered to trick us into overeating. Goldhamer and Lisle posit that humans have the same fundamental drives as other animals: we seek pleasure, avoid pain, and conserve energy. This "motivational triad" spurred early humans to prize foods that were the tastiest, safest, and easiest to get, and it's no coincidence that the tastiest foods—the ones that triggered a release of dopamine in the brain—were also the most calorically dense. Dopamine was nature's way of ensuring our forebears would fill themselves on a relatively few sources of nutrients rather than foraging all day for lots of undense foods low in nutrition. So long as humans were gatherers and scavengers who only rarely got their hands on anything fattier than a nut or more densely sugared than a berry, the motivational triad served them brilliantly. It's the reason our ancestors could eat to satiation without becoming overweight or obese as we do.

But eventually humans learned to hunt efficiently, then to domesticate animals and crops, and finally to hyper-refine the products from their fields and beasts by stripping them of fiber and nutrients and making them even more calorically dense. Today our diet is vastly fattier, more sugary, and saltier than anything we evolved to eat, but it tastes awfully good to people whose palates have been habituated to it. The dopamine rush that was once so useful in our evolution now encourages us to stuff ourselves with pizza and Oreos, and because junk like that is so very dense, we can cram a lot of it into our stomachs before our brains figure out we've over-eaten. That can't happen on lettuce. Pack your stomach to the brim with greens, and you'll have consumed about a hundred calories. Pack it with a McDonald's Combo Meal, and you'll have topped a thousand.

As Goldhamer and Lisle see it, we didn't become a "fat, sick, and miserable" race because we have no willpower or don't exercise enough or weren't loved enough by our parents. We're fat, sick, and miserable because we're doing what nature designed us to do: eat the densest, most delicious foods we can get our hands on with the least effort. This is the pleasure trap, and it's why no one wants a carrot once they've had Krispy Kreme.

Breaking free of the pleasure trap, they argue, is also a question of biology more than of fortitude or self-esteem. Research has shown that when an eater of fatty foods switches to less fatty foods, it can take up to three months before her taste buds deem the new food tasty. In Goldhamer and Lisle's experience, the only patients who can endure three months of eating food they don't like are ones whose pain, debility, or fear of death have reached an apex. For everyone else, the two clinicians have an answer, which, as you've no doubt guessed, is to fast. In days, fasting resets the taste buds and returns the internal compass to true north. To Goldhamer, this capacity of the taste buds to "neuroadapt" is a biomechanism of consummate beauty, and it's so powerful it apparently works against addictions stronger than food. His smokers, for instance, usually stop complaining about cravings after just two or three days of fasting and are "amazed how much easier it was to give up the cigarettes while fasting than it ever was the twenty-five times they've tried while eating."

But although Goldhamer's SOS-free, minimally processed vegan diet becomes more flavorful with reset taste buds, his patients still stumble. For many, the hardest part is not the minimally processed veganism but the SOS-freedom, which, however, Goldhamer believes is just as important. Salt, he says, may be noncaloric, but it sends blood pressure soaring and triggers a dopamine release that prompts us to eat a whole bag of chips instead of the handful we intended. Oils also trigger a dopamine release and at four thousand calories per pound are the densest food on earth. (It takes six thousand olives, stripped of their fiber, water, and most nutrients, to make a liter of oil.) That kind of density makes oily foods especially easy to overeat before our bodies have figured out they've had too much. Goldhamer has no truck with even cold-pressed olive oil, which, he says, may be healthier than butter, coconut oil, or hot-pressed olive oil, but "healthier doesn't mean it's healthy, just not as unhealthy as whatever it's being compared to." He has similar problems with sugar, each pound of which is condensed from thirty pounds of cane with nearly all the nutrition stripped out—the perfect compound to make our insulin do cartwheels.

The good news, Goldhamer has found, is once people's taste buds adapt to healthy food, they don't miss the salt, oil, and sugar. Fruits like berries are plenty sweet, they can taste the salt in vegetables like celery, and they require nothing fattier than a few nuts or half an avocado—which was just how I experienced it. The bad news, as he warns his patients, is "the world is designed to make you fat, sick, and miserable." Temptation lurks everywhere, from the Toblerone at the checkout counter to the Pepsi in the office vending machine to the brisket at the family barbecue. Many of his patients, on returning home, think they can dabble in such fare only to find their taste buds quickly rehabituated to it, after which unprocessed plants no longer taste so fine. Social pressures reinforce the problem, and the pressures are worse, Goldhamer believes, for women.

"If you're a woman," he said, "and you lose fifty pounds and you go back to work, do the other women go, 'Oh, dear, we're so happy for you. What can we do to support you in your new habits?' Or do you walk in the room, and they go, 'Oh here she comes, that bitch'? Believe me, they're going to bring you cupcakes."

Men, less physically critiqued, have it easier, but no one has it easy. Research has shown that for even the most successful diets, no more than 10 or 20 percent of people keep their lost weight off for even a year, and after two or three years that number falls to 2 or 3 percent. A study Goldhamer's team was working on has preliminarily found that 30 percent of TrueNorth's patients maintain their weight loss for a year. If that number is verified in peer review, it will be both an astounding success and a sad testament to how tight a snare the pleasure trap is.

Goldhamer isn't overflowing with ideas about how to increase that 30 percent, nor about how to spread his diet to more people. It is, he believes, simply a hard sell, as he discovered rather literally in an exchange two decades ago with a marketer at a large publishing house where *The Pleasure Trap* was under consideration. As Goldhamer told the story, the marketer was himself snared in the pleasure trap.

"He was about four hundred pounds, just huge, and he said, 'You've got to stop with this "pleasure's bad" stuff and start telling people to drink red wine and eat dark chocolate.'" He pointed to the Atkins diet books, which had sold millions of copies by telling people to eat fat.*

---

* Not long later, Dr. Robert Atkins dropped dead at the age of seventy-two from what may have been his second heart attack, although because his widow would not allow an autopsy, the cause of death will never be known.

"We can't say that," Goldhamer protested. "It's not true."

"Do you want to tell the truth," the marketer returned, "or do you want to sell books?"

When Goldhamer said they wanted to do both, the marketer nearly came unhinged.

"You're not going to sell books telling people they can't have anything," he sneered. "Get the fuck out of here and quit wasting our time."

The editor who had brought the book to her colleagues told Goldhamer they threw food at her at the next lunch meeting.

The Pleasure Trap will never sell millions of copies, but it recently surpassed a hundred thousand, a respectable showing for a practically unpublicized book from an obscure publisher. As Alvise Cornaro learned four centuries earlier with his *Discourses on the Sober Life*, some people are willing to trade indulgence for longevity, and a substantial share of them will even buy a book telling them how to do it.

*   *   *

In our stay at TrueNorth I met a woman, who called to mind another, who together suggested to me that Goldhamer was right to demand radical change of his sick patients. The woman at TrueNorth was a retired middle school teacher from Decatur, Alabama, who had topped four hundred pounds when she first came to the clinic eighteen months earlier. All her adult life she had been obese, and on three separate occasions over forty years she had lost and regained more than a hundred pounds. She rattled off her variant of what I came to think of as the TrueNorth chart: high blood pressure, cardiovascular disease, diabetes, acid reflux, gout, sleep apnea, restless legs, attention deficit disorder, depression, orthopedic woes, and much more that I wasn't able to jot down. For decades she was never out of pain. But one day a niece on "a weird hippie diet"—all plants, not one of them fried—got her to watch the 2011 documentary *Forks Over Knives*, the gentle battle hymn of the plant-based health movement. Steeped in the research of T. Colin Campbell and the cardiologist Caldwell Esselstyn, the movie has turned viewers vegan by the thousand.

The teacher was dumbfounded to learn that what she was eating might be the cause of her ailments, and she began to change her diet. Eventually she turned up at TrueNorth, stayed seven weeks, fasted most of them, got off all nine of her medications, and lost most of her diseases. Later she came back for two more fasts. On one of her travels she realized as she sat down on an airplane that she no longer needed the seatbelt extender she had requested for decades. She cried half the flight.

Her reforms didn't rid her of all her ills. Her gout still flared, and her joints creaked. "You're going to pay a price for sixty years of damaging your body," she said. But she had lost 220 pounds and had kept them off longer than she'd ever kept off weight before. She praised Jesus and Goldhamer, not necessarily in that order.

The woman she brought to my mind was a Seattleite I had met at Buchinger Wilhelmi. She was obese, fatigued, and had a sheaf of other health problems she didn't care to divulge, but she was radiant with hope that the tests the Buchinger doctors were running would turn up new avenues to fix her. She was, however, completely mystified by her obesity.

"It's not what I eat," she said, "so it must be something else."

The teacher from Alabama had told herself the same thing for years—"It's not what I eat"—and it was a phrase I, too, knew well from when I was thirty pounds heavier. I'm sure millions of other overweight people tell themselves the same. Goldhamer didn't countenance the sentence.

"Of *course* it's what you eat," he said. "And I'll prove it to you. Come do a medically supervised, water-only fast, and I guarantee you will lose weight." Physics demands it, just as physics says you cannot gain weight if you don't overeat. Moreover, according to Goldhamer, virtually everyone who adhered to an SOS-free, minimally processed vegan diet lost roughly two pounds a week until they reached a healthy weight. For all the considerable merits of Buchinger Wilhelmi, I feared the Seattleite would never hear a message like that in Überlingen, and until she did, I imagined she'd have a hell of a time taking the weight off and getting her health back.

*　*　*

Although my sample size is small, I can say with some confidence that if you visit a renowned fasting clinic, you're unlikely to escape without having to weather a patch of pseudoscientific or New Age claptrap that will make your eyeballs somersault and your brain mewl. At TrueNorth it came not from reincarnated Quebeckers but from the staff at educational lectures. Many of these talks were grounded in sturdy research or insightful practice, but a few simply whomperjawed Jennifer and me. One doctor said that while vaccines were an enormous boon that had cut childhood mortality, if you got vaccinated when you were under great stress, it might prove to be the drop that caused your cup to overflow and leave you with autism. I was speechless, and Jennifer, who has no tolerance for the madness of anti-vaxxers, nearly checked out of the clinic on the spot. I doubt any myth in medicine has been more thoroughly debunked. At another lecture, a young chiropractor-in-training whose stock in trade was a tossed salad of alternative-health catchphrases told us that meditation lengthened the life-prolonging telomeres on the ends of our DNA "by connecting them to godsource." He neglected to offer a citation.

But for my money the winner of the inanity stakes was a lecture on reflexology, a practice premised on the sound idea that if you apply pressure to certain points on the hands, feet, and ears, you can elicit good feelings in other parts of the body. Unfortunately, reason and reflexology take their leave of each other there. The reflexologist told us with utmost earnestness that we each had what amounted to a sensory map of the body invisibly imprinted on the surface of our hands, feet, and ears and that pressing on a certain part of the map could evoke a pointed reply in the corresponding part of the body, a bit like putting a needle in a voodoo doll. The maps were so specific that a practitioner of her talent could stimulate into action a patient's hypothalamus or liver or the adrenal gland of her choice. There isn't the slightest science or even convincing anecdote to support these marvelous notions, which she topped with an illuminating disquisition on shamanic journeying. If I got it right, by rhythmically drumming she could enter one of two spirit worlds, upper or lower, where amiable animalic guides led her on healing journeys. I looked around the room to make sure none of my fellow fasters had a glass of Flavor Aid in front of them. Some might as well have because afterward a handful always extolled even the looniest of talks as "just amazing" or "awesome." They were amazing and awesome alright.

Having heard much of a similar nature at Buchinger Wilhelmi and having slogged through whole marshes of it while reading the "literature" for this book, I think I understand the problem. Once you discover your doctor has been wrong about the cause and cure of your disease, you are primed to ask what else the authorities have missed. It's a healthy question, the very essence of scientific inquiry, but to arrive at the right answer requires a judicious weighing of evidence, and that is a skill, I'm sorry to say, that lies far beyond the ken of many fasters. At both clinics and online, I encountered a large number of fasters who happily swallowed just about any unorthodoxy, no matter how nonsensical, simply because the experts said it couldn't be. I shouldn't have been surprised. In America the same percentage of people—twenty—believe in Bigfoot and the Big Bang, forty percent of us think humans and dinosaurs coexisted, and nearly sixty percent think dreams can foretell the future. The numbers are only a little better in other countries. The fasters I came across were, in other words, an accurate sampling of a larger populace ill versed in rational discernment.

Since Goldhamer's own lectures were deeply rooted in evidence and he was clearly at pains to show fasting wasn't quackery, I asked him about some of the codswallop his staff was ladling out. He said he knew of no science to support either the vaccine theory of autism or reflexology, save for the clinical observation that people feel good when their ears, hands, or feet are pressed.

"And shamanic journeying?" I said.

His head fell into his hands.

"Oh god," he muttered. "Who's talking shamanic journeying?"

When he had recovered, he said he was in the process of reevaluating the clinic's educational program, but with more than fifty hours of talks to fill each month, it was slow going. He added that TrueNorth had recently started a Roku channel, but until the reevaluation was further along, no lectures except his own were being broadcast live. I took him to mean he was worried his staff might say something batshit crazy over the airwaves.

*   *   *

My fast came off without incident, the only faint drama provided by my weight. On the fourth day, when I dipped below 125 pounds, I joined the ranks of the clinically underweight, those with a body-mass index south of 18.5. TrueNorth didn't routinely fast people much beyond that, not from fear of starvation—at a BMI of 18 or even 17, most people still have weeks of fat reserves—but from fear of illness. The faster who became badly sick with so small a cache might get into trouble if his appetite disappeared, his sickness lingered, and he continued to wither. But since I had no complications and wanted to fast as long as possible to right whatever had gone awry in my gut, my doctor let me press on. When I broke the fast after nine days, the scale read 119 pounds, for a BMI of 17.6. I was all knobs and angles.

My gastrointestinal troubles, having disappeared with my food, were good enough to stay away as I refed. But after two joyously ungaseous weeks they returned, albeit not as potently as before. I was disappointed until I realized the partial failure would give this chronicle verisimilitude, that my claims for fasting would ring truer if the practice hadn't cured every last one of my ailments. A week later, though, the gut troubles redisappeared, and I mourned the loss to the literature of fasting for approximately eight seconds. Since then, the disturbance has flared in times of stress and calmed down once I have, a useful if odiferous barometer of my psychological health. I'm crossing fingers my next long fast will do in the unrest for good.

Beyond fatigue, Jennifer had neither struggle nor triumph to report of her fast—she is a great disappointment to a writer in search of material. But a few days after getting home, her physical therapist said her injured shoulder seemed less inflamed and moved more freely than before, although it was of course impossible to say whether the cause was her fast or not using the shoulder for two sluggy weeks.

The transformation of her taste buds, however, was beyond doubt. Before going to TrueNorth, she had halfheartedly tried the SOS-free vegan diet I'd been eating, but back in Boulder she took to it with a relish that surprised us both. Now she began each day with a voluptuous salad that became the joy of her mornings, she had no trouble abandoning the dairy and eggs she had long been attached to (she'd never been a meat eater), and her desk-drawer stash of Peanut Butter M&Ms and Pringles has yet to be replenished. Three months after the fast, she had a recidivous moment at a Walgreens cash register and walked out with three boxes of Good & Plenty, the licorice pieces made by Hershey. But by the time she made it home, she realized they sounded good only in her memory, not in her present, and threw them in the trash unopened.

Goldhamer didn't ask his patients to follow his diet forever, only for the same fifty years he asked of himself, at which point we were free to reevaluate. The first patient he ever counseled thus recently came back for a thirty-year follow-up. The man, now eighty-five, was a house painter, and his original complaint all those years ago had been an arthritic shoulder that kept him from painting ceilings.

"Back then he complained like crazy about the restrictive nature of the diet," Goldhamer said, "but he did it. When I saw him this time, it had been fourteen years since I'd seen him, so I said, 'What's wrong?' He says, 'Nothing.' I examine him. He's right. He's doing great for an eighty-five-year-old. He says, 'The diet seems to be working. I'm alive, and all my friends are dead. All my crew is dead.'"

His son, who had painted ceilings for him, refused to do the diet and died at sixty of cardiac arrest. Now the old man painted the ceilings himself. At the end of his appointment, he scheduled a follow-up with Goldhamer for fourteen years hence, when he would be ninety-nine. After that, he said, even though it wouldn't quite have been fifty years, he couldn't make any promises.

MORAL MALPRACTICE

Much of what passes for medicine today is malpractice, morally if not legally. What other word can we apply to doctors who reject a superior treatment for childhood epilepsy, rheumatoid arthritis, diabetes, and a number of other illnesses in favor of prescriptions and procedures that enrich themselves more than their patients? What other word for a profession that habitually treats the symptoms of disease when the cause could be severed at the root? Conventional physicians often scoff at osteopaths, chiropractors, and naturopaths for not practicing evidence-based medicine, but it is they who ignore the smashingly clear evidence that the body wants to heal itself and through fasting and diet frequently can.

Their blindness is curious. Every doctor accepts that a skin wound, if left alone and kept free of infection, will scar over and regenerate the dermis and epidermis. Many doctors even understand that had evolution not equipped our ancestors with this healing mechanism, we wouldn't be here today. But tell ten doctors that an equivalent process goes on beneath the skin and if left alone long enough it can often fix what ails, and nine will look at you as if you've grown antlers.

I cast no blame on physicians who have never heard the sort of evidence presented in this book. It's not taught in medical school and is almost never discussed at conferences or over the clinic water cooler. Their ignorance, though a blight, is understandable. But the physician who hears and dismisses the evidence is another story. I have in mind a certain doctor of a fibromyalgia patient who, having received his diagnosis and poked around the internet, said to the doctor that since conventional medicine had no remedy for his disease, and since there were many compelling claims that fasting had ameliorated or cured it in others, and since science had even elucidated mechanisms that might explain how fasting could achieve such reversals, wouldn't it be worth trying a prolonged fast? The doctor all but snorted him out of her office and in so doing aligned herself with the homeopath, the faith healer, and every other practitioner who ignores evidence-based medicine when the evidence doesn't suit her chosen creed. If my experience and that of many people I interviewed for this book are anything to go by, doctors like her are in the broad majority of the profession.

Powerful forces abet their bullheadedness. Upton Sinclair had it right that it's difficult to get a man to understand a thing when his salary depends on his not understanding it, and today the salaries that impede fasting are not just those of doctors. The staggeringly wealthy trusts that make drugs and medical devices and the only slightly less opulent corporations that run hospitals and clinics exist to create money first, health second. Every schizophrenic who forswears clozapine and every hypertensive who weens off Zestril is no less their enemy than the bicyclist is to the oil conglomerate. None of these corporations conspires against fasting. They don't have to. Each has only to reject threats to its profits as fastidiously as any other business, and fasting is manifestly a threat. Profit in our sickcare system flows not, as in fasting, from addressing the cause of disease, let alone preventing it in the first place, but from treating its symptoms in the already ill. The system's foundations are rubble, and if we are ever to replace sickcare with healthcare, they must be recast.

A few scientists, as we've seen, are doing some of the remedial work. The sciences themselves are no strangers to the corruption of profit, but academia still has a space for dispassionate evaluation, and cures that generate little wealth continue to emerge from laboratories and get published in scholarly journals. In our information-rich age, the discoveries about fasting are genies that can't be stuffed back into their lamps, and with time they will only multiply. The future may yet be bright for the science of fasting.

Individuals have a small but important say over whether therapeutic fasting spreads or contracts. Every time a patient asks a doctor if fasting or dietary change might heal with less harm than a statin or steroid, an angioplasty or bypass, medicine takes a small step forward. Merely to ask the question is to educate the doctor (especially if the patient hands her a fine book on the topic) and simultaneously registers a small protest on behalf of her time, the *sine qua non* of supervised fasting and dietary change. Doctors' time is the truly controlled substance of Western medicine, the commodity that medical corporations most detest dispensing, and thousands of small demands for more of it are surely a prerequisite for systemic change.

But individual nicks won't divert so powerful and self-perpetuating a system as for-profit Western medicine. Only collective action can do that. No sizable group exists to say a word for fasting, but allied groups in the vegan-health movement have been tilting against the sickcare system for decades and have of late been gaining a little ground. Might I suggest to the leaders of that movement—which, after all, shares fasting's premise that the body, naturally tended, can often maintain or recover its health—that they have little to lose and much to gain by adding fasting to their herbivorous agenda? Doing so would not only give practitioners another powerful remedy but in time could bring many of fasting's unorganized enthusiasts into the movement's ranks.

Finally, a small but growing contingent of doctors harbors the same doubts about medicine that Isaac Jennings did two centuries ago, and they could yet wield great influence. Much of this book can be read as a plea to them not only to educate themselves about the body's ability to heal itself (the TrueNorth Health Center, to repeat, trains doctors without charge to supervise fasts) but to bring fasting into their practices and add their voices to the fasting and vegan movements. Doing so will not be as lucrative as telling a patient her disease is beyond cure and sending her away after ten minutes with a couple of scripts. But the doctor who enables the diabetic to throw away his needle, who helps the arthritic set aside her walker, or who frees a child from a lifetime of seizures might just find the compensation sufficient.

ACKNOWLEDGMENTS

Many thanks to my energetic agent, the savvy and good-hearted Maxwell Sinsheimer, for suggesting I expand my earlier thoughts on fasting into a book and for supplying much good advice along the way. Thanks also to Jamison Stoltz, my editor at Abrams Press, for putting my words between two covers (and at quite some length, at that) and for many thoughtful editorial suggestions; to Margaret Moore for extraordinarily diligent copy-editing; and to Alane Salierno Mason at W. W. Norton for probing early questions that helped shape the direction of the book. A decade ago, Jofie Ferarri-Adler, now of Avid Reader Press, and Christopher Beha of *Harper's* helped me find a home for my first journalistic foray into fasting, for which I remain grateful.

My deep appreciation goes to everyone I interviewed for this book but especially to Françoise Wilhelmi de Toledo of the Buchinger Wilhelmi Clinic, who gave her time generously and helped me think through many aspects of fasting.

A hearty thank you to my neuroscientist brother-in-law, Michael Hendricks, for reading portions of the draft and saving me from multiple crimes against science. The remaining errors are of my own muddled devising.

To Federico Garza, *un abrazo fuerte* for helping translate tricky Spanish passages.

I owe a great debt to Matthieu Ricard, a Buddhist monk I've not had the pleasure of meeting but whose book *Happiness*, which I came across during the writing of this one, helped me find the equanimity to see the task through.

Warmest of thanks to Jake Ramsey and Noah Gershon for keeping the house renovation humming while I neglected carpentry for research and writing.

The gratitude that knows no bounds goes of course and as always to my wife Jennifer Hendricks, who saw me through many lows and highs, both literary and physical, all while writing her own book, seeing her students through four pandemic semesters, and paying the bills that my work emphatically does not. She's a wonder, that one.

SOURCES ON DIET

The research showing good health flows from a diet of minimally processed plants is vast. Below are some of the leading experts who have put the science before the public in a clear, accessible way and who have provided ample scholarly citations for curious readers. I've listed a few of their representative works as well as their websites and affiliated organizations. Their lectures and interviews are easily found online. I don't agree with all of their conclusions, and they don't always speak with unanimity among themselves, but any of their works would be a good place for the newcomer to start educating herself about the science of nutrition. For a quick overview, see the excellent 2011 documentary *Forks Over Knives*, www .forksoverknives.com.

Barnard, Dr. Neal. *Dr. Neal Barnard's Program for Reversing Diabetes*; *Your Body in Balance*; *The Vegan Starter Kit*. Physicians Committee for Responsible Medicine. www.pcrm.org.

Campbell, Prof. T. Colin. *The China Study*; *Whole*; *The Future of Nutrition*. T. Colin Campbell Center for Nutrition Studies. www.nutrition studies.org.

Davis, Brenda, R.D. *Nourish*; *Becoming Vegan*. www.brendadavisrd.com.

Davis, Dr. Garth. *Proteinaholic*.

Esselstyn, Dr. Caldwell. *Prevent and Reverse Heart Disease*. www.dress elstyn.com.

Fontana, Prof. Luigi. *The Path to Longevity*.

Greger, Dr. Michael. *How Not to Die*; *How Not to Diet*. NutritionFacts.org. www.nutritionfacts.org.

Hill, Simon, M.Nutr. *The Proof Is in the Plants*. The Proof Podcast. www.theproof.com.

Kahn, Dr. Joel. *The Plant-Based Solution*; *Your Whole Heart Solution*. www.drjoelkahn.com.

Longo, Prof. Valter. *The Longevity Diet*. www.valterlongo.com.

McDougall, Dr. John. *The Starch Solution*; *The Healthiest Diet on the Planet*. www.drmcdougall.com.

Ornish, Dr. Dean. *Reversing Heart Disease*; *Undo It!*; *The Spectrum*. www.deanornish.com.

Sherzai, Drs. Dean and Ayesha. *The Alzheimer's Solution*; *The 30-Day Alzheimer's Solution*. www.teamsherzai.com.

NOTES

To economize space, where multiple facts or quotations from different pages of one source appear near one another in my writing, I have grouped them under a single endnote, with the page numbers in the note appearing in the order the relevant material appears in my text. Thus: Francis Bacon, *The Historie of Life and Death* (I. Okes, 1638), 264, 38, 216.

x **"In the sciences"**: Johann Wolfgang von Goethe and Johann Peter Eckermann, *Conversations of Goethe*, trans. John Oxenford (George Bell, 1875), 47–48.

PROLOGUE

3 **In one study**: A. Goldhamer et al., "Medically supervised water-only fasting...," *Journal of Manipulative and Physiological Therapeutics*, vol. 24,5 (2001), 335–39, doi:10.1067/mmt.2001.115263.

6 **Goldhamer and Klaper wrote**: A. Goldhamer et al., "Water-only fasting and an exclusively...," *BMJ Case Reports*, vol. 2015 (2015), bcr2015211582, doi:10.1136/bcr-2015-211582.

6 **The editor, who held**: T. Myers et al., "Follow-up of water-only fasting...," *BMJ Case Reports*, vol. 2018 (2018), bcr2018225520, doi:10.1136/bcr-2018 -225520.

CHAPTER 1

9 **Henry S. Tanner**: For Tanner, see Robert A. Gunn, *Forty Days Without Food!* (Albert Metz, 1880); Alva A. Gregory, *Rational Therapy* (Palmer-Gregory

College, 1913), 58ff; Linda Burfield Hazzard, *Scientific Fasting* (Grant, 1927), 15ff; Hillel Schwartz, *Never Satisfied* (Anchor, 1986), 119ff; and newspaper dispatches during his 1880 fast.

9 **"not over particular":** "The Empty Man," *Minneapolis Tribune*, July 20, 1880, 1.

11 **dispatch to the *Chicago Medical Times*:** Moyer's dispatch was first published locally, e.g. in "Voluntary Starvation," *Minneapolis Tribune*, Nov. 28, 1877, 4.

11 **Mollie Fancher:** For Fancher, see Michelle Stacey, *The Fasting Girl* (Tarcher/ Putnam, 2002); Schwartz, *Never Satisfied*, 115ff.

12 **"They would like":** "Dr. Tanner's Fast," *Saturday Review* (London), July 24, 1880, 111.

13 **After two days, he felt:** For daily details of Tanner's fast, see above works and "Tanner's Triumph," *Boston Daily Globe*, Aug. 8, 1880, 5; P. H. Vander Weyde, "A Condensed History of Dr. Tanner's Recent Fast," *Scientific American*, suppl. 244, Sep. 4, 1880, 3890ff; "The Long Fast Finished," *New York Times*, Aug. 8, 1880, 1; and daily dispatches, esp. of *Minneapolis Tribune*.

14 **"a fraud":** "Tough Old Tanner," *Louisville Courier-Journal*, July 8, 1880, 3.

15 **"A strong minded female":** "The Fasting Doctor," *Minneapolis Tribune*, July 26, 1880, 2.

15 **"What woman, this weather":** "A Stomach's Revenge," *Minneapolis Tribune*, July 23, 1880, 2.

15 **"rude almost without":** Gunn, *Forty Days*, 95–96.

16 **Dr. Smock:** "A Stomach's Revenge," *Minneapolis Tribune*.

16 **Dr. W. B. Lee:** "For Forty Days," *Daily Constitution* (Atlanta), July 23, 1880, 1.

16 **A medical student in:** "Thirty-Nine," *Minneapolis Tribune*, Aug. 6, 1880, 2.

16 **James H. Rindley:** "Emulating Tanner," *New York Times*, Aug. 11, 1880, 5.

16 **Signor Goldschmidt:** "Imitators of Tanner," *British Medical Journal*, vol. 2, 1026 (1880), 354.

16 **Charles Livingston:** "The Other Fasting Idiot," *Washington Post*, Sep. 13, 1880, 1; "Livingston's Fast Broken," *Chicago Daily Tribune*, Sep. 19, 1880, 13.

16 **"Think what a saving":** "Dr. Tanner's Fast—Cui Bono?" *Scribner's Monthly*, Oct. 1880, 937.

16 **Reuben Kelsey:** "Other Starvation Cases," *Philadelphia Inquirer*, July 21, 1880, 3.

16 **"all physicians who"**: "Tanner's Task," *Minneapolis Tribune*, July 17, 1880, 2.

16 **"I am about giving up"**: "A Human Riddle," *Minneapolis Tribune*, July 19, 1880, 2.

16 **"a smiling, good-humored"**: "Half Completed," *Minneapolis Tribune*, July 18, 1880, 2.

17 **In his youth, Tanner had**: "Will Be Buried Alive," *Chicago Tribune*, Feb. 17, 1889, 25.

17 **"he generously invited"**: "A Stomach's Revenge," *Minneapolis Tribune*.

17 **"The whole thing is"**: "Dr. Tanner," *Chicago Daily Tribune*, Sep. 16, 1881, 11.

17 **"The first source"**: "Dr. Tanner's Fourth Week," *St. Louis Post-Dispatch*, July 21, 1880, 2.

18 **"The thing that makes"**: "Dr. Tanner," *Chicago Daily Tribune*.

18 **"the scientific results"**: "The Fast Ended," *Minneapolis Tribune*, Aug. 8, 1880, 1.

19 **One lecturess accused**: "Dr. Tanner Contradicts a Lecturer," *Sun* (Baltimore), Aug. 17, 1880, 1.

19 **The spring in Central Park**: Vander Weyde, "Condensed History."

19 **"that whoever had a surplus"**: "Beyond Comprehension," *Minneapolis Tribune*, July 21, 1880, 2.

19 **"there is hardly"**: "Dr. Tanner's Fast—Cui Bono?" *Scribner's*.

19 **"Even the Presidential"**: "Triumph of Dr. Tanner," *Sun* (Baltimore), Aug. 9, 1880, 1.

20 **"for the next 11 days"**: "A Rival in Cincinnati," *New York Times*, July 28, 1880, 2.

20 **"for several years been"**: "Another Case of Fasting," *New York Times*, Aug. 11, 1880, 2.

20 **"he will begin"**: "For Forty Days," *Daily Constitution*.

21 **"His worst battles"**: "The Fast Ended," *Minneapolis Tribune*.

21 **"Your experiment watched"**: Gunn, *Forty Days*, 102.

21 **"great pluck"**: Gunn, *Forty Days*, 105.

22 **"It is not thought"**: "The Fast Ended," *Minneapolis Tribune*.

22 **"Judge of their surprise"**: "The Long Fast Finished," *New York Times*.

23 **"We are inclined"**: "Dr. Tanner's Fast," *Kansas City Review of Science and Industry*, Sep. 1880, 285.

23 **"he felt like":** "The Long Fast Finished," *New York Times.*

24 **"It may be of use":** "The Fasting Man," *St. Louis Post-Dispatch*, July 24, 1880, 9.

24 **"An excitement to Americans":** Untitled editorial, *Times of India*, Aug. 23, 1880, 2.

24 **"Dr. Tanner may not":** "Dr. Tanner's Great Fast," *Scientific American*, Sep. 4, 1880, 144.

24 **"We have been disposed":** Robert A. Gunn, "Dr. Tanner's Fast and Its Lessons," *The Medical Tribune*, Aug. 15, 1880, 465–66.

25 **"the body to use up":** "The Tanner Fast," *St. Louis Courier of Medicine and Collateral Sciences*, Aug. 1880, 129–30.

25 **Dr. Peter Henri Van der Weyde:** P. H. Van der Weyde, "Dr. Tanner's Blood After Starvation," *The Medical Tribune*, Aug. 15, 1880, 462ff; "Effect of Starvation on the Blood," *Scientific American*, Aug. 28, 1880, 128; "Dr. Tanner's Fast," *Cincinnati Medical Advance*, Sep. 1, 1880, 162.

25 **"This ragged appearance":** Van der Weyde, "Effect of Starvation," 128.

25 **In a typical person:** "The Long Fast Finished," *New York Times.*

CHAPTER 2

28 **One brilliant and frankly:** Steve Hendricks, "Starving Your Way to Vigor," *Harper's*, Mar. 2012, 27–38.

28 **Scientists have hunted:** M. Lewis and J. Sealy, "Coastal complexity," *PloS One*, vol. 13,12 (2018), e0209411, doi:10.1371/journal.pone.0209411.

29 **A possible exception:** A. Bartsiokas and J. Arsuaga, "Hibernation in hominins from Atapuerca . . . ," *L'Anthropologie* vol. 124,5 (2020), 102797; Robin McKie, "Early humans may have survived the harsh winters by hibernating," *Guardian*, Dec. 20, 2020.

29 **so similar to those in yeast:** W. Liu et al., "From Saccharomyces cerevisiae to human," *Biomedical Reports*, vol. 7,2 (2017), 153–58, doi:10.3892/br .2017.941.

31 **"They entertain high hopes":** F. Carod-Artal and C. Vázquez-Cabrera, "Tratamiento de las cefaleas entre los aborígenes de Tierra de Fuego," [Treatment of headaches among the aborigines of Tierra de Fuego], *Revista Neurología*, vol. 47,7 (2008), 374–79, doi:10.33588/rn.4707.2008481.

32　**Fasting first emerges:** For Indian religions, see Karen Armstrong, *Buddha* (Penguin, 2004).

32　**"It was by fasts":** The Mahabharata of Krishna-Dwaipayana Vyasa Translated Into English Prose: Anuçasana Parva (Bhārata, 1893), 525–26.

35　**"While the body":** Kong Meng San Phor Kark See Monastery, *Buddhism for Beginners*, 3rd ed. (Awaken, 2010) 37–38.

36　**Some scholars think Buddhists:** L. Wilson, "Ascetic practices," in *Encyclopedia of Buddhism*, ed. Robert E. Buswell Jr. (Macmillan Reference, 1994), 33.

36　**Jainism:** James Laidlaw, "A life worth leaving: fasting to death . . . ," *Economy and Society*, vol. 34,2 (2005), 178–99, doi:10.1080/03085140500054545; James Laidlaw, *Riches and Renunciation* (Oxford Univ. Pr., 1995); Whitny Melissa Braun, *Sallekhanā* (PhD diss., Claremont Graduate Univ., 2015); Paul Dundas, *The Jains* (Routledge, 2003).

37　*Sallekhana*—**starvation unto death:** Laidlaw, "A life"; Braun, *Sallekhanā*; M. Sethi, "Ritual death in a secular state," *South Asian History and Culture*, vol. 10,2 (2019), 136–51, doi:10.1080/19472498.2019.1609261.

38　**Today somewhere between:** Sethi, "Ritual death"; Julie McCarthy, *Morning Edition*, "Fasting To The Death" NPR, Sep. 2, 2015.

38　**The American writer:** Neil Genzlinger, "Sue Hubbell, Who Wrote of Bees . . . ," *New York Times*, Oct. 18, 2018.

39　**"When I am going to make":** Paul Contino, *"Zhuangzhi,"* in *Finding Wisdom in East Asian Classics*, ed. William Theodore De Bary (Columbia Univ. Pr., 2011), 86–87.

40　**Early Taoists seem:** Stephen Eskildsen, *Asceticism in Early Taoist Religion* (SUNY Pr., 1998), 10, 43ff.

40　**Confucianism gave fasting:** Edward Slingerland, ed., *Analects* (Hackett, 2003); James Legge, *The Life and Teachings of Confucius* (J. B. Lippincott, 1867).

40　**On the other side:** Robert B. Pippin, "Introduction," in *Thus Spake Zarathustra*, ed. Adrian del Caro and Robert B. Pippin (Cambridge Univ. Pr., 2006); Denise Soufi, "Fasting," in *Encyclopædia Iranica*, updated 2012, online.

CHAPTER 3

42　**"Not even a Jew":** Suetonius, *The Lives of the Twelve Caesars: The Life of Augustus*, book 2 (Loeb Classical Library, 1913), online.

42 **"Let the meal":** Eliezer Diamond, *Holy Men and Hunger Artists* (Oxford Univ. Pr., 2004), 117.

43 **By the start of the Christian:** Veronika E. Grimm, *From Feasting to Fasting* (Routledge, 1996), 132; Rudolph Arbesmann, "Fasting and Prophecy in Pagan and Christian Antiquity," *Traditio*, vol. 7 (1951), 41–42; Darrell L. Bock, *Luke* (Baker Academic, 1994), section 18:12, online; Kent Berghuis, *Christian Fasting* (Biblical Studies, 2002), 54–61, online.

44 **"disfigure their faces":** Matthew 6:16–18.

45 **"Can you make":** Luke 5:34–35.

45 **This isn't at first:** Diamond, *Holy Men*, 97–98; Arbesmann, "Fasting and Prophecy," 5–6.

45 **Priests sometimes fasted:** Richard Finn, *Asceticism in the Graeco-Roman World* (Cambridge Univ. Pr., 2009), 15–16.

45 **After Achilles's understudy:** Rana Saadi Liebert, *Tragic Pleasure from Homer to Plato* (Cambridge Univ. Pr., 2017), 97, discussing Homer, *Iliad*, book 19:320–21.

45 **After Achilles avenges:** Homer, *Iliad*, book 24:31, 641–42, trans. A. T. Murray (Harvard Univ. Pr., 1924), online.

45 **The other widespread:** Grimm, *From Feasting*, 40; Joseph F. Wimmer, *Fasting in the New Testament* (Paulist, 1982), 23; Finn, *Asceticism*, 17; Jenifer Neils, "Women: Women in Greece," in *The Oxford Encyclopedia of Ancient Greece and Rome*, ed. Michael Gagarin (Oxford Univ. Pr., 2010).

46 **The yarn was spun:** Carl A. Huffman, "Pythagoras and the Pythagoreans," in *The Oxford Encyclopedia of Ancient Greece and Rome*, ed. Michael Gagarin (Oxford Univ. Pr., 2010); Christopher Riedweg, *Pythagoras* (Cornell Univ. Pr., 2012), 20.

46 **Hippocrates:** For Hippocrates and the Hippocratic Corpus, see G. E. R. Lloyd, ed., *Hippocratic Writings* (Penguin, 1983).

47 **After five disputatious centuries:** Vivian Nutton, *Ancient Medicine* (Routledge, 2004), 79ff; *In Our Time*, "The Four Humours," BBC Radio 4, Dec. 20, 2007.

47 **"boiled puppies":** Laurence M. V. Totelin, *Hippocratic Recipes* (Brill, 2009), 198.

47 **"Spasms are cured":** *Aphorisms*, section 6:39, in Lloyd, *Hippocratic Writings*, 230.

47 **"the place and season":** *Aphorisms*, section 1:2, in Lloyd, *Hippocratic Writings*, 206.

48 **One of the more thoughtful:** In *Regimen in Acute Diseases*, see passages 35, 41, 47 in Lloyd, *Hippocratic Writings*, 195, 197, 198–99.

49 **"The patient suffering":** Karl G. Kühn, *Claudii Galeni: Opera Omnia* (C. Cnobloch, 1821), 239–40 (Galen quoting Erasistratus), trans. for author by Joseph Miller, Mar. 25, 2020.

49 **"fasting, if taken":** *Aphorisms*, section 1:3, in Lloyd, *Hippocratic Writings*, 206.

49 **"dire consequences":** Grimm, *From Feasting*, 48–49.

49 **No Hippocratic author:** D. Cárdenas, "Let not thy food be confused . . . ," *e-SPEN Journal*, vol. 8,6 (2013), e260–62, doi:10.1016/j.clnme.2013.10.002.

49 **a character in a German novel:** Johann Michael von Loën, *The Honest Man at Court*, trans. John R. Russell (Camden House, 1997), 90.

49 **Methodism:** For Methodism, see Nutton, *Ancient Medicine*, 194–95; Erwin H. Ackerknecht, *A Short History of Medicine* (Johns Hopkins Univ. Pr., 2016), 55; Danielle Gourevitch, "The Paths of Knowledge," in *Western Medical Thought from Antiquity to the Middle Ages*, ed. Mirko D. Grmek (Harvard Univ. Pr., 2002), 114; C. Webster, "Heuristic Medicine," *Isis*, vol. 106,3 (2015), 657–58; D. Leith, "The *Diatritus* and Therapy in Graeco-Roman Medicine," *Classical Quarterly*, vol. 58,2 (2008), 581–600.

50 **Aulus Cornelius Celsus:** For Celsus, see "Aulus Cornelius Celsus," *Britannica* (Encyclopedia Britannica), online; Aulus Cornelius Celsus, *Of Medicine*, trans. James Greive (Univ. Pr. [Edinburgh], 1814), books 2:16 and 3:25, 71, 136ff.

50 **Galen:** For Galen, see *In Our Time*, "Galen," BBC Radio 4, Oct. 10, 2013; Han Baltussen, "Galen," in *The Oxford Encyclopedia of Ancient Greece and Rome* (Oxford Univ. Pr., 2010), online; P. N. Singer, "Galen," in *The Stanford Encyclopedia of Philosophy*, ed. Edward N. Zalta (Stanford Univ., 2016), online; Susan P. Mattern, *The Prince of Medicine* (Oxford Univ. Pr., 2013); Susan P. Mattern, *Galen and the Rhetoric of Healing* (Johns Hopkins Univ. Pr., 2008).

51 **"I could no longer":** Mattern, *Prince of Medicine*, 239–42; Mattern, *Galen*, 75.

52 **"Galen could have come"**: Mark Twain, "A Majestic Literary Fossil," *The Complete Works of Mark Twain* (Harper, 1925), 330.

53 **"For more than two thousand"**: David Wootton, *Bad Medicine* (Oxford Univ. Pr., 2006), 70, 2.

53 **Plato:** For Plato, see Julia Annas, "Plato," in *Oxford Classical Dictionary* (Oxford Univ. Pr., 2005), online; Richard Kraut, "Plato," in *The Stanford Encyclopedia of Philosophy*, ed. Edward N. Zalta (Stanford Univ., 2017), online.

54 **teachings of Jesus:** John 5:28–29, 6:39–40. Jesus's view on the afterlife was a continuation of the Old Testamentary view, as in Isaiah 26:19.

54 **"The authors of our"**: Plato, *Timaeus*, section 8, trans. Benjamin Jowett (Project Gutenberg eBook 1572), online; Grimm, *From Feasting*, 99.

54 **Unfortunately, a priggish Alexandrian:** Grimm, *From Feasting*, 28–33.

55 **"a plotter against"**: D. Winston, "Philo and the Rabbis on sex and the body," *Poetics Today*, vol. 19,1 (1998), 48, 58.

55 **"This is apparently"**: Berghuis, *Christian Fasting*, 32.

55 **"Others," Philo wrote:** Grimm, *From Feasting*, 31.

56 **"ate their food"**: Acts 2:46–47.

56 **Paul warned of "liars"**: 1 Timothy 4:3.

56 **"warring against the law"**: Romans 7:22–24.

56 **He, too, called for:** Grimm, *From Feasting*, 65–66; H. Musurillo, "The Problem of Ascetical Fasting in the Greek Patristic Writers," *Traditio*, vol. 12 (1956), 47ff; Gilles Herrada, "The Mysterious Fate of Homosexuality," in *Integral Voices on Sex, Gender, and Sexuality*, ed. Sarah E. Nicholson and Vanessa D. Fisher (SUNY Pr., 2014), 109.

56 **The Christians' fast days:** *The Didache* section 8:1, in Thomas O'Loughlin, *The Didache* (Baker Academic, 2010), 166.

57 **Tertullian:** For Tertullian, see Grimm, *From Feasting*, 114–39; Finn, *Asceticism*, 65–66.

57 **"Abstention from food"**: Grimm, *From Feasting*, 129.

58 **This was the immensely:** Grimm, *From Feasting*, 156.

58 **"amazed to see"**: William Harmless, *Desert Christians* (Oxford Univ. Pr., 2004), 64, 168.

58 **The Antony of Athanasius radiated:** Berghuis, *Christian Fasting*, 125–26.

59 **"It releases sin."**: Diamond, *Holy Men*, 96–97.

59 **In Babylonia, probably:** Bava Metzia 33a, *The William Davidson Talmud* (Sefaria), online.

59 **"But I meant to sin!":** Grimm, *From Feasting*, 26.

60 **A sort of poor man's:** Finn, *Asceticism*, 59.

60 **The paschal fast:** For the paschal fast, see in *The New Schaff-Herzog Encyclopedia of Religious Knowledge*, ed. Samuel M. Jackson (Funk and Wagnalls, 1909): Hans Achelis, "Fasting," vol. 4, 281–84; P. Drews, "Holy Week," vol. 5, 333–36; "Lent," vol. 5, 448. Also Arbesmann, "Fasting and Prophecy," 46; Finn, *Asceticism*, 154–55.

61 **Fasting caught Christians' fancy:** Giles Constable, "Attitudes Toward Self-Inflicted Suffering in the Middle Ages," The Ninth Stephen J. Brademas, Sr., Lecture (Hellenic College Pr., 1982), 11–12; Teresa M. Shaw, *The Burden of the Flesh* (Fortress Pr., 1998), 163.

61 **When Macarius of Alexandria:** Arbesmann, "Fasting and Prophecy," 34.

62 **Another monk by the name:** Palladius, "Heron," in *The Lausiac History of Palladius*, ed. W. K. Lowther Clarke (Macmillan, 1918), 106–7.

62 **At the Egyptian monastery:** Andrew Jotischky, *A Hermit's Cookbook* (Continuum, 2011), 28, 32–33.

62 **"A king who wants":** Jotischky, *A Hermit's Cookbook*, 43.

62 **The extreme end:** Arbesmann, "Fasting and Prophecy," 35.

62 **Battheus of Edessa:** Walter Vandereycken and Ron van Deth, *From Fasting Saints to Anorexic Girls* (Athlone, 1994), 22.

62 **Adolius of Tarsus:** Arbesmann, "Fasting and Prophecy," 34.

62 **Simeon the Stylite:** For Simeon, see Andrew T. Crislip, *From Monastery to Hospital* (Univ. of Michigan Pr., 2005), 96ff; Herbert Thurston, "Simeon Stylites the Elder, Saint," in *Catholic Encyclopedia*, vol. 13 (Robert Appleton, 1912), 795; Musurillo, "Ascetical Fasting," 33.

64 **Misogyny, of course:** 1 Timothy 2.

64 **Not only did fasting:** Helène Whittaker, "Women and fasting in early Christianity," in *Gender, Cult, and Culture in the Ancient World from Mycenae to Byzantium*, ed. Lena Larsson Lovén and Agneta Strömberg (Paul Åströms Förlag, 2003), 110; Shaw, *Burden of the Flesh*, 85; Sebastian P. Brock and Susan Ashbrook Harvey, *Holy Women of the Syrian Orient* (Univ. of California Pr., 2008), 142ff.

64   **"The virginal eyes":** Shaw, *Burden*, 251.

64   **"When sleep comes":** Sharman Apt Russell, *Hunger* (Basic, 2005), 45.

64   **The harsh calls:** Shaw, *Burden*, 9, 25, 242.

65   **Jerome of Stridon:** For Jerome, see Grimm, *From Feasting*, 157–79; Shaw, *Burden*, 96–112.

66   **"harms man by dulling":** Grimm, *From Feasting*, 101.

66   **"Observe what fasting":** Andrew Crislip, *Thorns in the Flesh* (Univ. of Pennsylvania Pr., 2012), 62.

67   **"brings peace for body":** Musurillo, "Ascetical Fasting," 19.

67   **"her face was pale":** Crislip, *Thorns*, 101.

67   **John Chrysostom:** For Chrysostom, see Wendy Mayer and Pauline Allen, *John Chrysostom* (Routledge, 1999); Shaw, *Burden*, 130–40.

67   **"For when the heart":** Musurillo, "Ascetical Fasting," 6–7, 15, 17–18.

68   **"If only everyone":** Berghuis, "Christian Fasting," 107.

68   **Cassian, incidentally, was fascinated:** Shaw, *Burden*, 114; Finn, *Asceticism*, 127.

CHAPTER 4

69   **The odds of developing:** Michael Greger, *How Not to Diet* (Flatiron Books, 2019), 38.

69   **One study found those:** E. Pedditzi et al., "The risk of overweight/obesity in mid-life . . . ," *Age and Ageing*, vol. 45,1 (2016), 14–21, doi:10.1093/ageing/afv151.

69   **90 percent greater:** M. Loef and H. Walach, "Midlife obesity and dementia," *Obesity* (Silver Spring), vol. 21,1 (2013), E51–55, doi:10.1002/oby.20037.

69   **and at just about any age:** For the link between overweight and poor thinking, see Greger, *How Not to Diet*, 39–40.

69   **In an analysis:** R. Caleyachetty et al., "Metabolically healthy obese and incident cardiovascular . . . ," *Journal of the American College of Cardiology*, vol. 70,12 (2017), 1429–37, doi:10.1016/j.jacc.2017.07.763; Sarah Boseley, "No such thing as 'fat but fit' . . . ," *Guardian*, May 17, 2017.

70   **At a BMI of 24.5:** Greger, *How Not to Diet*, 46.

70   **and at a BMI of 25:** L. Fontana and F. Hu, "Optimal body weight for health . . . ," *Aging Cell*, vol. 13,3 (2014), 391–400, doi:10.1111/acel.12207.

70 **"You are perfect":** Jack Kornfield, *The Wise Heart* (Bantam, 2008), 20 (ellipsis in original).

75 **There is evidence:** G. Cahill Jr. and R. Veech, "Ketoacids? Good medicine?" *Transactions of the American Clinical and Climatological Association*, vol. 114 (2003), 149–61.

76 **Dr. Françoise Wilhelmi de Toledo:** Françoise Wilhelmi de Toledo and Hubert Hohler, *Therapeutic Fasting* (Thieme, 2012), 84.

CHAPTER 5

85 **In the tale:** Margaret Wade Labarge, *A Baronial Household of the Thirteenth Century* (Barnes & Noble, 1980), 169.

85 **"It is the nature":** Bridget Ann Henisch, *Fast and Feast* (Pennsylvania State Univ. Pr., 1976), 41.

86 **The gentler pole:** Christina Lee, "Reluctant Appetites," in *Saints and Scholars*, ed. Stuart McWilliams (D. S. Brewer, 2012), 171; Rudolph M. Bell, *Holy Anorexia* (Univ. of Chicago Pr., 1985), 120–21; Ken Albala, "The Ideology of Fasting in the Reformation Era," in *Food and Faith in Christian Culture*, ed. Ken Albala and Trudy Eden (Columbia Univ. Pr., 2011), 43.

86 **In Siena in the High:** Augustine Thompson, *Cities of God* (Pennsylvania State Univ. Pr., 2005), 282.

86 **By one scholarly reckoning:** Elisheva Baumgarten, *Practicing Piety in Medieval Ashkenaz* (Univ. of Pennsylvania Pr., 2014), 58.

86 **The most devout:** Caroline Walker Bynum, *Holy Feast and Holy Fast* (Univ. of California Pr., 1988), 37ff.

87 **In 1287, when the Archbishop:** Henisch, *Fast and Feast*, 46–47.

87 **So obstinately did monks:** Bynum, *Holy Feast*, 42.

87 **During strict fasts:** Albala, "Ideology of Fasting," 47.

87 **More-plebeian households:** Henisch, *Fast and Feast*, 44.

87 **Dispensations had appeared:** Lee, "Reluctant Appetites," 185; Albala, "Ideology of Fasting," 45–46; David Grumett and Rachel Muers, *Theology on the Menu* (Routledge, 2010), 56.

88 **Clare of Assisi:** For Clare, see Bynum, *Holy Feast*, 15, 99–101, 193; Bell, *Holy Anorexia*, 123–27.

89 **"In Advent and Lent":** Bynum, *Holy Feast*, 210.

89 **Benvenuta Bojani:** For Benvenuta, see Bell, *Holy Anorexia*, 128.

89 **Catherine of Siena:** For Catherine, see Bell, *Holy Anorexia*, 22–53; Bynum, *Holy Feast*, 165–80.

90 **"Don't be afraid!":** R. Kiely, "The Saint Who Lost Her Head," in *Religion and the Arts*, vol. 8,3 (2004), 305.

91 **they also shared other attributes:** Bynum, *Holy Feast*, 204.

92 **In one study of the 261:** Bell, Holy Anorexia, x.

92 **One of the earliest took place:** Walter Vandereycken and Ron van Deth, *From Fasting Saints to Anorexic Girls* (Athlone, 1994), 27.

93 **Inquisitors often rigged:** Vandereycken and van Deth, *Fasting Saints*, 38.

93 **In 1573, the Dutchman:** Gregory Zilboorg and George W. Henry, *A History of Medical Psychology* (W. W. Norton, 1941), 209ff; Bynum, *Holy Feast*, 92; Vandereycken and van Deth, *Fasting Saints*, 61.

93 **As recently as 2004, Pope John:** Vandereycken and van Deth, *Fasting Saints*, 29.

94 **"A diet attempted":** Henisch, *Fast and Feast*, 29.

94 **"If thou faste":** Arthur Brandeis, ed., *Jacob's Well* (Keegan Paul, 1900), 143.

94 **They were encouraged:** Bynum, *Holy Feast*, 263–65.

94 **"Fast is medicine":** Bynum, *Holy Feast*, 44.

95 **In fourteenth-century England:** Grumett and Muers, *Theology*, 53.

95 **"At Rome they":** Henisch, *Fast and Feast*, 47.

95 **the truly telling blow:** For Froschauer and Zwingli, see Albala, "Ideology of Fasting," 41ff; David Gentilcore, *Food and Health in Early Modern Europe* (Bloomsbury Academic, 2016), 99; Grumett and Muers, *Theology*, 54–56.

96 **With dizzying swiftness:** For the Reformation, see Albala, "Ideology of Fasting," 48–50; Alec Ryrie, "The Fall and Rise of Fasting in the British Reformations," in *Worship and the Parish Church in Early Modern Britain*, ed. Natalie Mears and Alec Ryrie (Ashgate, 2013), 100–102; Grumett and Muers, *Theology on the Menu*, 31, 53ff.

96 **The idea had precedent:** Grumett and Muers, *Theology on the Menu*, 30.

96 **In the earliest days of Plymouth:** Henry K. Rowe, "Fast-Day," in *The New Schaff-Herzog Encyclopedia of Religious Knowledge*, vol. 4, ed. Samuel M. Jackson (Funk and Wagnalls, 1909), 279–80.

96 **Other colonies followed suit:** Hillel Schwartz, *Never Satisfied* (Doubleday, 1986), 117.

97 **George Washington proclaimed:** John C. Fitzpatrick, ed., *The Writings of George Washington*, vol. 14 (US Government Printing Office, 1936), 369.

97 **Abraham Lincoln called:** Roy P. Basler, ed., *Collected Works of Abraham Lincoln*, vol. 6 (New Brunswick, 1955), 156–57.

97 **The civic fast days:** Rowe, "Fast-Day," 279–80; R. Marie Griffith, *Born Again Bodies* (Univ. of California Pr., 2004), 30.

97 **"public humiliation, prayer":** Woodrow Wilson, "Proclamation 1445—Decoration Day, 1918," in Gerhard Peters and John T. Woolley, ed., The American Presidency Project, Univ. of California Santa Barbara, online.

97 **There was, however, a succedaneum:** Harry S. Truman, "National Day of Prayer, 1952," Proclamations, Harry S. Truman Library & Museum, online.

97 **"The rich Papist":** Sydney Watts, "Enlightened Fasting," in *Food and Faith in Christian Culture*, ed. Ken Albala and Trudy Eden (Columbia Univ. Pr., 2011), 107.

98 **One doctor in the 1820s:** Vandereycken and van Deth, *Fasting Saints*, 105–8.

98 **Despite their regular exposure:** Joan Jacobs Brumberg, *Fasting Girls* (Vintage, 2000), 64.

98 **Sarah Jacob:** For Jacob, see John Cule, *Wreath on the Crown* (Gomerian, 1967); Brumberg, *Fasting Girls*, 65–73.

99 **In 1916, nearly four decades:** Michelle Stacey, *The Fasting Girl* (Tarcher/Putnam, 2002), 307.

100 **Alvise Cornaro's *Discourses*:** Gerald J. Gruman, "The Rise and Fall of Prolongevity Hygiene 1558–1873," *Bulletin of the History of Medicine*, Jan. 1, 1961, 224. Decent online editions of *Discourses on the Sober Life* are Alvise Cornaro, *The Art of Living Long*, trans. William F. Butler (Springer, 2005); Luigi Cornaro, *Discourses on the Sober Life* (Thomas Y. Crowell, 1916).

100 **According to one biographer:** Greg Critser, "Foreword," in Alvise Cornaro, *Writings on the Sober Life* (Univ. of Toronto Pr., 2014), x.

100 **"I accustomed myself ":** Cornaro, *Art of Living*, 7, 10, 12, 17, 33.

100 **Each day he ate:** His ounces may have been "short" ounces, in which case his twelve and fourteen ounces were more like ten and twelve of ours, or

284 grams of food and 333 grams of wine. For his diet, see Marisa Milani, "Introduction," in Alvise Cornaro, *Writings on the Sober Life* (Univ. of Toronto Pr., 2014), 22–23; Critser, "Foreword," xi.

101 **"is the confident"**: Milani, "Introduction," 13, 22.

102 **To bolster his case**: Critser, "Foreword," xx.

102 **Francis Bacon, lord chancellor**: Francis Bacon, *The Historie of Life and Death* (I. Okes, 1638), 264, 38, 216.

103 **"health and long life"**: William Temple, "Of health and long life," *The Works of Sir William Temple*, vol. 3 (S. Hamilton, 1814), 286.

103 **As a young man, Fernel**: Ragnar Granit, "Jean Fernel," in *Complete Dictionary of Scientific Biography* (Encyclopedia.com, updated 2018), online.

103 **"for it works"**: Henry Mason, *Christian Humiliation* (John Clarke, 1625), 157–63.

104 **Friedrich Hoffmann**: For Hoffmann, see Steve Naragon, "Hoffmann, Friedrich (1660–1742)," in *The Bloomsbury Dictionary of Eighteenth Century German Philosophers*, ed. Heiner F. Klemme and Manfred Kuehn (Bloomsbury, 2016), 346–48.

104 **Among Hoffmann's four hundred**: Friedrich Hoffmann, *Gründliche Anweisung, wie ein Mensch vor dem frühzeitigen Tod und allerhand Arten Krankheiten durch ordentliche Lebens-Art sich verwahren könne* [*Thorough Instruction on How a Person Can Protect Himself from Premature Death and All Kinds of Diseases Through an Orderly Way of Life*], vol. 5 (Renger, 1719), 400–60. Because Hoffmann's fasting chapter has never been translated from the eighteenth-century German, I have instead translated from the modern version republished as Friedrich Hoffmann, *Wie man manche schwere Krankheit durch Mäßigkeit und Fasten kurieren kann* [*How Temperance and Fasting Cure Certain Serious Illnesses*] (Jungborn Rudolf Just, 1926), 3, 8, 24–25, 27, 33–34, 40–41.

CHAPTER 6

107 **One such observance**: Edward Miller, "Remarks on the Effects of Abstinence at the Approach of Acute Diseases," *Medical Repository*, vol. 1,2 (1797), 194, 197, 199, 203.

109 **"this cheap, simple":** Cornelius C. Blatchly, "An Essay on the beneficial use of occasional Fasting," *Medical Repository*, new series vol. 4 (1818), 246.

109 **Isaac Jennings:** For Jennings, see I. Jennings, *Philosophy of Human Life* (Jewett, Proctor & Worthington, 1852), 28–39; Isaac Jennings, *Medical Reform* (Oberlin Pr., 1847), 222; Isaac Jennings, *The Tree of Life* (Miller, Wood, 1867), 186.

111 **"His uprightness and":** Samuel Orcutt and Ambrose Beardsley, "Isaac Jennings, M. D.," *The History of the Old Town of Derby, Connecticut, 1642–1880* (Springfield, 1880), 603.

112 **It was a rude start:** Howard Markel, *PBS NewsHour*, "Dec. 14, 1799: The excruciating final hours of President George Washington," Dec. 14, 2014; D. Morens, "Death of the president," *New England Journal of Medicine*, vol. 341,24 (1999), 1845–50.

114 **"hypothesize about the":** James C. Whorton, *Nature Cures* (Oxford Univ. Pr., 2002), 11.

114 **"there is but one":** Paul Starr, *The Social Transformation of American Medicine* (Basic, 2017), 42.

114 **"always treat nature":** Whorton, *Nature Cures*, 6.

114 **"How often," one thoughtful:** E. D. F(enner), "Homaeopathy, Allopathy, and 'Young Physic,'" *New-Orleans Medical and Surgical Journal*, vol. 2,1 (1845), 761.

115 **"The patient treated":** Robert B. Sullivan, "Sanguine Practices," *Bulletin of the History of Medicine*, vol. 68,2 (1994), 225.

115 **Samuel Thomson:** For Thomson, see Whorton, *Nature Cures*, 39–45; James C. Whorton, *Crusaders for Fitness* (Princeton Univ. Pr., 1982), 24.

116 **Sylvester Graham:** For Graham, see Whorton, *Crusaders*, 43, 47; Whorton, *Nature Cures*, 86–87, 93–94; Hillel Schwartz, *Never Satisfied* (Doubleday, 1986), 25–26.

116 **"GLUTTONY and *not starvation*":** Sylvester Graham, "Excessive Alimentation," *Graham Journal of Health and Longevity*, May 26, 1838, 162.

117 **"You are not":** William Cobbett, *A Year's Residence in the United States of America*, 3rd ed. (J. M. Cobbett, 1822), 198.

117 **"You Yankees load":** Whorton, *Crusaders*, 26–27.

117 **(correct, as it turned out):** See "Sources on Diet" in this book.

118 **nonetheless achieve "wonderful effects":** Sylvester Graham, *Lectures on the Science of Human Life* (Horsell, Aldine, 1849), 194, 62.

118 **Dr. William Alcott:** James C. Whorton, "'Christian Physiology,'" *Bulletin of the History of Medicine*, vol. 49,4 (1975), 466–81.

119 **Edward Kittredge:** For Kittredege, see Herbert M. Shelton, *Natural Hygiene* (Dr. Shelton's Health School, 1968), chap. 28, online.

120 **"prolonged fasting"—which he:** George Miller Beard, *Eating and Drinking*, 2nd ed. (G. P. Putnam, 1871), 124–25.

121 **"that the mischief":** Ralph Waldo Emerson, "New England Reformers," lecture, Mar. 3, 1844, EmersonCentral.com.

121 **"Some men seem":** Whorton, *Crusaders*, 72.

121 **In the end, heroic medicine:** David Wootton, *Bad Medicine* (Oxford Univ. Pr., 2007), 149, 167.

121 **"I firmly believe":** Oliver Wendell Holmes, *Currents and Counter-Currents in Medical Science* (Ticknor and Fields, 1861), 39.

122 **Popularized by a Liverpool surgeon:** Thomas Morris, "Do no harm," *Thomas Morris* (blog), Aug. 19, 2019.

122 **"The amount of death":** Starr, *Social Transformation*, 55.

122 **One of those methods:** Wootton, *Bad Medicine*, 143, 181–83; Starr, *Social Transformation*, 54; Whorton, *Nature Cures*, 15.

123 **"The mortality amongst":** Wootton, *Bad Medicine*, 183.

123 **To understand why, we need:** Whorton, *Nature Cures*, 64; Starr, *Social Transformation*, 98.

124 **Its birthdate can be placed:** Wootton, *Bad Medicine*, 224.

125 **They seized the opportunity:** Starr, *Social Transformation*, 102; Whorton, *Nature Cures*, 135.

CHAPTER 7

126 **In the early 1980s, researchers:** C. Goodrick et al., "Effects of intermittent feeding upon . . . ," *Gerontology*, vol. 28,4 (1982), 233–41, doi:10.1159/000212538.

126 **lived 34 percent longer:** H. Sogawa and C. Kubo, "Influence of short-term repeated fasting . . . ," *Mechanisms of Ageing and Development*, 115,1–2 (2000), 61–71, doi:10.1016/s0047-6374(00)00109-3.

126 **lived 40 percent longer:** G. Roth et al., "Delayed loss of striatal dopamine receptors...," *Brain Research*, vol. 300,1 (1984), 27–32, doi:10.1016/0006 -8993(84)91337-4.

126 **To suss out the discrepancies:** Goodrick, "Effects of intermittent feeding."

126 **Mature rodents could:** C. Goodrick et al., "Differential effects of intermittent feeding...," *Journal of Gerontology*, vol. 38,1 (1983), 36–45, doi:10.1093 /geronj/38.1.36.

127 **The studies also tended:** K. Varady and M. Hellerstein, "Alternate-day fasting and chronic disease prevention," *American Journal of Clinical Nutrition*, vol. 86,1 (2007), 7–13, doi:10.1093/ajcn/86.1.7.

127 **In one of her studies:** K. Varady et al., "Short-term modified alternate-day fasting," *American Journal of Clinical Nutrition*, vol. 90,5 (2009), 1138–43, doi:10.3945/ajcn.2009.28380; S. Bhutani et al., "Improvements in coronary heart disease risk...," *Obesity* (Silver Spring), vol. 18,11 (2010), 2152–59, doi:10.1038/oby.2010.54.

128 **Varady was agreeably:** Anahad O'Connor, "Fasting Diets Are Gaining Acceptance," *New York Times* (China), Apr. 4, 2016; M. Klempel et al., "Dietary and physical activity adaptations...," *Nutrition Journal*, vol. 9 (2010), 35, doi:10.1186/1475-2891-9-35; Krista Varady, "Scientific Research Behind Intermittent Fasting," *SuperFastDiet* (blog), Dec. 6, 2017.

128 **Non-obese people, per other:** K. Varady et al., "Alternate day fasting for weight loss...," *Nutrition Journal*, vol. 12,1 (2013), 146, doi:10.1186/1475 -2891-12-146.

128 **In fact, on a range:** J. Trepanowski et al., "Effect of alternate-day fasting on weight loss...," *JAMA Internal Medicine*, vol. 177,7 (2017), 930–38. doi:10.1001/jamainternmed.2017.0936; B. Alhamdan et al., "Alternate-day versus daily energy restriction diets," *Obesity Science & Practice*, vol. 2,3 (2016), 293–302, doi:10.1002/osp4.52; Y. Cui et al., "Health effects of alternate-day fasting in adults," *Frontiers in Nutrition*, vol. 7 (2020), 586036, doi:10.3389 /fnut.2020.586036; J. Park et al., "Effect of alternate-day fasting on obesity...," *Metabolism: Clinical and Experimental*, vol. 111 (2020), 154336, doi:10.1016/j.metabol.2020.154336.

128 **Even better, mADF:** K. Varady and K. Gabel, "Safety and efficacy of alternate day fasting," *Nature Reviews Endocrinology*, vol. 15,12 (2019), 686–87, doi:10.1038/s41574-019-0270-y.

128 **the 5:2 diet:** Michael Mosley and Mimi Spencer, *The FastDiet* (Atria, 2015).

130 **In a yearlong study:** Trepanowski, "Effect of alternate-day fasting."

130 **Varady also learned:** O'Connor, "Fasting Diets."

130 **We have decades of research:** For the controversy over high-fat versus low-fat diets, see from the T. Colin Campbell Center for Nutrition Studies, online: Thomas Campbell, "Selling Fat: The Recipe for A Low-Carb Diet Book," May 3, 2016; T. Colin Campbell, "A Fallacious, Faulty and Foolish Discussion About Saturated Fat," Apr. 18, 2014; Susan Levin, "Oversaturation of Fat in the Media," Aug. 14, 2014.

130 **"literally eat whatever":** *Horizon*, "Eat, Fast and Live Longer," BBC, Aug. 6, 2012, at ca. 41:00.

130 **And even in those studies:** K. Varady et al., "Effects of weight loss via high fat . . . ," *Scientific Reports*, vol. 5 (2015), 7561, doi:10.1038/srep07561

134 **But a healthier diet:** N. Veronese et al., "Combined associations of body weight and lifestyle . . . ," *British Medical Journal* (Clinical research ed.), vol. 355 (2016), i5855, doi:10.1136/bmj.i5855; L. Fontana and F. Hu, "Optimal body weight for health and longevity," *Aging Cell*, vol. 13,3 (2014), 391–400, doi:10.1111/acel.12207.

CHAPTER 8

140 **Edward Hooker Dewey:** For Dewey, see Edward Hooker Dewey, *The True Science of Living* (Henry Bill, 1895), 29, 34, 65–67, 143–44, 148, 171–76, 179–81, 213; Edward Hooker Dewey, *The No-Breakfast Plan and the Fasting-Cure* (Dewey, 1900), 15, 17, 26, 32–35, 40, 117–26, 153–54, 181, 197–201.

141 **Yeo was a professor:** Gerald Frances Yeo, *A Manual of Physiology*, 4th American ed. (P. Blakiston, 1889), 418.

143 **"All that Dr. Dewey's":** "Food and Feeding," *British Medical Journal*, vol. 1,2563 (1910), 389.

144 **"A little starvation":** Mark Twain, "My Debut As A Literary Person," *Century*, Nov. 1899.

144 **Bernarr Macfadden:** For Macfadden, see Mark Adams, *Mr. America* (HarperCollins, 2010), prologue & chaps. 4–8, 9, 10, 12, 14–16, e-book.

146 **"disease is not sent":** R. Griffith, "Apostles of Abstinence," *American Quarterly*, vol. 52,4 (2000), 608.

148 **"every kind of dyspepsia":** Bernarr Macfadden, *Macfadden's Encyclopedia of Physical Culture*, vol. 3 (Physical Culture, 1920), 1224–25.

148 **"Your physicians have failed":** Macfadden, Macfadden's Encyclopedia, 1267.

148 **"Refuse to be an invalid!":** Bernarr Macfadden and Felix Oswald, *Fasting, Hydropathy and Exercise* (Physical Culture, 1900), 8.

149 **a Dr. William S. Wilkinson:** "Fiftieth Day of Doctor's Fast and He Walks Three Miles and Uses Indian Clubs," *Cincinnati Enquirer*, June 15, 1903, 1; Hillel Schwartz, *Never Satisfied* (Doubleday, 1986), 122.

149 **"Is prolonged fasting":** "Diseased?—Then Fast," *New York Tribune*, Mar. 15, 1903, 10.

151 **"I aimed at":** D. Rosner and G. Markowitz, "A short history of occupational safety . . . ," *American Journal of Public Health*, vol. 110,5 (2020), 622–28.

151 **historians of the Progressive Era:** Griffith, "Apostles," 629.

151 **But in fact *The Fasting Cure*:** Upton Sinclair, *The Fasting Cure* (Mitchell Kennerley, 1911), 7–8, 11 18–19, 21, 23–25, 35, 46, 51, 63.

153 **"It is difficult":** Upton Sinclair, *I, Candidate for Governor* (Univ. of California Pr., 1994), 109.

154 **"shallow and unscrupulous":** Sinclair, *Fasting Cure*, 35.

154 **"a wholesale believer":** James C. Whorton, *Crusaders for Fitness* (Princeton Univ. Pr., 1982), 197.

154 **"I look forward":** Sinclair, *Fasting Cure*, 46.

154 **Guillaume Guelpa:** For Guelpa, see R. Tattersall, "Fasting, purgation, autointoxication and diabetes," *Diabetes Digest*, vol. 9,1 (2010), 6–8; Thierry de Lestrade, *El ayuno como fuente de salud* [*Fasting as a Source of Health*], trans. Ramón Sala Gili (Milenio, 2014), 71–73.

155 **He may have been influenced:** Mahmood S. Mozaffari, ed., *New Strategies to Advance Pre/Diabetes Care*, vol. 3 (Springer, 2013), ix.

155 **"is never harmful":** G. Guelpa, "Starvation and Purgation in the Relief of Disease," *British Medical Journal*, vol. 2,2597 (1910), 1050.

155 **"scarcely received in":** Tattersall, "Fasting, purgation."

155 **Another eminent doctor:** "Reports of Societies: Disintoxication in Diabetes and Gout," *British Medical Journal*, vol. 2 (1921), 989.

155 **"The resulting benefits":** Edouard Berthollet, *Le Retour à la Santé par le Jeûne* [*The Return to Health by Fasting*] (Genillard, 1950), 114–28, online excerpt at Jeune-et-Randonnee.com.

156 **He hypothesized that:** A. Mazur, "Why were 'starvation diets' promoted for diabetes . . . ," *Nutrition Journal*, vol. 10 (2011), 23, doi:10.1186/1475-2891-10-23.

156 **We have little research:** S. Furmli et al., "Therapeutic use of intermittent fasting for people . . . ," *BMJ Case Reports*, vol. 2018 (2018), bcr2017221854, doi:10.1136/bcr-2017-221854.

156 **a diet of minimally refined plants:** Michael Greger, *How Not to Die* (Flatiron, 2015), 100–21; Neal D. Barnard, *Dr. Neal Barnard's Program for Reversing Diabetes* (Rodale, 2008).

157 **"a half dozen cases":** Dewey, *No-Breakfast*, 176.

158 **In a paper published:** Elizabeth E. Bailey et al., "The use of diet in the treatment of epilepsy," *Epilepsy & Behavior*, vol. 6 (2005), 4–8; de Lestrade, *El ayuno*, 74.

158 **"as long as they":** H. Conklin, "Cause and Treatment of Epilepsy," *Journal of the American Osteopathic Association*, vol. 22,1 (1922), 12, 14; "Fasting Urged by Osteopath as Cure of Epilepsy," *San Francisco Chronicle*, July 5, 1922, 5.

158 **"Discomfort of the patient":** "Chicago Association Meeting," *The Osteopathic Physician*, vol. 31,1 (1917), 28.

158 **He estimated he cured:** Conklin, "Cause and Treatment," 12.

159 **Henry Howland . . . H. Rawle Geyelin:** For Howland and Geyelin, see "Section on Medicine," *Medical Record*, vol. 99,24 (1921), 1037–39.

160 **Then again, Geyelin:** William G. Lennox and Stanley Cobb, *Epilepsy* (Williams and Wilkins, 1928), 130–31; James W. Wheless, "History and Origin of the Ketogenic Diet," in *Epilepsy and the Ketogenic Diet*, ed. C. E. Stafstrom and J. M. Rho (Humana, 2004), 37.

161 **The first big discovery:** For fasting and ketogenic diet as anti-epileptic therapy, see Bailey, "Use of diet"; Wheless, "History and Origin"; James W. Wheless, "History of the ketogenic diet," *Epilepsia*, vol. 49, suppl. 8 (2008), 3–5, doi:10.1111/j.1528-1167.2008.01821.x.

161 **In 1925, a Mayo team:** M. Peterman, "The ketogenic diet in epilepsy," *JAMA*, vol. 84,26 (1925), 1979–83, doi:10.1001/jama.1925.02660520007003.

162 **On rare occasion:** W. Lennox and S. Cobb, "Studies in Epilepsy: VIII. The Clinical Effect of Fasting," *Archives of Neurology and Psychiatry*, vol. 20,4 (1928), 771–79, doi:10.1001/archneurpsyc.1928.02210160112009.

162 **"an emergency procedure":** Lennox and Cobb, "Studies in Epilepsy," 779.

162 **By 1930, less than a decade:** Bailey, "Use of diet," 6.

163 **"For most patients":** Bailey, "Use of diet," 6.

CHAPTER 9

164 **Herbert Macgolfin Shelton:** For Shelton, see Jean A. Oswald, *Yours for Health* (Franklin, 1989), 24, 28, 36–38, 40–41, 51–52, 59–60, 68–69, 75, 83, 89, 94, 96, 98, 103–4, 111–14, 117–18, 128–30, 138; Alec Burton, "Foreword," in Herbert M. Shelton, *Fasting Can Save Your Life*, 2nd ed. (National Health Association, 2009), online.

165 **"the courses of measles":** Herbert M. Shelton, *Fasting Can Save Your Life*, 2nd ed. (National Health Association, 2009), chap. 17, online.

166 **A young woman from White Plains:** Shelton, *Fasting Can Save*, chap. 34.

166 **"Of course he didn't":** Shelton, *Fasting Can Save*, chap. 34.

166 **"I have seen cancerous":** Jean A. Oswald and Herbert M. Shelton, *Fasting for the Health of It* (Franklin, 1983), 168–69.

167 **"I am not 'scientific'":** Herbert Shelton, "I am not Scientific," *Hygienic Review*, Sep. 1946, online.

167 **"*Science* stubbornly clings":** Herbert M. Shelton, "Foreword to The Fifth Edition," in *The Science and Fine Art of Fasting*, 5th ed. (National Hygiene, 1978), 1.

168 **One fasting "doctor,":** Gregg Olsen, *Starvation Heights* (Three Rivers, 2005).

168 **Gerald Benesh was twice:** Oswald, *Yours for Health*, 97; "Clinic Operator Jailed," *Cincinnati Enquirer*, Oct. 15, 1952, 36.

169 **Christopher Gian-Cursio was arrested:** Oswald, *Yours for Health*, 92–93; "$500 Bail Forfeit Ordered in Case Of 'Naturopath,'" *Democrat and Chronicle* (Rochester), Oct. 1, 1953, 30.

169 **By one count, Gian-Cursio:** "The Christopher Gian-Cursio Collection," H. J. Lutcher Stark Center for Physical Culture and Sports, Univ. of Texas, online.

170 **One was of a thirty-nine-year-old:** Oswald and Shelton, *Fasting for the Health*, 172; Shelton, *Fasting Can Save*, chap. 32.

170 **A thirty-eight-year-old optometrist:** Oswald and Shelton, *Fasting for the Health*, 173–74; Shelton, *Fasting Can Save*, chap. 20.

171 **"a twisted and distorted":** Shelton, *Fasting Can Save*, chap. 22.

171 **One of his more successful:** Oswald and Shelton, *Fasting for the Health*, 174–75; Shelton, *Fasting Can Save*, chaps. 1, 21.

171 **There were other successes:** For the reversals of sexual disorders, nasal polyps, and retinitis pigmentosa, see Oswald and Shelton, *Fasting for the Health*, 166–77.

172 **Shelton also claimed reversals:** Shelton, *Fasting Can Save*, chap. 8; Oswald and Shelton, *Fasting for the Health*, 177–99.

173 **In one of the fatal cases:** For the death of William Carlton under Virginia Vetrano, see Petition for Writ of Certiorari, *Shelton v. Carlton*, 467 U.S. 1206 (No. 83-1628); Brief in Opposition to Certiorari, *Shelton v. Carlton*, 467 U.S. 1206 (No. 83-1628); *Carlton v. Shelton*, 722 F.2d 203 (5th Cir. 1984). Vetrano's other victims were Armand John Gilbert, Keith V. Ellis, and Joy Michelle Bristo.

CHAPTER 10

176 **Otto Buchinger:** For Buchinger, see Otto Buchinger, *La cura por el ayuno* [*The Fasting Cure*], trans. Carlota Romero and Elinor Gisela Thomas (Lidiun, 1988); interviews by author of Françoise Wilhelmi de Toledo, Überlingen, Germany, Nov. 2020.

178 **"But whatever the essence":** Buchinger, *La cura*, 15.

182 **"the most contemplative":** Buchinger, *La cura*, 41.

188 **I was happy she didn't:** Andreas Michalsen, *The Nature Cure* (Viking, 2019), 30ff.

188 **"Allow yourself to enjoy":** Françoise Wilhelmi de Toledo and Hubert Hohler, *Therapeutic Fasting* (Thieme, 2012), 59.

191 **"Better to ask me":** Françoise Wilhelmi de Toledo, *El arte de ayuno* [*The Art of Fasting*] (Maeva, 2018), 69.

191 **Still, some illnesses proved:** For the illnesses Buchinger fasted, see Buchinger, *La cura*, 78–79, 83–85, 87–89.

193 **"Whoever doesn't turn"**: Buchinger, *La cura*, 107–8.

193 **Like Shelton, he never**: Buchinger, *La cura*, 81, 93–94.

194 **Such contents might explain**: Buchinger, *La cura*, 48.

195 **Johann Glauber**: For Glauber, see John T. Young, *Faith, Medical Alchemy and Natural Philosophy* (Ashgate, 1998), 183–216.

196 **"Usually 4 to 7 stools"**: Buchinger, *La cura*, 47.

199 **"the cure of the body"**: Buchinger, *La cura*, 1.

199 **A *New York Times* correspondent**: Cathy Horyn, "Famine or Feast?" *T: The New York Times Style Magazine*, Nov. 16, 2014, 101.

203 **There was little research**: R. Huber et al., "Effects of abdominal hot compresses on . . . ," *BMC Gastroenterology*, vol. 7 (2007), 27, doi:10.1186/1471-230X-7-27.

CHAPTER 11

204 **"indistinguishable from young"**: Charles Manning Child, *Senescence and Rejuvenescence* (Univ. of Chicago Pr., 1915), 156–57.

204 **Eight years later, Sergius Morgulis**: Sergius Morgulis, *Fasting and Undernutrition* (E. P. Dutton, 1923), 199–200.

204 **"approximately one-half"**: Margarete M. Kunde, "The After Effects of Prolonged Fasting on the Basal Metabolic Rate," *Journal of Metabolic Research*, 1923, vol. 3, 443.

205 **Given the rejuvenation**: T. Brailsford Robertson et al., "The influence of intermittent starvation and . . . ," *Australian Journal of Experimental Biology and Medical Science*, vol. 12,1 (1934), 33–45.

205 **"a rugged old man"**: "Scientist's Scientist," *Time*, Feb. 10, 1941.

206 **"His hands are like"**: "Has an Appetite for Hardware, Glass and Gravel," *San Francisco Examiner*, Apr. 30, 1933, 76.

206 **In those experiments, Carlson**: A. Carlson and F. Hoelzel, "Apparent prolongation of the life span . . . ," *Journal of Nutrition*, vol. 31 (1946), 363–75, doi:10.1093/jn/31.3.363.

206 **Carlson and Hoelzel speculated**: A. J. Carlson and F. Hoelzel, "Nutrition, senescence, and rejuvenescence," *Public Health Reports* (Washington), vol. 67,2 (1952), 129–30.

207 **Cornell professor Clive McCay**: C. McCay and M. Crowell, "Prolonging

the Life Span," *Scientific Monthly*, vol. 39,5 (1934), 405–14; C. McCay et al., "The effect of retarded growth upon . . . ," *Nutrition* (Burbank), vol. 5,3 (1989), 155–71.

208 **The other force:** Sharman Apt Russell, *Hunger* (Basic, 2005), 113–36.

208 **Don Kendrick was a professor:** D. Kendrick, "The effects of infantile stimulation and . . . ," *Developmental Psychobiology*, vol. 6,3 (1973), 225–34, doi:10.1002/dev.420060307.

209 **In June of 1965, a Scotsman:** W. Stewart and L. Fleming, "Features of a successful therapeutic fast of 382 days' duration," *Postgraduate Medical Journal*, vol. 49,569 (1973), 203–9, doi:10.1136/pgmj.49.569.203.

210 **The revival began with:** W. Bloom, "Fasting as an introduction to the treatment of obesity," *Metabolism: Clinical and Experimental*, vol. 8,3 (1959), 214–20.

210 **A twenty-year-old woman:** D. Collison, "Total fasting for up to 249 days" (letter), *Lancet*, vol. 289,7481 (1967), 112.

210 **A thirty-year-old Glaswegian:** W. Stewart et al., "Massive obesity treated by intermittent fasting," *American Journal of Medicine*, vol. 40,6 (1966), 967–86, doi:10.1016/0002-9343(66)90209-9.

210 **Clinicians who gave their fasters:** F. Fawzy et al., "Psychotherapy as an adjunct to supervised fasting for obesity," *Psychosomatics*, vol. 25,11 (1984), 821–29, doi:10.1016/S0033-3182(84)72943-4.

210 **So did fasters who made:** G. Duncan et al., "Correction and control of intractable obesity," *JAMA*, vol. 181 (1962), 309–12, doi:10.1001/jama.1962.03050300029006.

210 **Their view of fasting:** P. Cubberley, "Lactic acidosis and death . . . ," *New England Journal of Medicine*, vol. 272 (1965), 628–30, doi:10.1056/NEJM196503252721208; G. Duncan et al., "Contraindications and therapeutic results of fasting in obese patients," *Annals of the New York Academy of Sciences*, vol. 131,1 (1965), 632–6, doi:10.1111/j.1749-6632.1965.tb34826.x; I. Spencer, "Death during therapeutic starvation for obesity," *Lancet*, vol. 291,7555 (1968), 1288–90, doi:10.1016/s0140-6736(68)92299-x; L. Hermann and M. Iversen, "Death during therapeutic starvation," *Lancet*, vol. 2,7561 (1968), 217, doi:10.1016/s0140-6736(68)92649-4; A. Kahan and A. Porter, "Death during therapeutic starvation" (letter), *Lancet*, vol. 291,7556 (1968), 1378–79.

211 **Recent research suggests:** Interview by author of Alan Goldhamer, Santa Rosa, California, June 8, 2021.

212 **Unfortunately, their preferred "fast":** Marjolijn Bijlefeld and Sharon K. Zoumbari, "Liquid Protein Diets," in *Encyclopedia of Diet Fads*, 2nd ed. (Greenwood, 2014), 123; Nadine Brozan, "The Liquid Protein Diet Controversy," *New York Times*, May 18, 1977, 50.

212 **In fact, although the body:** Goldhamer interview; interviews by author of Françoise Wilhelmi de Toledo, Überlingen, Germany, Nov. 2020.

213 **Between 1979 and 1988, a handful:** L. Sköldstam et al., "Effect of fasting and lactovegetarian diet on rheumatoid arthritis," *Scandinavian Journal of Rheumatology*, vol. 8,4 (1979) 249–55, doi:10.3109/03009747909114631; A. Udén et al., "Neutrophil functions and clinical performance . . . ," *Annals of the Rheumatic Diseases*, vol. 42,1 (1983), 45–51, doi:10.1136/ard.42.1.45; I. Hafström et al., "Effects of fasting in disease activity, neutrophil function . . . ," *Arthritis & Rheumatology*, vol. 31,5 (1988), 585–92, doi:10.1002/art.1780310502.

214 **Kjeldsen-Kragh, a conventional:** J. Kjeldsen-Kragh et al., "Controlled trial of fasting and one-year . . . ," *Lancet*, vol. 338,8772 (1991), 899–902, doi:10.1016/0140-6736(91)91770-u.

215 **To all appearances, fasting:** I. Choi et al., "A diet mimicking fasting promotes regeneration . . . ," *Cell Reports*, vol. 15,10 (2016), 2136–46, doi:10.1016/j.celrep.2016.05.009.

215 **In pilot trials in humans:** R. de Cabo and M. Mattson, "Effects of intermittent fasting on health, aging, and disease," *New England Journal of Medicine*, vol. 381,26 (2019), 2541–51, doi:10.1056/NEJMra1905136.

215 **Fasting enjoyed one other:** For the Abrahamses and the Charlie Foundation, see "Ketogenic Diet Pioneer Reunites with Charlie Abrahams," Johns Hopkins Children's Center, Apr. 1, 2008, online; James W. Wheless, "History and Origin of the Ketogenic Diet," in *Epilepsy and the Ketogenic Diet*, ed. C. E. Stafstrom and J. M. Rho (Humana, 2004), 40ff; Melissa Hendricks, "High Fat and Seizure Free," *Johns Hopkins Magazine*, Apr. 1995, online; Travis Christofferson and Dominic D'Agostino, "The Origin (and future) of the Ketogenic Diet," parts 1–3, Robb Wolf (website), Sep. 24–Oct. 7, 2015.

218 **drugs don't work for nearly 40 percent:** Z. Chen et al., "Treatment outcomes

in patients with newly...," *JAMA Neurology*, vol. 75,3 (2018), 279–86, doi:10.1001/jamaneurol.2017.3949.

218 **Nudged by the Charlie Foundation:** Jim Abrahams, "Mrs. Kelly," The Charlie Foundation, July 9, 2014, online.

218 **In 2008, British researchers:** E. Neal et al., "The ketogenic diet for the treatment of childhood epilepsy," *Lancet. Neurology*, vol. 7,6 (2008), 500–506, doi:10.1016/S1474-4422(08)70092-9.

218 **Scientists are still working:** I. Meira et al., "Ketogenic diet and epilepsy," *Frontiers in Neuroscience*, vol. 13 (2019), 5, doi:10.3389/fnins.2019.00005.

218 **The ketone beta-hydroxybutyrate:** S. Anton et al., "Flipping the metabolic switch," *Obesity* (Silver Spring), vol. 26,2 (2018), 254–68, doi:10.1002/oby.22065.

218 **It could have to do:** de Cabo and Mattson, "Effects of intermittent fasting"; M. Mattson et al., "Intermittent metabolic switching, neuroplasticity and brain health," *Nature Reviews. Neuroscience*, vol. 19,2 (2018), 63–80, doi:10.1038/nrn.2017.156.

219 **In 2005, more than a decade:** K. Mastriani et al., "Evidence-based versus reported epilepsy management practices," *Journal of Child Neurology*, vol. 23,5 (2008), 507–14, doi:10.1177/0883073807309785.

220 **For the first twelve or so:** Mark P. Mattson, Maria Buchinger Prize Lecture, 18th Congress of the Medical Society for Fasting and Nutrition, Überlingen, Germany, 2019, at 1:07:20.

220 **The increase is a sign:** For fasting metabolism, see Mattson, "Intermittent metabolic switching"; de Cabo and Mattson, "Effects of intermittent fasting."

220-221 **In one experiment, rat hearts:** Y. Kashiwaya et al., "Control of glucose utilization in working perfused rat heart," *Journal of Biological Chemistry*, vol. 269,41 (1994), 25502–14, https://pubmed.ncbi.nlm.nih.gov/7929251/.

221 **Even short fasts reduce inflammatory:** The Real Truth About Health, "Can Fasting Save Your Life, By Author: Alan Goldhamer, D.C.," YouTube, July 6, 2020, at 52:30; L. Hanlin et al., "Fasting reduces plasma interleukin-6...," *Brain, Behavior, and Immunity*, vol. 49, suppl. (2015), e22, doi:10.1016/j.bbi.2015.06.093; I. Alam et al., "Recurrent circadian fasting (RCF) improves blood pressure...," *Journal of Translational Medicine*, vol. 17,1 (2019), 272, doi:10.1186/s12967-019-2007-z; K. Speaker et al., "A single bout of

fasting (24 h) . . . ," *Mediators of Inflammation*, vol. 2016 (2016), 1698071, doi:10.1155/2016/1698071; Satchin Panda, *The Circadian Code* (Rodale, 2018), 201.

221 **Fasting mice, for example:** D. Lavin et al., "Fasting induces an anti-inflammatory effect . . . ," *Obesity* (Silver Spring), vol. 19,8 (2011), 1586–94, doi:10.1038/oby.2011.73.

221 **Fasting also generates antioxidants:** T. Arumugam et al., "Age and energy intake interact to modify . . . ," *Annals of Neurology*, vol. 67,1 (2010), 41–52, doi:10.1002/ana.21798.

221 **Recent research has also proven:** M. Mattson et al., "Meal frequency and timing in health and disease," *PNAS*, vol. 111,47 (2014), 16647–53, doi:10.1073/pnas.1413965111; M. Hatori et al., "Time-restricted feeding without reducing caloric . . . ," *Cell Metabolism*, vol. 15,6 (2012), 848–60, doi:10.1016/j.cmet.2012.04.019; Andreas Michalsen, *The Fasting Fix* (Viking, 2020), 185–86.

222 **Contrary to wide belief:** Michael Greger, *How Not to Die* (Flatiron, 2015), 100–121; Neal D. Barnard, *Dr. Neal Barnard's Program for Reversing Diabetes* (Rodale, 2008).

222 **Once the part is dissolved:** Panda, *Circadian Code*, 207.

222 **"When once we":** Herbert M. Shelton, *Fasting and Sun Bathing*, 3rd ed. (Dr. Shelton's Health School, 1950), chap. 15, online.

223 **In one promising experiment:** I. Madorsky et al., "Intermittent fasting alleviates the neuropathic . . . ," *Neurobiology of Disease*, vol. 34,1 (2009), 146–54, doi:10.1016/j.nbd.2009.01.002.

223 **In a simple but telling:** K. Matt et al., "Influence of calorie reduction on DNA repair . . . ," *Mechanisms of Ageing and Development*, vol. 154 (2016), 24–29, doi:10.1016/j.mad.2016.02.008.

223 **The best of them help:** Marilyn Hair and Jon Sharpe, "Fast Facts About the Human Microbiome," Center for Ecogenetics and Environmental Health, Univ. of Washington, online; Z. Kho and S. Lal, "The human gut microbiome," *Frontiers in Microbiology*, vol. 9 (2018), 1835, doi:10.3389/fmicb.2018.01835.

224 **If we refeed on plants:** Wilhelmi de Toledo interviews.

224 **We now know, for example:** Wilhelmi de Toledo interviews.

224 **Scientists have multiple names:** Michalsen, *Fasting Fix*, 273–74.

224 **In other studies:** Luigi Fontana, *The Path to Longevity* (Hardie Grant, 2020), 51.

CHAPTER 12

226 **Valter Longo:** For Longo, see Valter Longo, *The Longevity Diet* (Avery, 2018), 25–36, 96–137, 154, 180; Valter Longo, lectures, Congress of the Medical Society for Fasting and Nutrition, Überlingen, Germany, 2013, 2015, online; interview by author of Valter Longo, telephone, Nov. 19, 2011.

226 **Roy Walford:** For Walford, see Thomas H. Maugh II, "Roy Walford, 79," *Los Angeles Times*, May 1, 2004; Terrell Tannen, "Roy Walford," *Lancet*, vol. 363,9425 (2004), 2003, doi:10.1016/S0140-6736(04)16428-3; Gary Taubes and David Fukumoto, "Staying Alive," *Discover*, Jan. 31, 2000.

227 **The results were fantastic:** J. Most et al., "Calorie restriction in humans," *Ageing Research Reviews*, vol. 39 (2017), 36–45, doi:10.1016/j.arr.2016.08.005; R. Walford et al., "The calorically restricted low-fat nutrient-dense . . . ," *PNAS*, vol. 89,23 (1992), 11533–7, doi:10.1073/pnas.89.23.11533; R. Walford et al., "Calorie restriction in biosphere 2," *Journals of Gerontology. Series A, Biological Sciences and Medical Sciences*, vol. 57,6 (2002), B211–24, doi:10.1093/gerona/57.6.b211.

230 **When he bathed his yeast:** M. Mirisola et al., "Serine- and threonine/valine-dependent activation . . . ," *PLoS Genetics*, vol. 10,2 (2014), e1004113, doi:10.1371/journal.pgen.1004113.

232 **Other colleagues found similar:** V. Longo, "Mutations in signal transduction proteins increase . . . ," *Neurobiology of Aging,* vol. 20,5 (1999), 479–86, doi:10.1016/s0197-4580(99)00089-5.

233 **When Kenyon knocked out:** C. Kenyon, "The first long-lived mutants," *Philosophical transactions of the Royal Society of London. Series B, Biological Sciences*, vol. 366,1561 (2011), 9–16, doi:10.1098/rstb.2010.0276; C. Kenyon, "The Plasticity of Aging," *Cell*, vol. 120,4 (2005), 449–60, doi:10.1016/j.cell.2005.02.002.

234 **In 1957, a young Israeli:** For the Larons and the doctors and scientists who studied them, see Gary Taubes, "Rare Form of Dwarfism Protects Against

Cancer," *Discover*, Mar. 26, 2013, online; Peter Bowes, "An experimental eating regime may slow aging . . . ," *Quartz*, Apr. 12, 2016, online.

237 **In 1990, Guevara-Aguirre:** A. Rosenbloom et al., "The little women of Loja," *New England Journal of Medicine*, vol. 323,20 (1990), 1367–74. doi:10.1056 /NEJM199011153232002.

238 **Over the next decade:** J. Guevara-Aguirre et al., "Growth hormone receptor deficiency is associated . . . ," *Science Translational Medicine*, vol. 3,70 (2011), 70ra13, doi:10.1126/scitranslmed.3001845.

239 **When researchers created mutant:** Martin Holzenberger, "IGF-1 Receptors in Mammalian Longevity," in *Endocrine Aspects of Successful Aging*, ed. P. Chanson et al. (Springer, 2004), 35–48.

243 **In 1988, a cadre of young:** I. Siegel et al., "Effects of short-term dietary restriction on survival of mammary ascites tumor-bearing rats," *Cancer Investigation*, vol. 6,6 (1988), 677–80, doi:10.3109/07357908809078034.

243 **Cancer does not thrive:** Michalsen, *Fasting Fix*, 175; S. de Groot et al., "Effects of short-term fasting on cancer treatment," *Journal of Experimental & Clinical Cancer Research*, vol. 38,1 (2019), 209, doi:10.1186/s13046-019 -1189-9.

243 **Building on this:** C. Lee et al., "Fasting cycles retard growth of tumors and . . . ," *Science Translational Medicine*, vol. 4,124 (2012), 124ra127, doi:10.1126/scitranslmed.3003293; C. Lee et al., "Reduced levels of IGF-I mediate differential . . . ," *Cancer Research*, vol. 70,4 (2010), 1564–72, doi:10.1158/0008-5472.CAN-09-3228.

244 **But where fasting really:** L. Raffaghello et al., "Starvation-dependent differential stress resistance . . . ," *Proceedings of the National Academy of Sciences*, vol. 105,24 (2008), 8215–20, doi:10.1073/pnas.0708100105.

245 **He ran the same experiment:** Carl Marziali, "Fasting weakens cancer in mice," USC News, Feb. 8, 2012, online; Lee, "Fasting cycles retard."

245 **"Would I be enthusiastic":** J. Couzin, "Can fasting blunt chemotherapy's debilitating side effects?" *Science*, vol. 321,5893 (2008), 1146–47, doi:10.1126/science.321.5893.1146a.

246 **In the end, Longo:** F. Safdie et al., "Fasting and cancer treatment in humans," *Aging*, vol. 1,12 (2009), 988–1007, doi:10.18632/aging.100114.

247 **The results, which Longo:** T. Dorff et al., "Safety and feasibility of fasting in . . . ," *BMC Cancer*, vol. 16 (2016), 360, doi:10.1186/s12885-016-2370-6.

247 **A later study by other:** K. Tinkum et al., "Fasting protects mice from lethal DNA damage . . . ," *PNAS*, vol. 112,51 (2015), E7148-54, doi:10.1073 /pnas.1509249112.

247 **In another experiment:** Lee, "Reduced levels of IGF-I."

249 **Once more they could:** C. Cheng et al., "Fasting-mimicking diet promotes Ngn3-driven . . . ," *Cell*, vol. 168,5 (2017), 775–88.e12, doi:10.1016/j .cell.2017.01.040.

249 **Next Longo put mice:** S. Di Biase et al., "Fasting-mimicking diet reduces HO-1 . . . ," *Cancer Cell*, vol. 30,1 (2016), 136–46, doi:10.1016/j.ccell.2016 .06.005; Emily Gersema, "Fasting-like diet turns the immune system against cancer," USC News, July 12, 2016, online.

250 **In Longo's first randomized:** M. Wei et al., "Fasting-mimicking diet and markers/risk factors . . . ," *Science Translational Medicine*, vol. 9,377 (2017), eaai8700, doi:10.1126/scitranslmed.aai8700.

250 **To date, hundreds of thousands:** Personal communications by author with Valter Longo, Oct. 2021.

250 **"as effective as fasting":** *Fasting*, directed by Doug Orchard (Doug Orchard, 2017), transcript at https://subslikescript.com/movie/Fasting-7813060.

251 **In 2019, when researchers:** J. Rahmani et al., "The influence of fasting and energy restricting . . . ," *Ageing Research Reviews*, vol. 53 (2019), 100910, doi:10.1016/j.arr.2019.100910.

251 **The fasters had more:** S. de Groot et al., "The effects of short-term fasting on tolerance . . . ," *BMC Cancer*, vol. 15 (2015) 652, doi:10.1186/s12885-015 -1663-5.

251 **In a trial in Berlin:** S. Bauersfeld et al., "The effects of short-term fasting on quality . . . ," *BMC Cancer*, vol. 18,1 (2018), 476, doi:10.1186/s12885-018 -4353-2; Michalsen, *Fasting Fix*, 177.

CHAPTER 13

253 **"'critical' situations before":** Otto Buchinger, *La cura por el ayuno* [*The Fasting Cure*], trans. Carlota Romero and Elinor Gisela Thomas (Lidiun, 1988), 53.

256 **Maria Buchinger:** For Maria Buchinger, see Clínica Buchinger Wilhelmi, ed., *Maria Buchinger* (Maeva, 2016); interviews by author of Françoise Wilhelmi de Toledo, Überlingen, Germany, Nov. 2020.

256 **"Famous people are":** Daniel Chu, "At the Buchinger Clinic in Spain, the Clients May Starve, but They Do It with Style," *People*, Aug. 4, 1986. See also Maria Pina, "Agosto en la Buchinger, donde los famosos pagan por no comer" ["August at the Buchinger, where the famous pay not to eat"], *El Mundo* (Madrid), Aug. 25, 2019.

259 **"there is nothing":** Buchinger, *La cura*, 52.

262 **Catherine Kousmine:** For Kousmine, see websites of La Fondation Dr C. Kousmine, www.kousmine.fr, and L'Association Kousmine Française, www .kousmine.fr; Wilhelmi de Toledo interviews.

263 **have since been corroborated:** T. Fiolet et al., "Consumption of ultra-processed foods and cancer risk," *British Medical Journal*, vol. 360 (2018), k322, doi:10.1136/bmj.k322; T. Colin Campbell, *The China Study*, revised ed. (BenBella, 2016).

264 **although not dairy:** Campbell, *China Study*; Neal Barnard, *The Cheese Trap* (Grand Central, 2017); Michael Greger, *How Not to Die* (Flatiron, 2015).

265 **"Analytic thinking is":** Buchinger, *La cura*, 20.

268 **Buchinger and other German:** Buchinger, *La cura*, 95; Jean A. Oswald and Herbert M. Shelton, *Fasting for the Health of It* (Franklin, 1983), 166; Herbert M. Shelton, *Fasting Can Save Your Life*, 2nd ed. (National Health Association, 2009), chap. 36, online.

268 **"our dear old mother":** Buchinger, *La cura*, 19.

269 **Her first foray was:** Françoise G. Wilhelmi de Toledo et al., "The Buchinger Klinik Programme for the treatment of obesity," in *Obesity in Europe 1993*, ed. H. Ditschuneit et al. (John Libbey, 1994), 289–93.

270 **In one trial, she reported:** S. Drinda et al., "Effects of periodic fasting on fatty liver index," *Nutrients*, vol. 11 (2019), 2601, doi:10.3390/nu11112601.

270 **And in an evaluation:** F. Wilhelmi de Toledo et al., "Safety, health improvement and well-being...," *PloS ONE*, vol. 14, 1 (2019), e0209353, doi:10 .1371/journal.pone.0209353.

272 **But I could find only:** A. Michalsen et al., "In-patient treatment for fibromyalgia," *Evidence-Based Complementary and Alternative Medicine*, vol. 2013

(2013), 908610, doi:10.1155/2013/908610; M. Oribe et al., "Fasting therapy in fibromyalgia," *Clinical Rheumatology and Related Research*, vol. 19,1 (2007), 24–30, doi:10.14961/cra.19.24.

275 **"Whoever fasts only"**: Buchinger, *La cura*, 15–16.

275 **"That man digs"**: Buchinger, *La cura*, 1–2.

277 **"The grocery, the tavern"**: Buchinger, *La cura*, 99.

278 **I was still reattaching:** This spurious idea of mixing amino acids was popularized by Frances Moore Lappé, who later retracted the claim, in her 1971 bestseller *Diet for a Small Planet*.

278 **It's true that in the:** M. Yang and T. Van Itallie, "Composition of weight lost during short-term weight reduction," *Journal of Clinical Investigation*, vol. 58,3 (1976), 722–30, doi:10.1172/JCI108519; Michael Greger, *How Not to Diet* (Flatiron, 2019), 273; W. Kephart et al., "The three-month effects of a ketogenic...," *Sports* (Basel) vol. 6,1 (2018), 1, doi:10.3390/sports6010001.

278 **systemically inflame the body:** F. Cândido et al., "Impact of dietary fat on gut microbiota...," *International Journal of Food Sciences and Nutrition*, vol. 69,2 (2018), 125–43, doi:10.1080/09637486.2017.1343286.

278 **narrow arteries:** S. Phillips et al., "Benefit of low-fat over low-carbohydrate diet...," *Hypertension* (Dallas), vol. 51,2 (2008), 376–82, doi:10.1161/HYPERTENSIONAHA.107.101824; L. Schwingshackl and G. Hoffmann, "Low-carbohydrate diets impair flow-mediated dilatation," *British Journal of Nutrition*, vol. 110,5 (2013), 969–70, doi:10.1017/S000711451300216X.

278 **lay waste to healthy intestinal bacteria:** Y. Zhang et al., "Altered gut microbiome composition in children...," *Epilepsy Research*, 145 (2018), 163–8, doi:10.1016/j.eplepsyres.2018.06.015; G. Brinkworth et al., "Comparative effects of very low-carbohydrate, high-fat...," *British Journal of Nutrition*, vol. 101,10 (2009), 1493–502, doi:10.1017/S0007114508094658.

278 **up to seventeen vitamins and minerals:** B. Zupec-Kania and M. Zupanc, "Long-term management of the ketogenic diet," *Epilepsia*, vol. 49, suppl. 8 (2008), 23–6, doi:10.1111/j.1528-1167.2008.01827.x; J. Calton, "Prevalence of micronutrient deficiency in popular diet plans," *Journal of the International Society of Sports Nutrition*, vol. 7 (2010), 24, doi:10.1186/1550-2783-7-24.

278 **cancer, gallbladder disease, stroke, diabetes, and dementia:** N. Bueno et al., "Very-low-carbohydrate ketogenic diet v. low-fat...," *British Journal of*

Nutrition, vol. 110,7 (2013), 1178–87, doi:10.1017/S0007114513000548; F. Sacks et al., "Dietary fats and cardiovascular disease," *Circulation*, vol. 136,3 (2017), e1–e23, doi:10.1161/CIR.0000000000000510; Sophia Mitrokostas, "7 reasons you shouldn't do the keto diet long-term," *Insider*, Mar. 26, 2019, online.

278 **headaches, constipation, diarrhea, atrial fibrillation:** American College of Cardiology, "Low-Carb Diet Tied to Common Heart Rhythm Disorder," press release, Mar. 6, 2019, online.

279 **leaky gut:** G. Wu et al., "Linking long-term dietary patterns with gut microbial enterotypes," *Science*, vol. 334,6052 (2011), 105–8, doi:10.1126/science .1208344.

279 **most alarmingly, early death:** H. Noto et al., "Low-carbohydrate diets and all-cause mortality," *PLoS ONE*, vol. 8,1 (2013), e55030, doi:10.1371 /journal.pone.0055030; S. Li, "Low carbohydrate diet from plant or animal sources . . . ," *Journal of the American Heart Association*, vol. 3,5 (2014), e001169, doi:10.1161/JAHA.114.001169; I. Bank et al., "Sudden cardiac death in association . . . ," *Pediatric Neurology*, vol. 39,6 (2008), 429–31, doi:10.1016/j.pediatrneurol.2008.08.013.

279 **In one trial, after just:** Greger, *How Not to Diet*, 106.

281 **A few weeks later:** F. Grundler et al., "Excretion of heavy metals and glyphosate . . . ," *Frontiers in Nutrition*, vol. 8 (2021), 708069, doi:10.3389 /fnut.2021.708069; personal communications to author from Buchinger Wilhelmi Clinic, Mar. 18 and Sep. 14, 2020.

281 **One of the few trials:** M. Imamura and T. Tung, "A trial of fasting cure for PCB-poisoned patients in Taiwan," *American Journal of Industrial Medicine*, vol. 5,1–2 (1984), 147–53; also under same title in *Progress in Clinical and Biological Research*, vol. 137 (1984), 147–53.

CHAPTER 14

283 **Henry Clark:** For Clark, see "Tanner's Fast Outdone," *Cincinnati Enquirer*, July 18, 1882, 7; "Forty-One Days' Fast," *San Francisco Chronicle*, July 22, 1882, 4; Charles Edward Page, *The Natural Cure of Consumption, Constipation . . .* (Fowler and Wells, 1884), 140–43; "A Long Fast," *Chicago Daily Tribune*, July 16, 1882, 9.

284 **"that his delightful":** "Tanner's Mental Experiences," *Minneapolis Tribune*, Dec. 28, 1890, 7.

285 **That organ was:** "Fasting as a Remedy for Insanity," *Phrenological Journal*, Oct. 1882, 214.

285 **Christoph Wilhelm Hufeland . . . Anton Müller . . . Benjamin Rush:** For Hufeland, Müller, and Rush, see Mary de Young, "Diet: Hunger Cure, or Famine Cure," in *Encyclopedia of Asylum Therapeutics, 1750–1950s* (McFarland, 2015), 76–77.

286 **Estella Kuenzel:** For Kuenzel, see Edward Hooker Dewey, *The No-Breakfast Plan and the Fasting-Cure* (Dewey, 1900), 141–45.

287 **"The results," the writer:** Bernarr Macfadden, *Macfadden's Encyclopedia of Physical Culture*, vol. 3 (Physical Culture, 1920), 1341.

287 **"when the insane":** Jean A. Oswald, *Yours for Health* (Franklin, 1989), 125.

287 **"her behavior was":** Jean A. Oswald and Herbert M. Shelton, *Fasting for the Health of It* (Franklin, 1983), 187.

288 **The pair also said:** "Nutrition, Senescence, And Rejuvenescence," *Public Health Reports*, vol. 67,2 (1952), 129–30; "Scientist's Scientist," *Time*, Feb. 10, 1941.

288 **For the longest time:** I. Sletten et al., "Total fasting in psychiatric subjects," *Canadian Psychiatric Association Journal*, vol. 12,6 (1967), 553–58, doi:10.1177/070674376701200604.

289 **"Fasting is an indispensable":** Leo Tolstoy, "The First Step," in *The Complete Works of Count Tolstoy*, vol. 19, ed. and trans. Leo Wiener (Dana Estes, 1905), 392.

289 **Yuri hadn't intended:** For Yuri Nikolayev's work, see Yuri S. Nikolayev, Голодание ради здоровья [*Fasting for Health*] (Don, 1990), 3, 11, 42–53, 60–65, 82–87, 100, 108, 119/120, online; Thierry de Lestrade, *El ayuno como fuente de salud* [*Fasting as a Source of Health*], trans. Ramón Sala Gili (Melenio, 2014), 83–130; A. Cott, "Controlled fasting treatment of schizophrenia in the USSR," *Schizophrenia*, vol. 3 (1971), 2–10; A. Cott, "Controlled fasting treatment for schizophrenia," *Journal of Orthomolecular Psychiatry*, vol. 3,4 (1974), 301–11; Allan Cott, *Fasting* (Hastings, 1997), 4; Allan Cott, *Fasting as a Way of Life* (Hastings, 1997), 74; Murray Seeger, "Soviet Cure-All: Eat Nothing for 30 Days," *Los Angeles Times*, Apr. 3, 1972, A1; D. Boehme,

"Preplanned fasting in the treatment of mental disease," *Schizophrenia Bulletin*, vol. 3,2 (1977), 288–96, doi:10.1093/schbul/3.2.288.

298 **For the most common:** Boehme, "Preplanned fasting."

299 **for a range of conditions:** A. Kokosov et al., *Therapeutic Starvation in Internal Diseases* (Lan, 1999), online excerpt at http://golodanie-da.ru/vnutrennie bolezyi.htm.

299 **In one retrospective study:** A. Kokosov and S. Osinin, "Fasting therapy for patients with bronchial asthma," Conference on Therapeutic Fasting, Ulan-Ude (2001), abstract posted online in "Fasting Therapy in the Internal Pathology," https://apache2.pum.edu.pl/~fasting/bur_ab.doc.

299 **Most of the patients maintained:** O. Baranova et al., "Efficiency of fasting therapy in patients with sarcoidosis of the lungs," Conference on Therapeutic Fasting, Ulan-Ude (2001), abstract posted online in "Fasting Therapy in the Internal Pathology," https://apache2.pum.edu.pl/~fasting/bur_ab.doc.

301 **The opening arose from:** For Allan Cott, see Allan Cott, *Fasting as a Way of Life*, 75–77; Allan Cott, *Fasting*, 35; de Young, "Diet," 78–79; Cott, "Controlled fasting" (1974); Cott, "Controlled fasting" (1971); Nikolayev, *Fasting*, 108/120; Boehme, "Preplanned fasting"; Seeger, "Soviet Cure-All."

302 **But this modest publicity:** E. Paterson, "The fasting cure," *Medical Post*, vol. 36,7 (2000), 38; Harold D. Foster, *What Really Causes Schizophrenia* (Trafford, 2003), discussing Dr. Abram Hoffer.

302 **A group of Japanese:** J. Suzuki et al., "Fasting therapy for psychosomatic diseases . . . ," *Tohoku Journal of Experimental Medicine*, vol. 118, suppl. (1976), 245–59, doi:10.1620/tjem.118.suppl_245; J. Suzuki et al., "Fasting therapy for psychosomatic disorders in Japan," *Psychotherapy and Psychosomatics*, vol. 31,1–4 (1979), 307–14, doi:10.1159/000287345; H. Yamamoto et al., "Psychophysiological study on fasting therapy," *Psychotherapy and Psychosomatics*, vol. 32,1–4 (1979), 229–40, doi:10.1159/000287392.

303 **In the 1980s and 1990s:** For fasting's effect on the brain, see R. de Cabo and M. Mattson, "Effects of intermittent fasting on health, aging, and disease," *New England Journal of Medicine*, vol. 381,26 (2019), 2541–51, doi:10.1056/NEJMra1905136; M. Mattson et al., "Intermittent metabolic switching, neuroplasticity and brain health," *Nature Reviews. Neuroscience*, vol. 19,2 (2018), 63–80, doi:10.1038/nrn.2017.156; S. Anton et al., "Flipping

the metabolic switch," *Obesity* (Silver Spring), vol. 26,2 (2018), 254–68, doi:10.1002/oby.22065.

303 **When scientists fasted vinegar flies:** Y. Hirano et al., "Fasting launches CRTC to facilitate . . . ," *Science*, vol. 339,6118 (2013), 443–46, doi:10.1126 /science.1227170.

303 **When researchers fasted mice:** A. Fontán-Lozano et al., "Caloric restriction increases learning consolidation . . . ," *Journal of Neuroscience*, vol. 27,38 (2007), 10185–95, doi:10.1523/JNEUROSCI.2757-07.2007.

303 **and when mice were fasted:** L. Li et al., "Chronic intermittent fasting improves cognitive . . . ," *PloS ONE*, vol. 8,6 (2013), e66069, doi:10.1371 /journal.pone.0066069.

303 **Old rats who ate:** R. Singh et al., "Late-onset intermittent fasting dietary restriction . . . ," *Age* (Dordrecht), vol. 34,4 (2012), 917–33, doi:10.1007 /s11357-011-9289-2.

303 **but in one ongoing experiment:** Mark P. Mattson, Maria Buchinger Prize Lecture, 18th Congress of the Medical Society for Fasting and Nutrition, Überlingen, Germany, 2019, at 44:39, citing work by Jake Mullins and Dimitrios Kapogiannis. See also K. Prehn et al., "Caloric restriction in older adults," *Cerebral Cortex*, vol. 27,3 (2017), 1765–78, doi:10.1093/cercor /bhw008.

304 **In mice with a mutation:** V. Halagappa et al., "Intermittent fasting and caloric restriction ameliorate . . . ," *Neurobiology of Disease*, vol. 26,1 (2007), 212–20, doi:10.1016/j.nbd.2006.12.019. See also Y. Kashiwaya et al., "A ketone ester diet exhibits anxiolytic . . . ," *Neurobiology of Aging*, vol. 34,6 (2013), 1530–39, doi:10.1016/j.neurobiolaging.2012.11.023.

304 **In mice who were fasted:** W. Duan and M. Mattson, "Dietary restriction and 2-deoxyglucose administration . . . ," *Journal of Neuroscience Research*, vol. 57,2 (1999), 195–206, doi:10.1002/(SICI)1097-4547(19990715)57:2 <195::AID-JNR5>3.0.CO;2-P.

304 **In a similar experiment in rhesus:** N. Maswood et al., "Caloric restriction increases neurotrophic factor . . . ," *PNAS*, vol. 101,52 (2004), 18171–76, doi:10.1073/pnas.0405831102; R. Love, "Calorie restriction may be neuroprotective in AD and PD," *Lancet Neurology*, vol. 4,2 (2005), 84, doi:10.1016 /S1474-4422(05)00985-3.

304 **In yet another experiment, mice:** W. Duan et al., "Dietary restriction normalizes glucose metabolism...," *PNAS*, vol. 100,5 (2003), 2911–16, doi:10.1073/pnas.0536856100.

304 **When scientists gave fasted mice:** T. Arumugam et al., "Age and energy intake interact to modify...," *Annals of Neurology*, vol. 67,1 (2010), 41–52, doi:10.1002/ana.21798; S. Manzanero et al., "Intermittent fasting attenuates increases in neurogenesis...," *Journal of Cerebral Blood Flow and Metabolism*, vol. 34,5 (2014), 897–905, doi:10.1038/jcbfm.2014.36.

304 **When researchers surgically concussed:** L. Davis et al., "Fasting is neuroprotective following traumatic brain injury," *Journal of Neuroscience Research*, vol. 86,8 (2008), 1812–22, doi:10.1002/jnr.21628.

304 **One group of scientists:** Mattson, "Intermittent metabolic switching."

305 **Among the very few studies:** I. Parikh et al., "Caloric restriction preserves memory and reduces...," *Aging*, vol. 8,11 (2016), 2814–26, doi:10.18632/aging.101094.

305 **A similar effect was demonstrated:** A. Willette et al., "Calorie restriction reduces psychological stress reactivity...," *Psychoneuroendocrinology*, vol. 37,7 (2012), 903–16, doi:10.1016/j.psyneuen.2011.10.006.

306 **fasting increases several mood-lifting molecules:** Andreas Michalsen, *The Fasting Fix* (Viking, 2020), 184.

CHAPTER 15

307 **Alan Goldhamer:** For Goldhamer, see interviews of Goldhamer: by author, Santa Rosa, California, June 8, 2021; Alan Goldhamer, "Dr. Alan Goldhamer Q & A," interview by Chef A. J., parts 1 & 2, YouTube, Jan. 25, 2017; Dillon Holmes, Well Your World, "Prolonged Water Fasting Q&A Dr. Alan Goldhamer," YouTube, Oct. 21, 2017; Rich Roll Podcast, episode 541, "The Crazy Benefits of Water-Only Fasting," Aug. 24, 2020. And see lectures by Goldhamer: TrueNorth Health Center, "The TrueNorth Health Story," DVD, ca. 2011; The Real Truth About Health, "Can Fasting Save Your Life, By Author: Alan Goldhamer, D.C." YouTube, July 6, 2020; INDTVUSA, "Alan Goldhamer, D.C.—Fasting Can Save Your Life," YouTube, July 14, 2018; SOUL Documentary, "Dr. Alan Goldhamer Talk at TrueNorth Health Center 12/30/19," YouTube, Dec. 30, 2019.

313 **T. Colin Campbell:** For Campbell, see Mark Huberman, "An Interview with T. Colin Campbell, Ph.D.," *Health Science* (spring 2016), National Health Association, 5–11.

315 **That fasting lowered:** F. G. Benedict, *A Study of Prolonged Fasting* (Carnegie Institution, 1915), 119–23; G. Duncan, "Intermittent fasts in the correction and control of intractable obesity," *Transactions of the American Clinical and Climatological Association*, vol. 74 (1962), 124.

315 **In 2001, the obscure but:** A. Goldhamer et al., "Medically supervised water-only fasting in the treatment of hypertension," *Journal of Manipulative and Physiological Therapeutics*, vol. 24,5 (2001), 335–39, doi:10.1067 /mmt.2001.115263.

315 **In 2002, Goldhamer and Campbell:** A. Goldhamer et al., "Medically supervised water-only fasting in the treatment of borderline hypertension," *Journal of Alternative and Complementary Medicine*, vol. 8,5 (2002), 643–50, doi:10.1089/107555302320825165.

316 **"High blood pressure cannot":** "Why High Blood Pressure is a 'Silent Killer,'" American Heart Association, updated Nov. 30, 2017, online.

319 **He reported that on:** A. Goldhamer, "Initial cost of care results in medically supervised . . . ," *Journal of Alternative and Complementary Medicine*, vol. 8,6 (2002), 696–97, doi:10.1089/10755530260511694.

320 **Klaper believes a healthy:** The Real Truth About Health, "Should Everyone Fast? How Often Should People Fast? . . . ," interview of Michael Klaper, You-Tube, Nov. 18, 2019, at 1:00 and 19:40.

320 **But Goldhamer worried:** Sharman Apt Russell, *Hunger* (Basic, 2005), 63.

321 **At the end of 2010, a thirty-three-year-old:** *(Un)Well*, episode 4, "Fasting," Netflix, 2020; Lynae Chambers, "Jonathan's Story," Jonathan Kamm (website), Nov. 10, 2019.

323 **"The doctor of fasting":** Otto Buchinger, *La cura por el ayuno* [*The Fasting Cure*], trans. Carlota Romero and Elinor Gisela Thomas (Lidiun, 1988), 41–42.

323 **In 2018, Gomet hiked:** *La Marche Sans Faim* [*The Walk Without Hunger*], directed by Damien Artero (Planète.D, 2019).

324 **When the ruby-throated:** Françoise Wilhelmi de Toledo and Hubert Hohler, *Therapeutic Fasting* (Thieme, 2012), 7, 33–34.

324 **A similar, earthbound tale:** F. Bertile et al., "The Safety Limits Of An Extended Fast," *Scientific Reports*, vol. 6 (2016), 39008 doi:10.1038/srep 39008.

324 **A devout man, Scott:** Jean A. Oswald and Herbert M. Shelton, *Fasting for the Health of It* (Franklin, 1983), 50, 88, 97.

CHAPTER 16

326 **One of the great uncelebrated:** For the circadian rhythms in this paragraph, see Satchin Panda, *The Circadian Code* (Rodale, 2018), 10–11, 145; "Timing of cancer radiation therapy may minimize hair loss, researchers say," press release, Salk Institute for Biological Studies, May 20, 2013.

326 **We have circadian rhythms:** Panda, *Circadian Code*, 11–12, 208.

328 **Researchers made the discovery:** A. Chaix et al., "Time-restricted eating to prevent and manage . . . ," *Annual Review of Nutrition*, vol. 39 (2019), 291–315, doi:10.1146/annurev-nutr-082018-124320.

329 **In a study published:** N. Reynolds Jr. and R. Montgomery, "Using the Argonne diet in jet lag prevention," *Military Medicine*, vol. 167,6 (2002), 451–53, doi:10.1093/milmed/167.6.451.

329 **Fortunately, a couple of decades:** Patrick J. Skerrett, "A 'Fast' Solution to Jet Lag, *Harvard Business Review*, May 12, 2009, online.

331 **This sort of discord:** Panda, *Circadian Code*, 6; Chaix, "Time-restricted eating."

332 **In 2012, he published:** M. Hatori et al., "Time-restricted feeding without reducing . . . ," *Cell Metabolism*, vol. 15,6 (2012), 848–60, doi:10.1016/j .cmet.2012.04.019.

332 **"completely protected" them:** Panda, *Circadian Code*, 95.

332 **Panda later put the sickly:** A. Chaix et al., "Time-restricted feeding is a preventative . . . ," *Cell Metabolism*, vol. 20,6 (2014), 991–1005, doi:10.1016/j .cmet.2014.11.001; Panda, *Circadian Code*, xvi.

332 **Panda also experimented:** Panda, *Circadian Code*, 96.

333 **In fact, the same week:** H. Sherman et al., "Timed high-fat diet resets circadian . . . ," *FASEB Journal*, vol. 26,8 (2012), 3493–502, doi:10.1096/fj.12 -208868.

333 **A group under Mark Mattson:** K. Stote et al., "A controlled trial of reduced

meal frequency . . . ," *American Journal of Clinical Nutrition*, 2007, vol. 85,4, 981–88, doi:10.1093/ajcn/85.4.981.

334 **Multiple large observational studies:** Michael Greger, "How Circadian Rhythms Affect Blood Sugar Levels," NutritionFacts.org, YouTube, Feb. 5, 2020.

335 **One of the more convincing studies:** D. Jakubowicz et al., "High caloric intake at breakfast vs. . . . ," *Obesity* (Silver Spring), vol. 21,12 (2013), 2504–12, doi:10.1002/oby.20460.

335 **The maxim was in fact:** Adelle Davis, *Let's Eat Right to Keep Fit* (Harcourt Brace, 1954), 19.

336 **This was demonstrated rather:** R. Carroll et al., "Diurnal variation in probability of death . . . ," *International journal of epidemiology*, vol. 41,6 (2012), 1821–28, doi:10.1093/ije/dys191.

336 **On the same principle, scientists:** Catharine Paddock, "Scientists may have found 'best time' to administer chemo drugs," *Medical News Today*, May 9, 2018, online; R. Dallmann et al., "Dosing-time makes the poison," *Trends in Molecular Medicine*, vol. 22,5 (2016), 430–45, doi:10.1016/j.molmed .2016.03.004; Michael Greger, *How Not to Diet* (Flatiron, 2019), 320.

336 **In 2010, Spanish researchers:** R. Hermida et al., "Influence of circadian time of hypertension . . . ," *Chronobiology International*, vol. 27,8 (2010), 1629–51, doi:10.3109/07420528.2010.510230; K. Kirley et al., "PURLs: BP meds: this simple change improves outcomes," *Journal of Family Practice*, vol. 61,3 (2012), 153–55.

336 **No matter what we do:** Panda, *Circadian Code*, 10–11, 38, 173–74.

337 **The best studied of our:** For the circadian regulation of insulin, see Chai, "Time-restricted eating."

338 **Every morning, blue light:** S. Panda, "Circadian physiology of metabolism," *Science*, vol. 354,6315 (2016), 1008–15, doi:10.1126/science.aah4967; Panda, *Circadian Code*, 198; C. Morris, "Endogenous circadian system and circadian misalignment . . . ," *PNAS*, vol. 112,17 (2015), E2225–34, doi:10.1073/pnas.1418955112; E. Poggiogalle et al., "Circadian regulation of glucose, lipid . . . ," *Metabolism: Clinical and Experimental*, vol. 84 (2018), 11–27, doi:10.1016/j.metabol.2017.11.017.

338 **In one experiment, researchers:** A. Bowen et al., "Diurnal variation in

glucose tolerance," *Archives of Internal Medicine*, vol. 119,3 (1967), 261–64, doi:10.1001/archinte.1967.00290210093007.

338 **This circadian shift in insulin:** T. Sonnier et al., "Glycemic control is impaired in the evening . . . ," *Journal of Diabetes and its Complications*, vol. 28,6 (2014), 836–43, doi:10.1016/j.jdiacomp.2014.04.001.

338 **In another trial, when healthy:** F. Kobayashi et al., "Effect of breakfast skipping on diurnal variation . . . ," *Obesity Research & Clinical Practice*, vol. 8,3 (2014), e201–98, doi:10.1016/j.orcp.2013.01.001.

338 **In a trial from 2015 in Spain:** C. Bandín et al., "Meal timing affects glucose tolerance, substrate . . . ," *International Journal of Obesity*, vol. 39,5 (2015), 828–33, doi:10.1038/ijo.2014.182.

338 **In another study of the same:** M. Lombardo et al., "Morning meal more efficient for fat loss . . . ," *Journal of the American College of Nutrition*, vol. 33,3 (2014), 198–205, doi:10.1080/07315724.2013.863169.

339 **When researchers at Japan's:** Y. Tsuchida, "Effects of a late supper on digestion . . . ," *Journal of Physiological Anthropology*, vol. 32,1 (2013) 9, doi:10.1186/1880-6805-32-9.

339 **In another study simulating late:** F. Scheer et al., "Adverse metabolic and cardiovascular consequences of circadian misalignment," *PNAS*, vol. 106,11 (2009), 4453–58, doi:10.1073/pnas.0808180106.

339 **And in another Japanese trial:** T. Yoshizaki et al., "Effects of feeding schedule changes on . . . ," *European Journal of Applied Physiology*, vol. 113,10 (2013), 2603–11, doi:10.1007/s00421-013-2702-z.

339 **Consider the renovations:** Marcelo Campos, "Leaky gut," *Harvard Health Blog*, Sep. 22, 2017, online; Panda, *Circadian Code*, 145, 175–76, 185, 201.

341 **In fact, to process a meal:** Michael Greger, "Eat More Calories in the Morning than the Evening," NutritionFacts.org, YouTube, Jan. 29, 2020.

341 **In a crossover trial published:** S. Bo et al., "Is the timing of caloric intake associated . . . ," *International Journal of Obesity* (London), vol. 39,12 (2015), 1689–95, doi:10.1038/ijo.2015.138.

342 **Research shows we can't:** Greger, "Eat More Calories."

342 **A bigger reason:** Panda, *Circadian Code*, 36–41, 98, 192–94.

343 **It's a myth, incidentally:** See "Sources on Diet" in this book.

343 **When surveyed, the average:** C. Marinac et al., "Prolonged nightly fasting

and breast cancer prognosis," *JAMA Oncology*, vol. 2,8 (2016), 1049–55, doi:10.1001/jamaoncol.2016.0164.

343 **but a smartphone app:** Panda's app is myCircadianClock. S. Gill and S. Panda, "A smartphone app reveals erratic...," *Cell Metabolism*, vol. 22,5 (2015), 789–98, doi:10.1016/j.cmet.2015.09.005; Panda, *Circadian Code*, 61, 97–98.

344 **"eating late at night":** Panda, *Circadian Code*, 103.

344 **a 2013 study from Harvard:** L. Cahill et al., "Prospective study of breakfast eating and...," *Circulation*, vol. 128,4 (2013), 337–43, doi:10.1161/CIRCULATIONAHA.113.001474.

344 **In 2004, researchers in China:** M. Wu et al., "Effects of meal timing on tumor progression in mice," *Life Sciences*, vol. 75,10 (2004), 1181–93, doi:10.1016/j.lfs.2004.02.014.

344 **Taken together, the four-:** E. Filipski et al., "Effects of light and food schedules on liver...," *Journal of the National Cancer Institute*, vol. 98,7 (2005), 507–17, doi:10.1093/jnci/dji083. Note correction to figure 2 in "Erratum," *Journal of the National Cancer Institute*, vol. 97,10 (2005), 780, doi:10.1093/jnci/dji138.

345 **In the 1990s and early 2000s:** J. Pierce et al., "Influence of a diet very high in vegetables...," *JAMA*, vol. 298,3 (2007), 289–98, doi:10.1001/jama.298.3.289.

345 **Nonetheless, when Patterson separated:** Marinac, "Prolonged nightly" (2016); C. Marinac et al., "Prolonged nightly fasting and breast cancer risk," *Cancer Epidemiology, Biomarkers & Prevention*, vol. 24,5 (2015), 783–89, doi:10.1158/1055-9965.EPI-14-1292.

345 **In a trial at Brigham Young:** J. LeCheminant et al., "Restricting night-time eating reduces daily...," *British Journal of Nutrition*, vol. 110,11 (2013), 2108–13, doi:10.1017/S0007114513001359.

345 **a similar, uncontrolled trial by Panda:** Gill, "A Smartphone App"; Panda, *Circadian Code*, 82.

345 **Italian researchers tested:** T. Moro et al., "Effects of eight weeks of time-restricted feeding...," *Journal of Translational Medicine*, vol. 14,1 (2016) 290, doi:10.1186/s12967-016-1044-0.

346 **In an American trial:** D. Lowe et al., "Effects of time-restricted eating

on weight...," *JAMA Internal Medicine*, vol. 180,11 (2020), 1491–99, doi:10.1001/jamainternmed.2020.4153.

346 **and she designed two trials:** E. Sutton et al., "Early time-restricted feeding improves insulin sensitivity...," *Cell Metabolism*, vol. 27,6 (2018), 1212–21. e3, doi:10.1016/j.cmet.2018.04.010; H. Jamshed et al., "Early time-restricted feeding improves 24-hour glucose...," *Nutrients*, vol. 11,6 (2019), 1234, doi:10.3390/nu11061234; E. Ravussin et al., "Early time-restricted feeding reduces appetite and...," *Obesity* (Silver Spring), vol. 27,8 (2019), 1244–54, doi:10.1002/oby.22518.

347 **The great flaw:** Greger, *How Not to Diet*, 151–52.

354 **In a study at the National Institute on Aging:** S. Mitchell et al., "Daily fasting improves health and survival...," *Cell Metabolism*, vol. 29,1 (2019), 221–28.e3, doi:10.1016/j.cmet.2018.08.011.

354 **strengthening synapses:** B. Martin et al., "Caloric restriction and intermittent fasting," *Ageing Research Reviews*, vol. 5,3 (2006), 332–53.

354 **reducing stress hormones:** Panda, *Circadian Code*, 125.

354 **building stronger immune systems:** Y. Cissé et al. "Time-restricted feeding alters the innate immune...," *Journal of Immunology*, vol. 200,2 (2018), 681–87, doi:10.4049/jimmunol.1701136.

354 **ravages of Huntington's disease:** H. Wang et al., "Time-restricted feeding improves circadian dysfunction...," *eNeuro*, vol. 5,1 (2018), e0431-17.2017, doi:10.1523/ENEURO.0431-17.2017; Panda, *Circadian Code*, 230.

354 **a handful of observational studies from the 1970s:** R. Sichieri et al., "A prospective study of hospitalization with gallstone...," *American Journal of Public Health*, vol. 81,7 (1991), 880–84, doi:10.2105/ajph.81.7.880; C. Williams and J. Johnston, "Prevalence of gallstones and risk factors in Caucasian...," *Canadian Medical Association Journal*, vol. 122,6 (1980), 664–68; J. P. Capron et al., "Meal frequency and duration of overnight fast," *British Medical Journal* (Clinical research ed.), vol. 283,6304 (1981), 1435, doi:10.1136/bmj.283.6304.1435.

355 **"the health benefits":** Panda, *Circadian Code*, 98.

355 **On the strength of such:** Panda, *Circadian Code*, xvii; "Regular fasting could lead to longer, healthier life," American Heart Association News, Nov. 25, 2019, online.

CHAPTER 17

356 **Christina Gore:** For Gore, see "Resolving a Sixteen-year Headache," *Health Science* (spring 2016), 26–28; Kevin Gianni, The Renegade Health Show, episodes 636 & 637, "16 Year Headache Gone after Water Fast," parts 7 & 8, YouTube, Aug. 17 & 18, 2010.

357 **Sarita Bhola:** For Bhola, see "Finding Good Health after Losing 85 Pounds," *Science* (summer 2016), 26–28.

358 **Gabrielle Kirby:** For Kirby, see *Gabrielle's Journey*, directed by Kevin Jacobsen (S. O. L. Productions, 2000).

359 **Gabrielle Fennimore:** For Fennimore, see "Resolving Ulcerative Colitis," TrueNorth Health Center, online.

361 **Drs. Dean Ornish and Caldwell Esselstyn:** Dean Ornish, *Dr. Dean Ornish's Program for Reversing Heart Disease* (Random House, 1990); Caldwell B. Esselstyn Jr., *Prevent and Reverse Heart Disease* (Avery, 2007).

367 **This is the problem at the heart:** Douglas J. Lisle and Alan Goldhamer, *The Pleasure Trap* (Healthy Living, 2003).

370n **Not long later, Dr. Robert Atkins:** David Mikkelson, "Dr. Robert Atkins' Death," Snopes, Feb. 11, 2004, online.

374 **In America the same percentage:** Christopher Ingraham, "Study: Americans are as likely to believe in Bigfoot as in the big bang theory," *Washington Post*, Oct. 24, 2014, online; Eric Mack, "Flintstone facts? 41 percent of Americans say people and dinosaurs co-existed," CNET, June 26, 2015, online.

INDEX